INTERNATIONAL DIETETICS AND NUTRITION TERMINOLOGY (IDNT) REFERENCE MANUAL:

Standardized Language for the Nutrition Care Process

Second Edition

INTERNATIONAL DIETETICS AND NUTRITION TERMINOLOGY (IDNT) REFERENCE MANUAL: Standardized Language for the Nutrition Care Process

Second Edition

ISBN: 978-0-88091-426-0

American Dietetic Association
120 South Riverside Plaza
Suite 2000
Chicago, IL 60606-6995
800/877-1600
www.eatright.org

The views expressed in this publication are those of the authors and do not necessarily reflect policies and/or official positions of the American Dietetic Association. Mention of product names in this publication does not constitute endorsement by the authors or the American Dietetic Association. The American Dietetic Association disclaims responsibility for the application of the information contained herein.

10 9 8 7 6 5 4 3 2

Table of Contents

Several additional resources, including the Nutrition Assessment Matrix, Nutrition Diagnosis and Etiology Matrix, and camera ready pocket guides for the complete standardized language, are available on ADA's website (http://www.eatright.org). Sign in as a member and select Nutrition Care Process from the sidebar.

Assessment

Diagnosis

Intervention

Monitoring & Evaluation

Resources

Edition: 2009

Standardized Language Committee

Standardized Language Committee

Chair
Nancy Lewis, PhD, RD, FADA
Committee Member 2005-2008

Vice Chair
Elise Smith, MA, RD, LD
Committee Member 2006-2008

Judy Beto, PhD, RD, LD, FADA
Committee Member 2006-2008

Jennifer L Bueche, PhD, RD, CDN
Committee Member 2007-2008

Claudia A. Conkin, MS, RD, LD
Committee Member 2006-2008

Donna A Israel, PhD, RD, LD, LPC, FADA
Committee Member 2005-2008

Melinda Zook-Weaver MS RD LD
Committee Member 2007-2008

Elizabeth Thompson, MPH, RD
QM Committee Liaison
Committee Member 2007-2008

Pam Charney, PhD, RD, CNSD
Research Committee Liaison 2007-2008
Committee Member 2003-2007

Jessie Pavlinac, MS, RD, CSR, LD
Evidence Based Practice Committee Liaison
Committee Member 2007-2008

Constance J Geiger, PhD, RD, CD
Ex-Officio/BOD 2007-2008

Staff Liaisons

Esther Myers, PhD, RD, FADA
Director of Scientific Affairs and Research
American Dietetic Association
E-mail: emyers@eatright.org

Kay B. Howarter, MS, RD, LD
Senior Research Manager, Evidence Analysis Library
American Dietetic Association
E-mail: khowarter@eatright.org

Pam Michael, MBA, RD
Director, Nutrition Services Coverage Team
American Dietetic Association
E-Mail: pmichael@eatright.org

Col Laurie E. Sweet, MHA, MS, RD, LD
Staff Liaison 2007-2008

For a complete list of contributors, consultants, and expert reviewers, please refer to ADA's website, www.eatright.org, in the Nutrition Care Process section.

Foreword

It is this belief in a power larger than myself and other than myself which allows me to venture into the unknown and even the unknowable. ~Maya Angelou

For many of us, the Nutrition Care Process is uncharted territory. Just a few years ago, I, along with other members of the Standardized Language Committee, was not certain where the process and its standardized language would take us or the profession. However, now that I have had a glimpse of the process, I see the possibilities—a clear language to document and research practice, as well as measurable outcomes to evaluate the impact of nutrition care.

However, this challenges every professional to step beyond talking about the Nutrition Care Process and begin using the Nutrition Care Process. It challenges dietetics professionals at every level to analyze their practice and look to the standardized language for consistent communication. The process challenges dietetics professionals to venture, a little bit, into the unknowable. Fortunately, the ADA has suggestions and resources for this new venture, making the seemingly unknowable a little less mysterious.

Customize the Nutrition Care Process For Your Practice

One of the most common misconceptions about the Nutrition Care Process and its standardized language is that all practitioners will use every standardized language term developed for the four steps—nutrition assessment, nutrition diagnosis, nutrition intervention, and nutrition monitoring and evaluation. Thankfully, as dietetics practitioners are discovering, they are likely using only portions of each standardized terminology list depending on their practice setting and patient population. The standardized language for nutrition diagnosis contains 60 diagnoses, of which, most practitioners will use about ten commonly and others now and then.

It is understandable that some practitioners find learning a new nutrition language daunting at the beginning; however, as practitioners find the terms that describe their practice, the process becomes much clearer. In fact, many of the ADA practice groups are reviewing the standardized language to determine the most commonly used terms by dietetics professionals within their area of practice. Reach out to others, engage with a practice group, an on-line network, or a colleague as you customize the Nutrition Care Process for your practice.

Engage with Other Professionals About the Nutrition Care Process Through Nutrition Screening and Referral

Screening and referral are the entry points for patients/clients into the Nutrition Care Process. Employ nutrition screening or referral—defined by your institution, facility, or organization—as the bridge for introducing the Nutrition Care Process and it standardized language to other professional colleagues. As you communicate about the Nutrition Care Process, it reinforces your value in the overall health care, community, or wellness realm. Because nutrition professionals do not typically complete nutrition screening, it is a perfect place to initiate a conversation with other professionals about what dietetics professionals are doing to document and research their impact. Registered dietitians familiar with the Nutrition Care Process will be more effective at developing nutrition screening and referral mechanisms that are cost effective and accurately identify patients/clients who might have a nutrition problem.

Embrace and Understand the Need for Validation of the Standard Language

Validate means to confirm or prove. It may seem impractical to establish a standardized language, ask dietetics professionals to use it, and then make changes to the language later. Why not make sure the language is accurate, and then use it? The only way to truly confirm or prove the validity of the language is to use it and accept that as science and practice evolve, changes will occur.

Edition: 2009

As with the ongoing updating of the American Medical Association Current Procedural Terminology (CPT) codes, ADA anticipates changes to the standardized language and will publish the *International Dietetics and Nutrition Terminology (IDNT) Reference Manual* on a regular basis. The nutrition diagnosis language is undergoing study in a number of research projects to validate the language, such as those that explore use in ambulatory or inpatient settings or by specific types of practice, e.g., nutrition support and oncology. The Dietitians Association of Australia has initiated a research study evaluating the face validity of the nutrition diagnoses. It is believed with all of the steps in the process articulated in standardized terms, that the dietetics community will pursue additional research to validate the language. Future modifications to the language will be made based on the research results.

Explore the Publications and Resources Developed by Colleagues

Dietetics practitioners across the country are implementing the Nutrition Care Process. *The International Dietetics and Nutrition Terminology Reference Manual, Second Edition,* provides extensive detail and explanation about the complete standardized language for the profession of dietetics. This publication is indeed a comprehensive reference manual with more detail than professionals will need to access daily. Therefore, the *Pocket Guide for the International Dietetics and Nutrition Terminology Reference Manual, Second Edition,* is a practical reference for professionals as they learn this new language for the profession.

At this time, two toolkits are available from ADA for the on-line Evidence-Based Nutrition Practice Guidelines, based upon evidence analyses: Adult Weight Management and Disorders Lipid Metabolism. They contain sample forms and examples incorporating standardized language terms in the Nutrition Care Process steps. These are available for purchase from ADA for dietetics practitioners to use at the Store tab at www.adaevidencelibrary.com. Dietetics practitioners will find additional Evidence-Based Guidelines for Critical Illness, Pediatric Weight Management, and Oncology. Evidence-Based Guidelines for many other topics are undergoing analyses. See the Evidence Analysis Library, at www.adaevidencelibrary.com, for further information.

Within the Nutrition Care Process section of the ADA website, www.eatright.org, are:

- Nutrition Assessment Matrix and the Nutrition Diagnosis Etiology Matrix
- Camera-ready pocket guides for the complete standardized language
- Complete list of Acknowledgements including expert reviewers
- Presentations and information on change management and the basics of the Nutrition Care Process
- Information on how the Nutrition Care Process is linked to quality management/performance improvement and reimbursement
- Presentations explaining the various components of the Nutrition Care Process and how to implement the steps and language into your daily practice
- Frequently asked questions about the Nutrition Care Process
- Patient/client and performance improvement case studies
- Sample policies, procedures, chart audit tools and other information to aid throughout the implementation process
- Policy and procedure for submitting additions or changes to the standardized language.

Whether you have been practicing dietetics for five years or twenty-five years, you no doubt recognize that the Nutrition Care Process is a revolution for the profession. Join me in implementing the Nutrition Care Process, and I promise you won't find it so mysterious.

Nancy Lewis, PhD, RD
Chair, Nutrition Care Process/
Standardized Language Committee 2007-2008

Publication Highlights

Publications Related to the Nutrition Care Process

Since the Nutrition Care Process and Model development, the American Dietetic Association (ADA) has printed several publications related to the Nutrition Care Process. *Journal of the American Dietetic Association* articles and publications have been issued regarding the Nutrition Care Process and Model since 2002. The original article published in the 2003 *Journal* described the complete Nutrition Care Process (1). This article was updated in 2007-2008 by a subcommittee of the Nutrition Care Process Standardized Language Committee and which was chaired by Annalynn Skipper, PhD, RD. Part one of the updated article has been published in the July 2008 issue of the *Journal* (2). The second part of the article will be published in the *Journal* within the following year

This publication contains all four steps in the Nutrition Care Process, with standardized taxonomies. It includes the debut of the nutrition assessment taxonomy, the combination of the nutrition assessment and nutrition monitoring and evaluation reference sheets, and a revision to some of the nutrition diagnoses. Various tools (e.g., reference sheets, camera-ready pocket guides) are included for practitioners to implement the process in their practice.

New in this Publication

Nutrition Assessment

The **Nutrition Assessment** section is **REVISED** and presents the nutrition assessment taxonomy for the profession of dietetics. This involves organization of the terms into Domains and Classes with resulting changes to the matrix, development of combined nutrition assessment and nutrition monitoring and evaluation reference sheets, and clarification related to nutrient intake that appears inadequate. Due to space considerations, in this edition the nutrition assessment matrix has been moved to the ADA website, www.eatright.org, in the Nutrition Care Process section.

Nutrition Assessment Domain Changes

The Five Domains remain the same as in previous publications, but the titles of two Domains were modified for clarity.

- **Revision of Food/Nutrition History to Food/Nutrition-Related History** since this Domain includes related items such as medication use and physical activity.
- **Revision of Physical Examination Findings to Nutrition-Focused Physical Findings** reflecting that these are findings observed during a nutrition-focused physical exam, reported by the patient/client, or found in the medical record.

Combined Nutrition Assessment and Nutrition Monitoring and Evaluation Terms

This edition contains combined nutrition assessment and nutrition monitoring and evaluation domains, classes, terms, and reference sheets; comparative standards for evaluating nutrient intake and weight; and information clarifying how to address findings that may be consistent with inadequate intake.

- **Consolidation of the domains, classes and terms.** Nutrition assessment and nutrition monitoring data have substantial overlap in identification and approach. In both steps, data elements are compared to either the nutrition prescription/goal or a reference standard. While dietetics practitioners use assessment data for identification of whether a nutrition problem or diagnosis exists, the same types of data are collected during assessment and reassessment for the purposes of monitoring and evaluation.
  - The domains, classes and terms have been consolidated. Further information regarding the changes is available later in this chapter. A mapping of nutrition monitoring and evaluation terms is available in the Nutrition Monitoring and Evaluation chapter.
  - The combined reference sheets distinguish between nutrition assessment indicators and nutrition monitoring and evaluation indicators by placing *** next to indicators only used for nutrition assessment. In some reference sheets, there are NO indicators with *** because all of the indicators are used for both nutrition assessment and nutrition monitoring and evaluation.

- **Development of comparative standards reference sheets.** During nutrition assessment and monitoring and evaluation, practitioners determine a patient/client's estimated nutrient needs and often use this information to compare and interpret a patient/client's estimated intake of one or more nutrients. Therefore, comparative standard reference sheets are included with this edition of the reference manual. One potential source for comparison of intake is the Dietary Reference Intakes (DRIs). A comparative standard reference sheet for Recommended Body Weight/Body Mass Index/Growth is also provided.
- **Addition of interpretive information for the Dietary Reference Intakes (DRIs).** The DRIs are one reference standard that dietetics professionals can use for comparison of estimated intake. Since all DRIs are for healthy individuals in a particular life stage and gender group, they may not be applicable standards for all clinical scenarios. Specific guidance on how to use the DRIs is included in this manual.

Clarification for Inadequate Intake

Some dietetics practitioners have raised questions about assessing a patient/client's intake as "inadequate." Critical to the understanding of this subject is the recognition of three issues:

- Because it is very difficult to measure a patient/client's intake even when enteral and/or parenteral nutrition is provided as the sole source of nutrition, it is recommended to consider additional data for assessment of nutritional status. Indeed, these measures are estimates of intake.
- The DRIs are established for healthy individuals. It is not clear how the DRIs should be interpreted in patients/clients with an illness, injury, disease, or other medical condition.
- Inadequate nutrient intake does not necessarily equate to nutrient deficiency.

As such, the Standardized Language Committee included a clarification statement that should be given professional consideration during nutrition assessment or reassessment when comparing estimated intake to the DRIs and prior to identifying and labeling a patient/client with the nutrition diagnosis of "Inadequate [substance] Intake" (e.g. inadequate vitamin intake, inadequate protein intake). The note is part of the definition for the ten nutrition assessment and monitoring and evaluation reference sheets related to nutrient intake and the eleven nutrition diagnoses with "Inadequate" in the label.

> *Note: Whenever possible, nutrient intake data should be considered in combination with clinical, biochemical, anthropometric information, medical diagnosis, clinical status, and/or other factors as well as diet to provide a valid assessment of nutritional status based on a totality of the evidence. (Dietary Reference Intakes. Applications in Dietary Assessment. Institute of Medicine. Washington, D.C.: National Academy Press; 2000.)*

The notation from the Institute of Medicine (IOM) advises combining intake data with clinical, biochemical, and other supporting information to complete a valid assessment of nutritional status. While it is acknowledged that inadequate intake is not synonymous with nutritional status, there may be an implied expectation that an inadequate intake over a period of time will lead to a change in nutritional status. The difficulty encountered is in the ability to accurately predict the consequences of intake due to a myriad of factors, such as scientific uncertainty about "nutrient requirements," individual differences, and inaccurate intake assessments.

Bioactive substances do not have established DRIs. They are not considered essential nutrients because inadequate intakes do not result in biochemical or clinical symptoms of deficiency. However, naturally occurring food components with potential risk or benefit to health are reviewed by the Food and Nutrition Board of the Institute of Medicine and, if sufficient data exist, reference intakes are established. Further, the nutrition assessment and monitoring and evaluation reference sheets note that the criteria for evaluation of intake must be the patient/client goal or nutrition prescription since there are no established minimum requirements or Tolerable Upper Intake Levels. The patient/client goal or nutrition prescription would be based upon an individual goal or research, for example, the ADA Disorders of Lipid Metabolism Evidence-Based Guideline. This guideline considers the evidence supporting intake of plant stanol/sterol esters in the presence of lipid disorders. It is available on the ADA Evidence Analysis Library. Therefore, the note added to the definition of Inadequate Bioactive Substance Intake is:

> *Note: Bioactive Substances are not included as part of the Dietary Reference Intakes, and therefore there are no established minimum requirements or Tolerable Upper Intake Levels. However, RDs can assess whether estimated intakes are adequate or excessive using the patient/client goal or nutrition prescription for comparison.*

Further information regarding use of the word "inadequate" in the Nutrition Care Process can be found in the chapters on nutrition diagnosis and nutrition monitoring and evaluation and on the ADA website, www.eatright.org, in the Nutrition Care Process section.

Nutrition Diagnosis

The **Nutrition Diagnosis** section is **REVISED**. The changes include reorganization of elements within the Signs/Symptoms table in individual nutrition diagnosis reference sheets and revisions and clarifications to individual nutrition diagnosis reference sheets.

Reorganization of the Sign/Symptoms Reference Sheet Table

The changes related to reorganization of the Signs/Symptoms in individual nutrition diagnosis reference sheets affect the grouping of the terms, but do not influence the content of the nutrition diagnosis. There are four components of a nutrition diagnosis reference sheet—definition, etiology, signs/symptoms, and references—which are described in detail later in this chapter. Briefly, dietetics practitioners gather pertinent signs/symptoms during nutrition assessment to assist in identifying and labeling a nutrition diagnosis. With the reorganization and classification of the nutrition assessment terms and indicators, there are changes in placement of the signs/symptoms within the nutrition diagnosis sheets:

- In some cases, signs/symptoms gathered during the nutrition assessment are moved from one assessment domain or category, such as Client History, to another domain, such as Food/Nutrition-Related History. Again, these changes do not affect the content of the nutrition diagnosis, just the organization of the sign/symptoms.

Revisions and Clarifications

Changes in the nutrition diagnoses include revisions and clarifications to individual nutrition diagnosis reference sheets. First, specific changes to nutrition diagnosis labels, etiologies, and signs/symptoms were completed based upon practitioner questions and feedback and Committee review. Second, in response to questions about how to label and document inadequate intake, a note was added to the definition of the eleven nutrition diagnoses associated with inadequate intake. Since the note reminds practitioners to include additional supporting evidence (e.g., biochemical data, anthropometric data), nutrition-focused physical findings were added to two of the nutrition diagnoses. A chart for guiding interpretation of the DRIs was also added to the publication. Third, to assist practitioners with identifying the etiology (E) of a problem for use in the PES statement, the Committee developed a Nutrition Diagnosis Etiology Matrix.

Evident Protein-Energy Malnutrition (NI-5.2):

- Revision of the Nutrition Diagnosis Label. The words "Evident Protein-Energy" were removed from the label, and this nutrition diagnosis is retitled Malnutrition (NI-5.2).
- Removal of the two signs/symptoms (biochemical measures) related to serum albumin. The following footnote is added to the nutrition diagnosis. In the past, hepatic transport protein measures (e.g. albumin and pre-albumin) were used as indicators of malnutrition. The sensitivity of these as nutrition indicators has been questioned. An ADA evidence-analysis project is evaluating the body of science.
- Modifications to the sign/symptoms (anthropometric measurements) of weight change in adults and growth rate in pediatrics were added for clarity.

Inadequate Fat Intake (NI-5.6.1):

- Addition of an etiology, Alteration in gastrointestinal tract structure and/or function, supporting signs/symptoms already listed in the nutrition diagnosis.

Inappropriate Intake of Food Fats (specify) (NI-5.6.3):

- Modification of the nutrition diagnosis label removing the word "food." The nutrition diagnosis includes inappropriate fat from any source, for example, food, EN/PN, formula, and intravenously.

Swallowing Difficulty (NC-1.1):

- Modification of an etiology to include altered suck, swallow, breathe patterns within the list of Motor causes for this nutrition diagnosis.

Altered Nutrition-Related Laboratory Values (specify) (NC-2.2):

- Addition of an etiology, Prematurity, as a potential cause/contributing factor for this nutrition diagnosis.

Underweight (NC-3.1):

- Addition of an etiology—Small for gestational age, intrauterine growth retardation/restriction and/or lack of progress/appropriate weight gain per day.

Food- and Nutrition-related Knowledge Deficit (NB-1.1):

- Addition of an etiology, Lack of understanding of infant/child cues to indicate hunger.

Excessive Exercise (NB-2.2):

- Excessive Exercise (NB-2.2) is now Excessive Physical Activity (NB-2.2) reflecting involuntary and voluntary physical activity/movement, and exercise.

- Modification of the definition to: Involuntary or voluntary physical activity or movement that interferes with energy needs, growth, or exceeds that which is necessary to achieve optimal health.

Inadequate Intake

As noted earlier, some dietetics practitioners have raised questions about the use of the nutrition diagnosis label "inadequate" when describing the intake of patients/clients. There is concern that this may pose an increased risk of litigation or legal exposure. Additional information regarding this issue can be found at www.eatright.org in the Nutrition Care Process section.

- The Standardized Language Committee clarification statement that is included on the nutrition assessment and monitoring and evaluation reference sheets is also included as part of the definitions for the eleven nutrition diagnoses with "Inadequate" in the label.

  Note: Whenever possible, nutrient intake data should be considered in combination with clinical, biochemical, anthropometric information, medical diagnosis, clinical status, and/or other factors as well as diet to provide a valid assessment of nutritional status based on a totality of the evidence. (Dietary Reference Intakes. Applications in Dietary Assessment. Institute of Medicine. Washington, D.C.: National Academy Press; 2000.)

- If a synonym, or alternate word with the same meaning, for the term "inadequate" is helpful or needed, an approved alternate is the word "suboptimal." Thus, a dietetics professional could use either the nutrition diagnosis label "Suboptimal Protein Intake" or "Inadequate Protein Intake."

Because nutrient intake data should be considered in combination with clinical, biochemical, and anthropometric information, medical diagnosis, and/or clinical status, two nutrition diagnoses, Inadequate Protein Intake NI-5.7.1 and Inadequate Fiber Intake NI-5.8.5, were revised. The Committee added signs/symptoms of nutrition-focused physical findings in addition to intake and client history data.

A document detailing all of the specific changes to the nutrition diagnoses, the year in which the review or change occurred, and the rationale, is available in the Nutrition Care Process and Model Resource section of ADA's website at www.eatright.org in the Nutrition Care Process section. Editorial changes, not affecting the content, are not included in this document.

Nutrition Intervention

The **Nutrition Intervention** standardized language is **unchanged** in this publication.

Nutrition Monitoring and Evaluation

The **Nutrition Monitoring and Evaluation** section is **REVISED** with the development of combined nutrition assessment and nutrition monitoring and evaluation reference sheets as discussed in the nutrition assessment section above.

Further changes:

- **Revision of some specific nutrition monitoring and evaluation terms and nutrition care indicators.** Some of the individual reference sheet terms and/or indicators were changed. All of the changes were made in an attempt to help dietetics practitioners best identify and document what specific markers (indicators) are needed to monitor and evaluate patient/client improvements.

- **Elimination of intervention-oriented reference sheets in the Behavior class.** Identification of nutrition assessment terms entailed careful examination of etiologies and nutrition diagnoses. This focus on etiologies lead to the decision to eliminate several intervention-oriented, behavior reference sheets in favor of realigning monitoring and evaluation indicators with reference sheets related to the root cause of the behavior. For example, the reference sheet "Ability to Prepare Food/Meals" was eliminated, but the concept was added to the "Food and Nutrition Knowledge" reference sheet, because lack of adequate knowledge may be the root cause of an inability to prepare food/snacks. This concept was also included on an expanded "Adherence" reference sheet, because the patient/client may know what to do, but has not exerted the energy needed to do it. Lack of finances, food storage or preparation facilities may be the barrier to preparing food/meals and these concepts are reflected on the "Safe Food/Meal Availability" reference sheet. Finally, the concept was included on the "Nutrition-Related Activities of Daily Living" reference sheet, since cognitive or physical limitations may be the main reason the patient/client is not able to prepare food/meals.

- **Additions to the Behavior class.** The following new reference sheets were added to the Behavior class: Avoidance Behavior, Bingeing and Purging Behavior, Mealtime Behavior. These provide standardized language to support nutrition assessment and nutrition monitoring and evaluation of these important behaviors.

Not Included in this Publication

Several items, while not available in the publication, are available on ADA's website, www.eatright.org in the Nutrition Care Process Section. These include the Nutrition Assessment Matrix, Nutrition Diagnosis Etiology Matrix, a document that contains the complete changes to the nutrition diagnoses, case studies, and the Scope of Dietetics Practice Framework, Standards of Practice in Nutrition Care and Updated Standards of Professional Performance, and the Standards of Practice in Nutrition Care Appendix.

Nutrition Assessment Matrix Revision

The nutrition assessment matrix is revised in the following ways:

- **Reorganization of individual assessment terms from one domain to another.** In some cases, assessment data from one domain, such as Client History, is moved to another domain, such as Food/Nutrition-Related History. These changes do not affect the overall content of the nutrition assessment matrix, but do affect where individual items are placed. Likewise, as noted in the next chapter on nutrition diagnosis, these changes do not affect the content of the nutrition diagnosis to which they belong, just the organization of the sign/symptoms.

- **Reorganization of individual assessment terms from one class within a domain to another class.** New classes within the domains of nutrition assessment were identified. The intent of the classes is to best group similar pieces of nutrition assessment data. This required substantial reorganization of the nutrition assessment terms and indicators into their appropriate classes. As an example, nutrition assessment terms related to a gap in knowledge were placed in the class Knowledge/Beliefs/Attitudes when previously these terms could have been in the matrix in three areas—intake different from recommended, food/nutrient knowledge and skill, and/or nutrition and health awareness.

- **Clear delineation of terms.** Each nutrition assessment term gathers separate information. As with the standardized language terms for other steps in the Nutrition Care Process, it is necessary to ensure that the terms are discrete. For purposes of communication and data collection, a term must describe one concept. If dietetics practitioners, through the use of standardized language and the Nutrition Care Process, are describing dietetics practice, clear delineation between terms must be achieved.

Nutrition Diagnosis Etiology Matrix

As part of the review and development of the nutrition assessment standardized language, the etiologies associated with each nutrition diagnosis were examined. There are two significant changes regarding the nutrition diagnosis etiologies.

- **Nutrition Diagnosis and Etiology Matrix development.** A matrix of the etiologies and the nutrition diagnosis with which they are associated is included in this chapter.

- **Refinement of the Etiologies for clarity.** In the First Edition, for example, Excessive Mineral Intake NI-5.10.2 includes the etiology Lack of knowledge about management of diagnosed genetic disorders altering mineral homeostasis. This etiology is rephrased to be consistent with the other nutrition diagnoses. It now reads, "Food and nutrition-related knowledge deficit concerning management of diagnosed genetic disorders altering mineral homeostasis." These edits represent changes for clarity and content was not changed unless indicated.

Details and the rationale for changes to the Nutrition Diagnoses are available in the Nutrition Care Process and Model Resource section of the ADA website, www.eatright.org, in the Nutrition Care Process section. Each nutrition diagnosis reference sheet that was modified includes a notation on the last page indicating the publication year in which it was updated, e.g., Updated: 2009 Edition. Editorial changes not affecting the content were not included in the document.

Case Studies published previously (currently available only via the ADA website under the Practice section, in the Nutrition Care Process and Model Resource section) have been REVISED to include the nutrition assessment standardized language. The *Scope of Dietetics Practice Framework, Standards of Practice in Nutrition Care and Updated Standards of Professional Performance,* and the *Standards of Practice in Nutrition Care Appendix* are also available on the ADA website, www.eatright.org, in the Practice section.

References

1. Lacey K, Pritchett E. Nutrition care process and model: ADA adopts road map to quality care and outcomes management. *J Am Diet Assoc.* 2003;103:1061-1072.
2. Writing Group of the Nutrition Care Process/Standardized Language Committee. Nutrition care process and model part I: The 2008 update. *J Am Diet Assoc.* 2008;108:1113-1117.

Nutrition Care Process Summary

Introduction

Continually emerging from the American Dietetic Association's (ADA) strategic plan are priority actions that guide committees, work groups, and taskforces in creating tools to advance the dietetics profession. In 2002, to achieve the Association's strategic goals of promoting demand for dietetics practitioners and help them be more competitive in the marketplace, the ADA Quality Management Committee appointed the Nutrition Care Model Workgroup. This Workgroup developed the Nutrition Care Process and Model, a systematic process describing how dietetics practitioners provide care to patients/clients (1).

The Nutrition Care Process (NCP)is designed to improve the consistency and quality of individualized care for patients/ clients or groups and the predictability of the patient/client outcomes. It is not intended to standardize nutrition care for each patient/client, but to establish a standardized process for providing care.

> **Special Note:** The terms **patient/client** are used in association with the NCP; however, the process is also intended for use with groups. In addition, family members or caregivers are an essential asset to the patient/client and dietetics practitioner in the NCP. Therefore, **groups, families, and caregivers** of patients/clients are implied each time a reference is made to patient/client.

There are four steps in the process:

- Nutrition Assessment
- Nutrition Diagnosis
- Nutrition Intervention
- Nutrition Monitoring and Evaluation

Three of the Nutrition Care Process steps are very familiar to dietetics practitioners and nutrition textbooks skillfully cover their content—nutrition assessment, nutrition intervention, and nutrition monitoring and evaluation. However, the Workgroup identified a less well-defined aspect of nutrition care: nutrition diagnosis. Further, it recognized that a standard taxonomy for the second step in the process would greatly enhance the profession's ability to document, communicate, and research the impact of nutrition care.

As a result, the ADA's Standardized Language Committee was formed to create a taxonomy for the profession's unique nutrition diagnosis language. The language was described during presentations at the 2005 Food and Nutrition Conference and Exhibition and made available in a publication at that meeting (2). The nutrition diagnosis language is undergoing study in a number of research projects. Future modifications to the language will be made based on research results.

The Standardized Language Committee has examined in-depth all four Nutrition Care Process steps, and published a standardized language for nutrition assessment, nutrition diagnosis, nutrition intervention, and nutrition monitoring and evaluation, which is available in this publication, the *International Dietetics and Nutrition Terminology Reference Manual, Second Edition*. Through the committee's exploration of nutrition monitoring and evaluation, it became clear that there was substantial overlap between nutrition assessment and nutrition monitoring and evaluation terms in both concept and approach. Many data points are the same or related; the data purpose and use, however, are distinct in these two steps.

The Committee has now drafted the standardized language terms, indicators, evaluation criteria, and patient/client examples for nutrition assessment. These terms, due to their overlap with nutrition monitoring and evaluation, appear on combined reference sheets. This illustrates how the nutrition assessment process identifies a nutrition problem, and reassessment identifies whether nutrition intervention is or is not working. Therefore, this publication illustrates a complete language for describing the Nutrition Care Process for nutrition practitioners and provides tools for practitioners to implement the process into their practice.

Edition: 2009

Nutrition Care Process Steps

Step 1. Nutrition Assessment

Nutrition assessment is a systematic method for obtaining, verifying, and interpreting data needed to identify nutrition-related problems, their causes, and significance. It is an ongoing, nonlinear, dynamic process that involves initial data collection, but also continual reassessment and analysis of the patient/client's status compared to specified criteria. From the nutrition assessment data, the dietetics practitioner is able to determine whether a nutrition diagnosis/problem exists. This step, while well known to dietetics practitioners, will be enhanced by use of standardized nutrition assessment language for communicating about patients/clients with similar problems.

The nutrition assessment terms were identified and grouped into five domains:

- Food/Nutrition-Related History
- Biochemical Data, Medical Tests, and Procedures
- Anthropometric Measurements
- Nutrition-Focused Physical Findings
- Client History

Nutrition assessment begins after a patient/client referral or as a result of positive nutrition screening when it is determined that the patient/client may benefit from nutrition care. Nutrition assessment leads to the appropriate determination of whether a nutrition diagnosis/problem exists. If so, the dietetics practitioner correctly diagnoses the problem and creates a PES (Problem, Etiology, Signs/Symptoms) statement in Step 2 of the NCP. In addition, dietetics practitioners develop the plan for continuation of care or convey the need for further information or testing. If upon the completion of an initial assessment or reassessment it is determined that a nutrition problem does not exist or cannot be modified by further nutrition care, discharge or discontinuation from the episode of nutrition care may be appropriate.

Standardized language will facilitate more effective comparison of nutrition assessment findings. To this end, the Standardized Language Committee has described the standardized language, data collection, and evaluation approach for nutrition assessment. Many opportunities for research exist in nutrition assessment, which will result in improved determinations of the most appropriate nutrition assessment data to use for individuals and populations in various practice settings.

Step 2: Nutrition Diagnosis

Nutrition diagnosis is a critical step between nutrition assessment and nutrition intervention. The purpose of a standardized nutrition diagnosis language is to describe nutrition problems consistently so that they are clear within and outside the profession. The standard language will enhance communication and documentation of nutrition care, and it will provide a minimum data set and common data elements for future research.

In simple terms, a nutrition practitioner identifies and labels a specific nutrition diagnosis (problem) that, in general, he or she is responsible for treating independently (e.g., excessive carbohydrate intake). With nutrition intervention, the nutrition diagnosis ideally resolves, or at least the signs and symptoms improve. In contrast, a medical diagnosis describes a disease or pathology of organs or body systems (e.g., diabetes). In some instances, such as the nutrition diagnosis Swallowing Difficulty NC-1.1, nutrition practitioners are labeling or diagnosing the functional problem that has a nutritional consequence. Nutrition practitioners do not identify medical diagnoses; they diagnose phenomena in the nutrition domain.

ADA's Standardized Language Committee developed a framework that outlines three domains within which the nutrition diagnoses/problems fall.

- Intake
- Clinical
- Behavioral-Environmental

Sixty nutrition diagnoses/problems have been identified. A reference sheet was developed and it describes each nutrition diagnosis and incorporates expert input and research feedback.

It is this step in the Nutrition Care Process that results in the documentation of the nutrition diagnosis statement or PES statement. This statement is composed of three distinct components: the problem (P), the etiology (E) and the signs and symptoms (S). The PES statement is derived from the clustering and synthesis of information gathered during nutrition assessment.

Step 3: Nutrition Intervention

Nutrition intervention is the third step in the Nutrition Care Process. Nutrition interventions are specific actions used to remedy a nutrition diagnosis/problem, and can be used with individuals, a group, or the community at large. These nutrition interventions are intended to change a nutrition-related behavior, environmental condition, or aspect of nutritional health. A dietetics practitioner collaborates, whenever possible, with the patient/client(s) and other health care providers during the nutrition intervention.

Nutrition intervention consists of two interrelated components—planning and implementation. Planning involves prioritizing the nutrition diagnoses; conferring with the patient, others, and practice guides and policies; jointly establishing goals; and defining the nutrition prescription and identifying specific nutrition intervention(s). Implementing the nutrition intervention is the action phase, which includes carrying out and communicating the plan of care, continuing the data collection, and revising the nutrition intervention, as warranted, based on the patient/client response. This step cannot be completed unless both components are in place to support the nutrition intervention.

The nutrition intervention is, almost always, aimed at the etiology (E) of the nutrition diagnosis/problem identified in the PES statement. In very specific instances, the nutrition intervention is directed at reducing/eliminating the effects of the signs and symptoms (S). Generally, the signs and symptoms form the basis for the next step in the Nutrition Care Process: nutrition monitoring and evaluation (Step 4).

Four domains of nutrition intervention have been identified.

- Food and/or Nutrient Delivery
- Nutrition Education
- Nutrition Counseling
- Coordination of Care

The terminology is defined and reference sheets for each specific nutrition intervention are available for use by the profession. It is believed that the information necessary for medical record documentation, billing, and the description of the nutrition interventions for research are included in the terminology.

A dietetics practitioner will note that while some interventions are closely related (e.g., education and counseling), the terms are intentionally separated to distinguish between them. Additionally, specific descriptors of a nutrition intervention encounter (i.e., interactions, visits, contacts, sessions) are provided to assist a dietetics practitioner with the details of his/her encounters with patient/client(s). Examples of descriptors include encounters with individuals or groups, face to face or electronically conducted encounters, and the degree to which the dietetics practitioner is responsible for the patient/client care, to name a few.

Step 4: Nutrition Monitoring and Evaluation

The purpose of nutrition monitoring and evaluation is to quantify progress made by the patient/client in meeting nutrition care goals. During the monitoring and evaluation process, nutrition care outcomes—the desired results of nutrition care—have been defined, and specific indicators that can be measured and compared to established criteria have been identified. Nutrition monitoring and evaluation tracks patient/client outcomes relevant to the nutrition diagnosis and intervention plans and goals.

Edition: 2009

Selection of appropriate nutrition care indicators is determined by the nutrition diagnosis and its etiology and signs or symptoms and the nutrition intervention used. The medical diagnosis and health care outcome goals, and quality management goals for nutrition also influence the nutrition care indicators are chosen. Other factors, such as practice setting, patient/client population, and disease state and/or severity affect indicator selection.

The nutrition monitoring and evaluation terms are combined with the nutrition assessment terms and organized in four domains. There are no nutrition care outcomes associated with the domain entitled Client History. Items from this domain are used for nutrition assessment only and do not change as a result of nutrition intervention.

- Food/Nutrition-Related History
- Biochemical Data, Medical Tests, and Procedures
- Anthropometric Measurements
- Nutrition-Focused Physical Findings

During this step, dietetics practitioners monitor the patient/client progress by determining whether the nutrition intervention is being implemented and by providing evidence that the nutrition intervention is or is not changing the patient/client behavior or nutrition/health status. Dietetics practitioners measure outcomes by selecting the appropriate nutrition care indicator(s) and comparing the findings with nutrition prescription/intervention goals, and/or reference standards. The use of standardized indicators and criteria increases the validity and reliability of the outcome data and facilitates electronic charting, coding, and outcomes measurement.

Implementation of the Nutrition Care Process and Future Directions

Publications and Resources

Dietetics practitioners across the country are implementing the Nutrition Care Process. This new *International Dietetics and Nutrition Terminology Reference Manual, Second Edition* provides extensive detail and explanation about the complete standardized language for dietetics.

Toolkits are now available from ADA for the on-line Evidence-Based Nutrition Practice Guidelines, based upon evidence analyses (3-4). They contain sample forms and examples incorporating standardized language terms in the Nutrition Care Process steps. These are available for purchase from ADA for dietetics practitioners to use at the Store tab at www.adaevidencelibrary.com. Dietetics practitioners may find useful the extensive resources, including patient/client case studies, provided on the ADA website, www.eatright.org, in the Nutrition Care Process section.

Members have completed numerous presentations and newsletter articles for national, state, and Dietetic Practice Group audiences, with more than 10,000 individuals reached through presentations thus far. ADA also facilitates a peer network of dietetics practitioners who are leading the way in implementing the Nutrition Care Process in their facilities and communities.

ADA is moving ahead in a variety of ways to implement the standardized language of the Nutrition Care Process. In addition to numerous association activities, there are applications in the broader dietetics and medical communities.

Billing for Nutrition Encounters

As appropriate to the situation and payer, registered dietitians may bill for their services provided during encounters with patients/clients. On January 1, 2001, ADA announced three new current procedural terminology codes (CPT) for medical nutrition therapy (MNT). The codes were recognized by the Centers for Medicare & Medicaid Services (CMS) and are included in the American Medical Association's (AMA) Current Procedural Terminology CPT book. Other CPT codes may be applicable for nutrition education and training. Check payer policies to determine codes applicable for dietetics professionals' nutrition education or nutrition counseling services.

97802 Medical nutrition therapy; initial assessment and intervention, individual, face-to-face with the patient, each 15 minutes
97803 Reassessment and intervention, individual, face-to-face with the patient, each 15 minutes
97804 Group (2 or more individual(s), each 30 minutes
CPT codes, descriptions and material only are copyright ©2000 American Medical Association. All Rights Reserved.

The medical nutrition therapy CPT codes best describe services that dietetics professionals provide to patients/clients receiving services for a particular chronic disease or condition, and the code descriptors are for 15-minute increments of time that the registered dietitian spends face to face with the patient/client. As noted earlier, registered dietitians typically provide multiple units of the code in their initial and follow up visits.

In addition, based on the nutrition practice guidelines, patient/client needs, interests and medical necessity, registered dietitians normally provide nutrition services over several encounters with the patient/client. Multiple visits are needed to help the patient/client achieve goals, desired behavior changes, and/or expected outcomes.

Refer to the ADA website, www.eatright.org, in the Nutrition Care Process section under Coverage and Reimbursement for extensive resources regarding Medicare and insurance coverage for nutrition services.

International Information Sharing and Standardized Medical Languages

In 2005, the ADA Foundation funded an ADA hosted meeting to expand the dialogue with other international dietetic associations about ADA's standardized nutrition diagnosis language and similar efforts other associations have made. The meeting also initiated a dialogue between the foremost medical informatics organizations and the international nutrition and dietetics community. As a result of this dialogue:

- A presentation regarding the Nutrition Care Process has been accepted at the XV International Congress of Dietetics, September 8-11, 2008 in Yokohama, Japan.
- The Dietitians Association of Australia has initiated a research study evaluating the face validity of the nutrition diagnoses.
- The Dutch Association of Dietitians (Nederlandse Vereniging van Diëtisten) has requested permission to use the nutrition diagnoses in their health care databases.

Indeed, as the world moves fully into electronic health care records, health informatics, and common databases, the international community of nutrition and dietetics practitioners have the opportunity to work in partnership with the medical informatics organizations to ensure that data elements critical to capturing nutrition care are included in databases and collected in a consistent way.

ADA is working toward including the concepts from the Nutrition Care Process and the specific terms in standards for electronic health records and incorporating these into standardized informatics languages and language systems, such as the Systematized Nomenclature of Medicine International (SNOMED), Logical Observation Identifiers Names and Codes (LOINC), and United Medical Language System (UMLS). ADA is working with these groups to let them know the direction that the Association is headed and to keep them appraised of progress. Thus far, the feedback from the database and informatics groups has been quite positive, and they have expressed a need for documenting the unique nature of nutrition services.

Summary

This publication is the first complete publication of standardized languages for all four steps in the Nutrition Care Process. From conception of the Nutrition Care Process in 2002 through its implementation now, the Standardized Language Task Force continues to update ADA's House of Delegates, the Board of Directors, and members through reports, articles, case studies, presentations, publications, and the ADA website.

However, to see the strategic goals of an increased demand for dietetics practitioners who are more competitive in the marketplace come to fruition, practitioners need to take a historic step by implementing the Nutrition Care Process today.

References

1. Writing Group of the Nutrition Care Process/Standardized Language Committee. Nutrition care process and model part I: The 2008 update. *J Am Diet Assoc*. 2008;108:1113-1117.

2. American Dietetic Association. *Nutrition Diagnosis: A Critical Step in the Nutrition Care Process*. Chicago, IL: American Dietetic Association; 2006.

3. American Dietetic Association. Disorders of Lipid Metabolism Toolkit. Available at: https://www.adaevidencelibrary.com/store.cfm. Accessed December 13, 2007.

4. American Dietetic Association. Adult Weight Management Evidence-Based Nutrition Practice Guideline, 2006. Available at: https://www.adaevidencelibrary.com/store.cfm. Accessed December 13, 2007.

SNAPshot
NCP Step 1. Nutrition Assessment

What is the purpose of Nutrition Assessment? The purpose is to obtain, verify, and interpret data needed to identify nutrition-related problems, their causes, and significance. It is an ongoing, nonlinear, dynamic process that involves initial data collection, but also continual reassessment and analysis of the patient/client's status compared to specified criteria. This contrasts with nutrition monitoring and evaluation data where dietetics practitioners use similar, or even the same, data to determine changes in patient/client* behavior or nutritional status and the efficacy of nutrition intervention.

How does a dietetics practitioner determine where to obtain Nutrition Assessment data? It depends on the practice setting. For individuals, data can come directly from the patient/client through interview, observation and measurements, a medical record, and the referring health care provider. For population groups, data from surveys, administrative data sets, and epidemiological or research studies are used. A nutrition assessment matrix that links nutrition assessment parameters with nutrition diagnoses is available to assist practitioners in identifying nutrition diagnoses.

How are Nutrition Assessment data organized? In five categories:

Food/Nutrition-Related History	Biochemical Data, Medical Tests, and Procedures	Anthropometric Measurements	Nutrition-Focused Physical Findings	Client History
Food and nutrient intake, medication/herbal supplement intake, knowledge, beliefs, food and supplies availability, physical activity, nutrition quality of life	*Lab data (e.g., electrolytes, glucose) and tests (e.g., gastric emptying time, resting metabolic rate)*	*Height, weight, body mass index (BMI), growth pattern indices/percentile ranks, and weight history*	*Physical appearance, muscle and fat wasting, swallow function, appetite, and affect*	*Personal history, medical/health/family history, treatments and complementary/alternative medicine use, and social history*

What is done with the Nutrition Assessment data? Nutrition assessment data (indicators) are compared to criteria, relevant norms and standards, for interpretation and decision-making. These may be national, institutional, or regulatory norms and standards. Nutrition assessment findings are documented in nutrition diagnosis statements and nutrition intervention goal setting.

Critical thinking during this step...
- Determining appropriate data to collect
- Determining the need for additional information
- Selecting assessment tools and procedures that match the situation
- Applying assessment tools in valid and reliable ways
- Distinguishing relevant from irrelevant data
- Distinguishing important from unimportant data
- Validating the data

Is there a standardized language or taxonomy for Nutrition Assessment? Yes. With the development of standardized languages for the other NCP steps, it was clear that a standard taxonomy for nutrition assessment would support a consistent approach to the NCP and enhance communication and research. The terms for nutrition assessment and nutrition monitoring and evaluation are now combined, as the data points are the same or related; however, the data purpose and use are distinct in these two steps.

Are dietetics practitioners limited to the Nutrition Assessment data included in the Matrix and used in the Nutrition Diagnoses? Nutrition assessment data listed in the nutrition diagnoses reference sheets are undergoing study and research to confirm (validate) which data are most relevant to specific nutrition diagnoses. However, based on their patient/client population, practice setting and purpose, dietetics practitioners may utilize the ADA process to add or modify standardized language terms.

Detailed information about this step can be found in the American Dietetic Association's International Dietetics and Nutrition Terminology (IDNT) Reference Manual: Standardized Language for the Nutrition Care Process, Second Edition.

*Patient/client refers to individuals, groups, family members, and/or caregivers.

Edition: 2009

Nutrition Care Process Step 1. Nutrition Assessment

Introduction

Nutrition Assessment is the first of four steps in the Nutrition Care Process (1). At its simplest, it is a systematic method for obtaining, verifying, and interpreting data needed to identify nutrition-related problems, their causes, and significance. While the types of data collected during nutrition assessment may vary among nutrition settings, the process and intention are the same. When possible, the assessment data are compared to reliable norms and standards for evaluation. Further, nutrition assessment initiates data collection, which is continued throughout the Nutrition Care Process and forms the foundation for nutrition reassessment and reanalysis of data in nutrition monitoring and evaluation.

What Is New in This Edition Related to Nutrition Assessment?

This edition presents a standardized language for nutrition assessment. Development of standardized language for the other three steps in the Nutrition Care Process highlighted the need for a standard taxonomy for nutrition assessment that would support a consistent approach to nutrition assessment and the Nutrition Care Process as well as enhance communication and research.

The changes include:

Nutrition Assessment Domain Changes

The five Domains remain the same as in previous publications, but the titles of two Domains were modified for clarity.

- **Revision of Food/Nutrition History to Food/Nutrition-Related History** since this Domain includes related items such as medication use and physical activity.

- **Revision of Physical Examination Findings to Nutrition-Focused Physical Findings** reflecting that these are findings observed during a nutrition-focused physical exam, reported by the patient/client, or found in the medical record.

Nutrition Assessment Matrix Revision

The nutrition assessment matrix is revised in the following ways and is now available online:

- **Reorganization of individual assessment terms from one domain to another.** In some cases, assessment data from one domain, such as Client History, is moved to another domain, such as Food/Nutrition-Related History. These changes do not affect the overall content of the nutrition assessment matrix, but do affect where individual items are placed. Likewise, as noted in the next chapter on nutrition diagnosis, these changes do not affect the content of the nutrition diagnosis to which they belong, just the organization of the sign/symptoms.

- **Reorganization of individual assessment terms from one class within a domain to another class.** New classes within the domains of nutrition assessment were identified. The intent of the classes is to best group similar pieces of nutrition assessment data. This required substantial reorganization of the nutrition assessment terms and indicators into their appropriate classes. As an example, nutrition assessment terms related to a gap in knowledge were placed in the class Knowledge/Beliefs/Attitudes when previously these terms could have been in the matrix in three areas—intake different from recommended, food/nutrient knowledge and skill, and/or nutrition and health awareness.

- **Clear delineation of terms.** Each nutrition assessment term gathers separate information. As with the standardized language terms for other steps in the Nutrition Care Process, it is necessary to ensure that the terms are discrete. For purposes of communication and data collection, a term must describe one concept. If dietetics practitioners, through the use of standardized language and the Nutrition Care Process, are describing dietetics practice, clear delineation between terms must be achieved.

The nutrition assessment matrix, due to space considerations, has been moved to the ADA website, www.eatright.org, in the Nutrition Care Process section.

Combined Nutrition Assessment and Nutrition Monitoring and Evaluation Terms

This edition contains combined nutrition assessment and nutrition monitoring and evaluation domains, classes, terms, and reference sheets; comparative standards for evaluating nutrient intake and weight; and information clarifying how to address findings that may be consistent with inadequate intake.

- Consolidation of the domains, classes and terms. Nutrition assessment and nutrition monitoring data have substantial overlap in identification and approach. In both steps, data elements are compared to either the nutrition prescription/goal or a reference standard. While dietetics practitioners use assessment data for identification of whether a nutrition problem or diagnosis exists, the same types of data are collected during assessment and reassessment for the purposes of monitoring and evaluation.

  - The domains, classes and terms have been consolidated. Further information regarding the changes is available later in this chapter. A mapping of nutrition monitoring and evaluation terms is available in the nutrition monitoring and evaluation chapter.

  - The combined reference sheets distinguish between nutrition assessment indicators and nutrition monitoring and evaluation indicators by placing *** after indicators only used for nutrition assessment. In some reference sheets, there are NO indicators with *** because all of the indicators are used for both nutrition assessment and nutrition monitoring and evaluation.

  - As a specific example of a change, the nutrition monitoring and evaluation reference sheet Glucose Profile was modified to Glucose/Endocrine Profile. The term and its definition was expanded to include indicators used for nutrition assessment for identification of endocrine disorders, such as thyroid stimulating hormone, while maintaining indicators used for both nutrition assessment and monitoring and evaluation such as fasting glucose and HgbA1c. Thyroid stimulating hormone*** is a nutrition assessment only indicator. In contrast to glucose, which is used for both nutrition assessment and nutrition monitoring and evaluation, thyroid stimulating hormone does not change as a result of nutrition intervention.

> **Note:** On the combined nutrition assessment and monitoring and evaluation reference sheets, indicators used only for nutrition assessment (those that do not change as a result of nutrition intervention) have *** after the indicator. In some reference sheets, there are NO indicators with *** because all of the indicators are used for both nutrition assessment and nutrition monitoring and evaluation.

- **Development of comparative standards reference sheets.** During nutrition assessment and monitoring and evaluation, practitioners determine a patient/client's estimated nutrient needs and often use this information to compare and interpret a patient/client's estimated intake of one or more nutrients. Therefore, comparative standard reference sheets are included with this edition of the reference manual. One potential source for comparison of intake is the Dietary Reference Intakes (DRIs). A comparative standard reference sheet for Recommended Body Weight/Body Mass Index/Growth is also provided.

- **Addition of interpretive information for the Dietary Reference Intakes (DRIs).** The DRIs are one reference standard that dietetics professionals can use for comparison of estimated intake. Since all DRIs are for healthy individuals in a particular life stage and gender group, they may not be applicable standards for all clinical scenarios. Specific guidance on how to appropriately use the DRIs is included in this manual on pages 35-37 within this section.

Clarification for Inadequate Intake

Some dietetics practitioners have raised questions about assessing a patient/client's intake as "inadequate." Critical to the understanding of this subject is the recognition of three issues:

- Because it is very difficult to measure a patient/client's intake even when enteral and/or parenteral nutrition is provided as the sole source of nutrition, it is recommended that additional data for assessment of nutritional status be considered. Indeed, these measures are estimates of intake.

- The DRIs are established for healthy individuals. It is not clear how the DRIs should be interpreted in patients/clients with an illness, injury, disease, or other medical condition.

- Inadequate nutrient intake does not necessarily equate to nutrient deficiency.

As such, the Standardized Language Committee included a clarification statement that should be given professional consideration during nutrition assessment or reassessment when comparing estimated intake to the DRIs and prior to identifying and labeling a patient/client with the nutrition diagnosis of "Inadequate [substance] Intake" (e.g. inadequate vitamin intake, inadequate protein intake). The note is part of the definition for the ten nutrition assessment and monitoring and evaluation reference sheets related to nutrient intake and the eleven nutrition diagnoses with "Inadequate" in the label.

> *Note: Whenever possible, nutrient intake data should be considered in combination with clinical, biochemical, anthropometric information, medical diagnosis, clinical status, and/or other factors as well as diet to provide a valid assessment of nutritional status based on a totality of the evidence. (Dietary Reference Intakes. Applications in Dietary Assessment. Institute of Medicine. Washington, D.C.: National Academy Press; 2000.)*

The notation from the Institute of Medicine (IOM) advises combining intake data with clinical, biochemical, and other supporting information to complete a valid assessment of nutritional status. While it is acknowledged that inadequate intake is not synonymous with nutritional status, there may be an implied expectation that an inadequate intake over a period of time will lead to a change in nutritional status. The difficulty encountered is in the ability to accurately predict the consequences of intake due to a myriad of factors, such as scientific uncertainty about "nutrient requirements," individual differences, and inaccurate intake assessments.

- If a synonym, or alternate word with the same meaning, for the term "inadequate" is helpful or needed, an approved alternate is the word "suboptimal." Thus, a dietetics professional could use either the nutrition diagnosis label "Suboptimal Protein Intake" or "Inadequate Protein Intake."

Bioactive substances do not have established DRIs. They are not considered essential nutrients because inadequate intakes do not result in biochemical or clinical symptoms of deficiency. However, naturally occurring food components with potential risk or benefit to health are reviewed by the Food and Nutrition Board of the Institute of Medicine and, if sufficient data exist, reference intakes are established. Further, the nutrition assessment and monitoring and evaluation reference sheets note that the criteria for evaluation of intake must be the patient/client goal or nutrition prescription because there are no established minimum requirements or Tolerable Upper Intake Levels. The patient/client goal or nutrition prescription would be based upon an individual goal or research, for example, the ADA Disorders of Lipid Metabolism Evidence-Based Guideline. This guideline considers the evidence supporting intake of plant stanol/sterol esters in the presence of lipid disorders. It is available on the ADA Evidence Analysis Library. Therefore, the note added to the definition of Inadequate Bioactive Substance Intake is:

> *Note: Bioactive Substances are not included as part of the Dietary Reference Intakes, and therefore there are no established minimum requirements or Tolerable Upper Intake Levels. However, RDs can assess whether estimated intakes are adequate or excessive using the patient/client goal or nutrition prescription for comparison.*

Further information regarding use of the word "inadequate" in the Nutrition Care Process can be found in the chapters on nutrition diagnosis and nutrition monitoring and evaluation and on the ADA website, www.eatright.org, in the Nutrition Care Process section.

Nutrition Care Process and Nutrition Assessment

Step 1, Nutrition Assessment, of the Nutrition Care Process forms the foundation for progressing through the other three steps in the process. It is a systematic method for obtaining, verifying, and interpreting data needed to identify nutrition-related problems, their causes, and significance. Nutrition assessment is an ongoing, nonlinear, dynamic process that involves initial data collection, but also continual reassessment and analysis of the patient/client's status compared to specified criteria.

Edition: 2009

Special Note: The terms **patient/client** are used in association with the NCP; however, the process is also intended for use with groups. In addition, family members or caregivers are an essential asset to the patient/client and dietetics practitioner in the NCP. Therefore, **groups, families, and caregivers** of patients/clients are implied each time a reference is made to patient/client.

Several data sources frequently contribute to a nutrition assessment, such as information gained from the referring health care provider or agency, patient/client interview, medical record, patient/client rounds, community-based surveys, administrative data, and epidemiological studies. Data sources may vary among nutrition settings.

Patients/clients enter the first step of the NCP, nutrition assessment, through two means, screening and referral, both of which are outside of the NCP. Read more about screening and referral in the Foreword.

Strong critical thinking skills are essential for selection, collection and interpretation of data relevant to patients/clients. Each patient/client presents a unique mix of factors, which impact the nutrition assessment approach. The nature of the individual or group and the practice setting/environment guide the appropriate selection of validated and reliable tools to use in data collection.

Critical Thinking Skills for Nutrition Assessment
- Determining appropriate data to collect
- Determining the need for additional information
- Selecting assessment tools and procedures that match the situation
- Applying assessment tools in valid and reliable ways
- Distinguishing relevant from irrelevant data
- Distinguishing important from unimportant data
- Validating the data

Results of a Nutrition Assessment

Nutrition assessment leads to the appropriate initial determination that a nutrition diagnosis/problem exists. Nutrition reassessment, leads to re-verification that a nutrition diagnosis/problem exists. If so, the dietetics practitioner labels the problem and creates a PES (Problem, Etiology, Signs/Symptoms) statement in Step 2 of the NCP.

Upon completion of an initial or reassessment, it is also possible that a nutrition problem may not be identified, further information or testing may be necessary to make a determination, or the problem may not be modifiable by further nutrition care and discharge or discontinuation from this episode of nutrition care may be appropriate.

As noted earlier, screening and referral are the typical entrance points into the Nutrition Care Process. A screening tool may provide some evidence of an emerging nutrition problem; however, thorough review of the patient/client assessment data may yield no nutrition problem. The same may be true of a referral. Other medical professionals or system protocols may prompt a referral of a patient/client to a nutrition professional, but a nutrition problem is not always present. At that point, it is incumbent on the professional to document the approach recommended, such as whether additional information/testing is needed or if discharge from nutrition care is appropriate.

Important: Based on the nutrition assessment/reassessment, the dietetics practitioner determines:
- IF a nutrition diagnosis/problem exists AND
- The plan for continuation of care, specifically, progression through the NCP, the need for additional information/testing prior to continuing in the process, or discharge from nutrition care.

Relationships

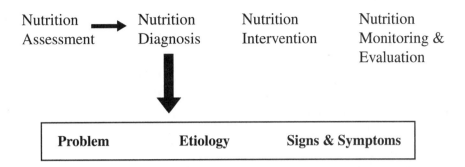

Dietetics practitioners use the data collected in the nutrition assessment to identify and label the patient/client's nutrition diagnosis using standard nutrition diagnostic terminology. Each nutrition diagnosis has a reference sheet that includes its definition, possible etiology/causes and common signs or symptoms identified in the nutrition assessment step.

Relationships

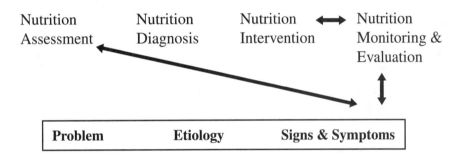

In addition, through nutrition reassessment, dietetics practitioners perform nutrition monitoring and evaluation to determine if the nutrition intervention strategy is working to resolve the nutrition diagnosis, its etiology, and/or signs and symptoms.

Nutrition Assessment Domains

In the development of the standardized nutrition diagnosis language, the following five domains of nutrition assessment data were identified—food/nutrition-related history; biochemical data, medical tests, and procedures; anthropometric measurements; nutrition-focused physical findings; and client history. Because the nutrition assessment forms the basis for identifying a nutrition diagnosis, these terms are reflected on each nutrition diagnosis reference sheet and the signs/symptoms are grouped by category of nutrition assessment data.

Following are some examples of data collected within each assessment domain; however, these examples are not all-inclusive:

> **Food/Nutrition-Related History** consists of food and nutrient intake, medication and herbal supplement intake, knowledge/beliefs/attitudes, behavior, factors affecting access to food and food/nutrition-related supplies, physical activity and nutrition quality of life.
>
>> **Food and nutrient intake** includes factors such as composition and adequacy of food and nutrient intake, meal and snack patterns, and current and previous diets and/or food modifications, and eating environment.

Edition: 2009

Medication and herbal supplement intake includes prescription and over-the-counter medications, including herbal preparations and complementary medicine products used.

Knowledge/beliefs/attitudes includes understanding of nutrition-related concepts and conviction of the truth and feelings/emotions toward some nutrition-related statement or phenomenon, along with readiness to change nutrition-related behaviors.

Behavior includes patient/client activities and actions which influence achievement of nutrition-related goals.

Factors affecting access to food and food/nutrition-related supplies includes factors that affect intake and availability of a sufficient quantity of safe, healthful food as well as food/nutrition-related supplies.

Physical activity and function includes physical activity, cognitive and physical ability to engage in specific tasks, e.g., breastfeeding and self-feeding.

Nutrition-related patient/client-centered measures consists of patient/client's perception of his/her nutrition intervention and its impact on life.

Note: Whenever possible, nutrient intake data should be considered in combination with clinical, biochemical, anthropometric information, medical diagnosis, clinical status, and/or other factors as well as diet to provide a valid assessment of nutritional status based on a totality of the evidence. (Dietary Reference Intakes. Applications in Dietary Assessment. Institute of Medicine. Washington, D.C.: National Academy Press; 2000.)

Anthropometric Measurements include height, weight, body mass index (BMI), growth pattern indices/percentile ranks, and weight history.

Biochemical Data, Medical Tests, and Procedures include laboratory data, (e.g., electrolytes, glucose, and lipid panel) and tests (e.g., gastric emptying time, resting metabolic rate).

Nutrition-Focused Physical Findings include findings from an evaluation of body systems, muscle and subcutaneous fat wasting, oral health, suck/swallow/breathe ability, appetite, and affect.

Client History consists of current and past information related to personal, medical, family, and social history.

Personal history includes general patient/client information such as age, gender, race/ethnicity, language, education, and role in family.

Patient/client/family medical/health history includes patient/client or family disease states, conditions, and illnesses that may have a nutritional impact.

Social history includes items such as socioeconomic status, housing situation, medical care support and involvement in social groups.

In addition to this reference, additional resources for nutrition assessment include *ADA's Pocket Guide to Nutrition Assessment* (3), and *ADA's Pocket Guide to Pediatric Nutrition Assessment* (4).

In regard to the Biochemical, Medical Tests, and Procedures category of nutrition assessment, the nutrition diagnoses may contain normal test levels and ranges only for guidance. Nutrition interventions should be individualized based on many factors, and laboratory values alone are not diagnostic. A nutrition diagnosis is assigned based on the clinical judgment of an appropriately educated, experienced individual.

Nutrition Assessment Components: Review, Cluster, and Identify

In the first step of the Nutrition Care Process, dietetics practitioners do the following three things—

- Review data collected for factors that affect nutritional and health status.
- Cluster individual data elements to identify a nutrition diagnosis as described in the nutrition diagnosis reference sheets.
- Identify standards by which data will be compared.

Review

Nutrition assessment indicators are clearly defined markers that can be observed and measured. Selected nutrition assessment data should be relevant to the patient/client's nutrition diagnosis, its etiology, and signs/symptoms. The data may also be relevant to the patient/client disease state, quality management goals for nutrition, and nutrition care and health care outcome goals.

Practitioners use nutrition assessment data to identify and provide evidence about a nutrition-related problem or diagnosis. Specific data elements or indicators may also be used by practitioners to monitor and evaluate progress made toward desired nutrition care outcomes, where the nutrition care outcome indicators provide information about the type and magnitude of progress made, when the nutrition problem is resolved, and what aspects of nutrition intervention are or are not working.

Cluster

Organized assessment data are clustered for comparison with the defining characteristics of suspected diagnoses as listed in the diagnosis reference sheets. One data element of the nutrition assessment may lead dietetics practitioners toward a particular nutrition diagnosis, but it is the clustering of data that results in identification of the correct nutrition diagnosis at that point in time.

Note: Defining characteristics are a typical cluster of signs and symptoms that provide evidence that a nutrition diagnosis exists. Signs are the observations of a trained clinician and symptoms are changes reported by the patient/client (1).

Identify

National, institutional, and/or regulatory standards are essential for nutrition assessment data comparison when available. For assessment data related to the intake of specific nutrients, comparative standards are available in this resource for guiding accurate documentation of a patient/client's nutrition recommendation and for comparison of the patient/client's estimates of intake or estimates of usual intake of one or more nutrients. Dietetics practitioners must identify the most appropriate reference standard or goal based upon, at a minimum, the following:

- Practice setting (e.g., inpatient or outpatient, long-term care, community)
- Age of the patient/client (e.g., pediatrics, geriatrics)
- Disease/injury state and severity (e.g., renal disease, diabetes, critical illness)

For example, HgbA1c is a valid measure of glucose status during a 60-90 day period. Therefore, it may be useful in assessing a patient/client's glucose status prior to a hospital admission, but is not relevant data for assessing an ICU patient/client with an acute elevation of blood glucose. This example illustrates the importance of appropriate nutrition assessment data selection and interpretation.

Each situation will be different depending upon the practice setting, population, and disease state and severity. Additional factors, such as regulations, care standards, and quality management goals, may also influence indicator selection and evaluation. Identification of the incorrect assessment data or misinterpretation of the data element may lead to an incorrect nutrition diagnosis. Moreover, the appropriate standards or criteria should be noted in the dietetics practitioner's policies and procedures or other documents for use in patient/client records, quality or performance improvement, or in formal research projects.

Edition: 2009

> **Nutrition Assessment Components Summary**
> - Review data collected for factors that influence nutritional and health status.
> - Cluster individual data elements to identify a nutrition diagnosis as described in the diagnosis reference sheets.
> - Identify standards by which data will be compared.

Nutrition Care Indicators

Nutrition care indicators are clearly defined markers that can be observed and measured. As noted previously, indicators gathered during nutrition assessment are clustered to identify and label a patient/client's nutrition diagnosis and its etiology and signs/symptoms. The indicators selected may also be used in the future to evaluate changes in the patient/client's nutrition diagnosis, disease state, quality management goals for nutrition, and health care outcome goals.

Nutrition care indicators include:

- Food and nutrient intake; medication use; growth and body composition; food and nutrition-related knowledge, attitudes and behaviors; food access; and functional capabilities such as physical activity
- Anthropometric data, such as growth pattern and weight history
- Laboratory values, such as HgbA1c, hematocrit, serum cholesterol
- Physical findings that are observed or obtained through interview or the medical record
- Personal and family medical history and social factors

Nutrition assessment reference sheets, combined with nutrition monitoring and evaluation reference sheets, define the nutrition care indicators that may be appropriate for assessment and monitoring and evaluation within a variety of practice settings.

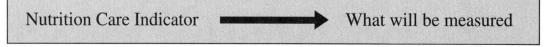

Nutrition Care Indicator ➡ What will be measured

Assessment of Nutrition Indicators

Dietetics practitioners make judgments comparing the actual value of the measured indicator to a science-based criteria or individualized goal.

Criteria

Two criteria are suggested for nutrition assessment. The same two criteria are used for monitoring and evaluation:

- Nutrition prescription or goal (e.g., a behavior has a goal not a nutrition prescription)
- Reference standard (e.g., national, institutional, and/or regulatory standards)

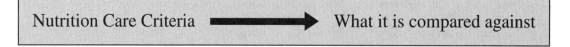

Nutrition Care Criteria ➡ What it is compared against

The nutrition prescription is the patient/client's individualized recommended dietary intake of energy and/or selected foods or nutrients based on current reference standards or dietary guidelines and the patient/client's health condition and nutrition diagnosis. For example, a patient of normal body weight has a serum LDL cholesterol of 150 mg/dL. His nutrition prescription is <30% calories from fat with <10% calories from saturated fat.

For biochemical measures such as LDL cholesterol, the criteria that may be used is the reference standard established by the National Heart Lung and Blood Institute of serum LDL <100 mg/dL.

Special Note: Laboratory parameters within the reference sheets are provided only for guidance.

- Laboratory values may vary depending on the laboratory performing the test.
- Scientific consensus concerning selection of biochemical tests, laboratory methods, reference standards, or interpretation of data does not always exist.
- Laboratory findings may be evaluated for their significance or lack of significance depending on the patient/ client population, disease severity, and/or treatment goals.
- Current national, institutional, and regulatory guidelines that affect practice should be applied as appropriate to individual patients/clients.

Reference standards, as noted previously, are national, institutional, and/or regulatory standards. Dietetics practitioners are familiar with reference standards for laboratory measures. Examples of other reference standards include:

- National standards for populations or patient/client groups or disease conditions, e.g., Dietary Reference Intakes (DRIs), Dietary Guidelines or guidelines for specific treatment or disease condition such as those developed by the American Society of Parenteral and Enteral Nutrition and/or the National Kidney Foundation.
- Institutional standards, e.g., established guidelines specifying how to evaluate weight change in geriatric patients/ clients.
- Regulatory standards, e.g., Omnibus Budget Reconciliation Act (OBRA) guidelines for long-term care, the Joint Commission standards.

Dietetics practitioners select the most appropriate reference standard or goal based upon the patient/client condition and patient care setting. Further, dietetics practitioners are responsible for understanding any defining parameters or limitations for reference standards used. The DRIs, for example, have very specific parameters for interpretation of estimated intake.

Assessment of Nutrient Intake

Dietetics practitioners must keep in mind that nutrient intake assessments are estimations. To begin with, data collection for nutrient intake is imprecise since it relies generally on patient/client estimations and reports of intake. Enteral and/or parenteral nutrition intake can be more precise if it is the sole source of nutrition and accurate records of enteral and/or parenteral nutrition delivery are available.

Once the data are collected, dietetics practitioners compare the estimated nutrient intake to a patient/client goal or a reference standard. Historically, the DRIs have been used for comparison of intake in a variety of populations since other specific reference standards are not always available. Practitioners must keep in mind that the DRIs have the following interpretation parameters:

- For evaluation of nutritional status, nutrient intake data should be combined with biochemical, clinical, anthropometric, medical diagnosis, and clinical data.
- The DRIs are established for healthy individuals. It is not clear how the DRIs should be interpreted in patients/ clients with an illness, injury, disease, or other medical condition.
- Estimations consistent with inadequate intake do not necessarily mean there is a nutrient deficiency.

The notation from the Institute of Medicine (IOM) advises combining intake data with clinical, biochemical, and other supporting information to complete a valid assessment of nutritional status. While it is acknowledged that inadequate intake is not synonymous with nutritional status, there may be an implied expectation that an inadequate intake over a period of time will lead to a change in nutritional status. The difficulty encountered is in the ability to accurately predict the consequences of intake due to a myriad of factors, such as, scientific uncertainty about "nutrient requirements," individual differences, and inaccurate intake assessments.

- If a synonym, or alternate word with the same meaning, for the term "inadequate" is helpful or needed, an approved alternate is the word "suboptimal." Thus, a dietetics professional could use either the nutrition diagnosis label "Suboptimal Protein Intake" or "Inadequate Protein Intake."

Edition: 2009

- The following note is part of the definition for the ten nutrition assessment and monitoring and evaluation reference sheets related to nutrient intake and the eleven nutrition diagnoses with "Inadequate" in the label.

  Note: Whenever possible, nutrient intake data should be considered in combination with clinical, biochemical, anthropometric information, medical diagnosis, clinical status, and/or other factors as well as diet to provide a valid assessment of nutritional status based on a totality of the evidence. (Dietary Reference Intakes. Applications in Dietary Assessment. Institute of Medicine. Washington, D.C.: National Academy Press; 2000.)

Bioactive substances do not have established DRIs. They are not considered essential nutrients because inadequate intakes do not result in biochemical or clinical symptoms of deficiency. However, naturally occurring food components with potential risk or benefit to health are reviewed by the Food and Nutrition Board of the Institute of Medicine and, if sufficient data exist, reference intakes are established. Further, the nutrition assessment and monitoring and evaluation reference sheets note that the criteria for evaluation of intake must be the patient/client goal or nutrition prescription since there are no established minimum requirements or Tolerable Upper Intake Levels. The patient/client goal or nutrition prescription would be based upon an individual goal or research, for example, the ADA Disorders of Lipid Metabolism Evidence-Based Guideline. This guideline considers the evidence supporting intake of plant stanol/sterol esters in the presence of lipid disorders. It is available on the ADA Evidence Analysis Library. Therefore, the note added to the definition of Inadequate Bioactive Substance Intake is:

  Note: Bioactive Substances are not included as part of the Dietary Reference Intakes, and therefore there are no established minimum requirements or Tolerable Upper Intake Levels. However, RDs can assess whether estimated intakes are adequate or excessive using the patient/client goal or nutrition prescription for comparison.

It is important to reiterate that dietetics professionals are given two criteria for use when assessing intake—the nutrition prescription/goal and the reference standards (e.g., national, institutional, and/or regulatory standards). Practitioners are not limited to using the DRIs as the criteria for comparison of nutrient intake data. In certain populations where other appropriate scientific information has emerged and reference standards are available, such as in renal disease, it may be appropriate to use an alternate reference standard instead of the DRIs.

Nutrition Assessment and Monitoring and Evaluation Reference Sheets

Following this introduction to nutrition assessment are combined Nutrition Assessment and Monitoring and Evaluation reference sheets.

Similarities between Nutrition Assessment and Monitoring and Evaluation

Dietetics practitioners familiar with the standardized language for nutrition monitoring and evaluation will find that the data described for nutrition assessment are quite familiar. In defining the nutrition monitoring and evaluation taxonomy, it was clear that there is substantial overlap between nutrition assessment and nutrition monitoring and evaluation terminology. Many data points assessed are used, through nutrition reassessment, in monitoring and evaluation.

Therefore, the domains, classes, terms, and reference sheets were combined for Nutrition Assessment and Nutrition Monitoring and Evaluation. The approach for collecting both types of data is the same. Practitioners first collect and record data and then interpret the data relative to some criteria, a goal or nutrition prescription or national, institutional, and/or regulatory standards. Further, dietetics practitioners assess and reassess data during monitoring and evaluation.

Some practitioners may believe that during an episode of nutrition care, nutrition assessment to nutrition monitoring and evaluation is a strictly linear process; however, this is not always the case. Dietetics professionals assess and reassess the patient/client during an episode of care to determine whether there are changes to the nutrition diagnosis, emergence of a new diagnosis, and progress because of nutrition intervention.

It is important to reiterate that while the data may be the same or related in these two steps, the purpose and use are distinct. The nutrition assessment data are needed to identify whether a nutrition-related problem exists and to establish a plan for continuation for care. The monitoring and evaluation data are necessary for evaluating the outcomes of nutrition interventions.

Differences between Nutrition Assessment and Nutrition Monitoring and Evaluation

Nutrition assessment includes a broader set of data elements or indicators since data may be assessed, but it may not be monitored for change after nutrition intervention. On the reference sheets, indicators practitioners use only for nutrition assessment have *** after the indicator. In some reference sheets, there are NO indicators with *** because all of the indicators are used for both nutrition assessment and nutrition monitoring and evaluation

One example of an indicator used only for nutrition assessment is body temperature. Practitioners include body temperature in a nutrition assessment if it is relevant to the patient/client's nutrition diagnosis and/or nutrition intervention. However, the practitioner cannot change the fever through nutrition intervention; therefore, body temperature is not included in nutrition monitoring and evaluation as an indicator of the impact of nutrition care. Another example of assessment only indicators not used in monitoring and evaluation are medical history data, since nutrition intervention does not influence the presence or absence of a medical diagnosis (or diagnoses).

Nutrition Assessment and Nutrition Monitoring and Evaluation Reference Sheet Content

The combined reference sheets contain eight distinct components:

- Definition of the nutrition assessment and monitoring and evaluation term
- The nutrition assessment and monitoring and evaluation indicators
- Measurement method or data sources recommended
- The nutrition interventions with which the nutrition assessment and monitoring and evaluation data are associated
- The nutrition diagnoses with which the nutrition assessment and monitoring and evaluation data are used
- The criteria for evaluation
- The patient/client nutrition assessment and monitoring and evaluation documentation example
- References

Following is a more complete description of the eight components of the combined nutrition assessment and nutrition monitoring and evaluation reference sheet.

The **Definition** defines the specific parameters of the term.

The **Indicators** identify the data elements that are evaluated to (a) determine the defining characteristics of the patient/client, (b) to measure change based upon nutrition intervention. Dietetics practitioners may or may not use all of the indicators associated with a term. Indicators practitioners use only for nutrition assessment have *** after the indicator. In some reference sheets, there are NO indicators with *** because all of the indicators are used for both nutrition assessment and nutrition monitoring and evaluation.

The **Measurement Method or Data Sources** identify some of the resources dietetics practitioners use to obtain nutrition assessment and nutrition monitoring and evaluation data.

The typical **Nutrition Interventions** with which the nutrition care outcomes are associated are listed.

The typical **Nutrition Diagnoses** associated with the term and indicators are listed.

Two **Criteria** are identified for comparison of the indicators: (a) goal/nutrition prescription, or (b) reference standard.

The **Patient/Client Example** includes sample nutrition assessment and monitoring and evaluation documentation. It describes only one of the indicators. As described earlier, depending on the practice setting (e.g., inpatient or outpatient, long-term care, community), patient/client (e.g., pediatrics, geriatrics), and disease state and severity, one or multiple indicators may be followed at a time.

References for measurement techniques and reference standards for common patient/client populations and settings. Dietetics practitioners are not limited to the references offered and are encouraged to use others pertinent to their patient/client and practice setting needs.

Edition: 2009

Once measurement techniques and criteria, as well as any other pertinent parameters, are identified, they should be noted in the dietetics practitioner's policies and procedures or other documents for use in patient/client records, quality or performance improvement, or in formal research projects.

Individual Patient/Client Example

Nutrition assessment and/or monitoring and evaluation term: Nutritional anemia profile

Nutrition care indicator: Serum ferritin

Criteria: Based on a reference standard: The patient/client's serum ferritin is 8 ng/mL, which is below (above, below, within) the expected limit for adult females.

Nutrition assessment and monitoring and evaluation documentation:

Initial nutrition assessment with patient/client	Patient/client's serum ferritin is 8 ng/mL, which is below the expected limit for adult females. Will monitor change in serum ferritin at the next appointment.
Reassessment after nutrition intervention	Goal/reference standard achieved as patient/client's serum ferritin is 10.9 ng/mL, within normal limits.

Group Example

Nutrition assessment and/or monitoring and evaluation term: Nutritional anemia profile

Nutrition care indicator: Hemoglobin

Criteria: Based on a reference standard: 20% or fewer of low-income women will have a hemoglobin level < 11.0 g/dL during the third trimester of pregnancy (Healthy People 2010).

Nutrition assessment and monitoring and evaluation documentation:

Initial nutrition assessment with population	44% of low-income black women have a hemoglobin level of < 11.0 g/dL during the third trimester of pregnancy. Monitor change in prevalence of low hemoglobin levels among low-income women.
Reassessment after nutrition intervention	Prevalence of anemia among low-income pregnant women is 29%. Significant progress made toward the Healthy People 2010 target, 20% or less, for prevalence of anemia.

These reference sheets will assist dietetics practitioners working in a variety of settings, with individuals and groups, when assessing and monitoring and evaluating nutrition care indicators.

Nutrition Assessment: Documentation

Documentation is recommended throughout the Nutrition Care Process and supports all of the steps. Quality documentation of the nutrition assessment step should be relevant, accurate, and timely. Inclusion of the following information would further describe quality nutrition assessment documentation:

- Date and time
- Pertinent data collected and comparison with standards, such as, estimated nutrient intake; Dietary Reference Intakes; patient/client perceptions, values, and motivation related to presenting problems; patient/client's level of understanding, food-related behaviors, and other nutrition care indicators for future nutrition monitoring and evaluation
- Reason for discharge/discontinuation if appropriate

Nutrition Assessment: Data Sources and Tools

To complete a patient/client's nutrition assessment, the following tools may be useful:

- Screening or referral form
- Patient/client interview
- Medical or health records
- Consultation with other caregivers including family members
- Community based surveys and focus groups
- Statistical reports, administrative data and epidemiological studies.

These tools can be used when patients are seen individually or in groups, or when the encounter is conducted by phone or via computer. Pooled data may be monitored and evaluated using tracking forms and computer software programs.

Summary

Nutrition assessment is the first step in the Nutrition Care Process, but it is used throughout each cycle of the Nutrition Care Process and is not an isolated event. Dietetics practitioners recognize that nutrition assessment is a dynamic process that develops throughout the Nutrition Care Process. For example, a dietetics practitioner may be in the middle of the nutrition education intervention when the client provides a new piece of information that may cause a modification of the nutrition diagnosis, PES statement, or even the nutrition intervention.

Future research will continue to shed light on the appropriate data to collect and their application in nutrition assessment with a patient/client. Moreover, as the profession utilizes nutrition assessment within the other steps of the Nutrition Care Process, the most valid and reliable assessment data to use in nutrition diagnosis, nutrition intervention, and nutrition monitoring and evaluation will also become evident.

References

1. Writing Group of the Nutrition Care Process/Standardized Language Committee. Nutrition care process and model part I: The 2008 update. *J Am Diet Assoc*. 2008;108:1113-1117.
2. US Preventive Services Task Force. Guide to Clinical Preventive Services, 2nd ed. Washington, DC: US Department of Health and Human Services, Office of Disease Prevention and Health Promotion; 1996.
3. Pamela Charney, Ainsley Malone, eds. *ADA Pocket Guide to Nutrition Assessment*, 2nd ed. Chicago, IL: American Dietetic Association; 2009.
4. Leonberg, BL. *ADA Pocket Guide to Pediatric Nutrition Assessment*. Chicago, IL: American Dietetic Association; 2008.

Edition: 2009

Nutrition Assessment and Monitoring and Evaluation Terminolog[...]

This is a combined list of Nutrition Assessment and Monitoring and Evaluation terms. Indicators that are shaded are used ONLY [...] assessment. The rest of the indicators are used for assessment and monitoring and evaluation.

FOOD/NUTRITION-RELATED HISTORY (FH)

Food and nutrient intake, medication/herbal supplement intake, knowledge/beliefs/attitudes and behavior, food and supply availability, physical activity, nutrition quality of life.

Food and Nutrient Intake (1)

Composition and adequacy of food and nutrient intake, meal and snack patterns, current and previous diets and/or food modifications, and eating environment.

Diet History (1.1)

Description of food and drink regularly provided or consumed, past diets followed or prescribed and counseling received, and the eating environment.

Diet order (1.1.1)

❑ General, healthful diet	FH-1.1.1.1
❑ Modified diet (*specify*) _____	FH-1.1.1.2
❑ Enteral nutrition order (*specify*) _____	FH-1.1.1.3
❑ Parenteral nutrition order (*specify*) _____	FH-1.1.1.4

Diet experience (1.1.2)

❑ Previously prescribed diets	FH-1.1.2.1
❑ Previous diet/nutrition education/counseling	FH-1.1.2.2
❑ Self-selected diet/s followed	FH-1.1.2.3
❑ Dieting attempts	FH-1.1.2.4

Eating environment (1.1.3)

❑ Location	FH-1.1.3.1
❑ Atmosphere	FH-1.1.3.2
❑ Caregiver/companion	FH-1.1.3.3
❑ Appropriate breastfeeding accommodations/facility	FH-1.1.3.4

Energy Intake (1.2)

Total energy intake from all sources, including food, beverages, supplements, and via enteral and parenteral routes.

Energy intake (1.2.1)

❑ Total energy intake	FH-1.2.1.1

Food and Beverage Intake (1.3)

Type, amount, and pattern of intake of foods and food groups, indices of diet quality, intake of fluids, breast milk and infant formula

Fluid/Beverage intake (1.3.1)

❑ Oral fluids amounts	FH-1.3.1.1
❑ Food-derived fluids	FH-1.3.1.2
❑ Liquid meal replacement or supplement	FH-1.3.1.3

Food intake (1.3.2)

❑ Amount of food	FH-1.3.2.1
❑ Types of food/meals	FH-1.3.2.2
❑ Meal/snack pattern	FH-1.3.2.3
❑ Diet quality index	FH-1.3.2.4
❑ Food variety	FH-1.3.2.5

Breast milk/infant formula intake (1.3.3)

❑ Breast milk intake	FH-1.3.3.1
❑ Infant formula intake	FH-1.3.3.2

Enteral and Parenteral Nutrition Intake (1.4)

Specialized nutrition support intake from all sources, e.g., enteral and parenteral routes.

Enteral and Parenteral Nutrition Intake (1.4.1)

❑ Access	FH-1.4.1.1
❑ Formula/solution	FH-1.4.1.2
❑ Discontinuation	FH-1.4.1.3
❑ Initiation	FH-1.4.1.4
❑ Rate/schedule	FH-1.4.1.5

Bioactive Substance Intake (1.5)

Alcohol, plant stanol and sterol esters, soy protein, psyllium and β-glucan, and caffeine intake from all sources, e.g., food, beverages, supplements, and via enteral and parenteral routes.

Alcohol intake (1.5.1)

❑ Drink size/volume	FH-1.5.1.1
❑ Frequency	FH-1.5.1.2
❑ Pattern of alcohol consumption	FH-1.5.1.3

Bioactive substance intake (1.5.2)

❑ Plant sterol and stanol esters	FH-1.5.2.1
❑ Soy protein	FH-1.5.2.2
❑ Psyllium and β-glucan	FH-1.5.2.3

Caffeine intake (1.5.3)

❑ Total caffeine	FH-1.5.3.1

Macronutrient Intake (1.6)

Fat and cholesterol, protein, carbohydrate, and fiber intake from all sources including food, beverages, supplements, and via enteral and parenteral routes.

Fat and cholesterol intake (1.6.1)

❑ Total fat	FH-1.6.1.1
❑ Saturated fat	FH-1.6.1.2
❑ Trans fatty acids	FH-1.6.1.3
❑ Polyunsaturated fat	FH-1.6.1.4
❑ Monounsaturated fat	FH-1.6.1.5
❑ Omega-3 fatty acids	FH-1.6.1.6
❑ Dietary cholesterol	FH-1.6.1.7
❑ Essential fatty acids	FH-1.6.1.8

Protein intake (1.6.2)

❑ Total protein	FH-1.6.2.1
❑ High biological value protein	FH-1.6.2.2
❑ Casein	FH-1.6.2.3
❑ Whey	FH-1.6.2.4
❑ Amino acids	FH-1.6.2.5
❑ Essential amino acids	FH-1.6.2.6

Carbohydrate intake (1.6.3)

❑ Total carbohydrate	FH-1.6.3.1
❑ Sugar	FH-1.6.3.2
❑ Starch	FH-1.6.3.3
❑ Glycemic index	FH-1.6.3.4
❑ Glycemic load	FH-1.6.3.5
❑ Source of carbohydrate	FH-1.6.3.6

Fiber intake (1.6.4)

❑ Total fiber	FH-1.6.4.1
❑ Soluble fiber	FH-1.6.4.2
❑ Insoluble fiber	FH-1.6.4.3

Micronutrient Intake (1.7)

Vitamin and mineral intake from all sources, e.g., food, beverages, supplements, and via enteral and parenteral routes.

Vitamin intake (1.7.1)

❑ A (1)	❑ Riboflavin (7)
❑ C (2)	❑ Niacin (8)
❑ D (3)	❑ Folate (9)
❑ E (4)	❑ B6 (10)
❑ K (5)	❑ B12 (11)
❑ Thiamin (6)	❑ Multivitamin (12)
❑ Other (specify) _____ (13)	

Mineral/element intake (1.7.2)

❑ Calcium (1)	❑ Potassium (5)
❑ Chloride (2)	❑ Phosphorus (6)
❑ Iron (3)	❑ Sodium (7)
❑ Magnesium (4)	❑ Zinc (8)
❑ Multi-mineral (9)	
❑ Multi-trace element (10)	
❑ Other, (specify) _____ (11)	

Medication and herbal supple[...]

Prescription and over the counter m[...] ing herbal preparations and compl[...] products used.

Medication and herbal supplements (2.1)

❑ Medications, specify prescription or OTC	FH-2.1.1
❑ Herbal/complementary products (*specify*)	FH-2.1.2
❑ Misuse of medication (*specify*)	FH-2.1.3

Knowledge/Beliefs/Attitudes (3)

Understanding of nutrition-related concepts and conviction of the truth and feelings/emotions toward some nutrition-related statement or phenomenon, along with readiness to change nutrition-related behaviors.

Food and nutrition knowledge (3.1)

❑ Area(s) and level of knowledge	FH-3.1.1
❑ Diagnosis specific or global nutrition-related knowledge score	FH-3.1.2

Beliefs and attitudes (3.2)

❑ Conflict with personal/family value system	FH-3.2.1
❑ Distorted body image	FH-3.2.2
❑ End-of-life decisions	FH-3.2.3
❑ Motivation	FH-3.2.4
❑ Preoccupation with food	FH-3.2.5
❑ Preoccupation with weight	FH-3.2.6
❑ Readiness to change nutrition-related behaviors	FH-3.2.7
❑ Self-efficacy	FH-3.2.8
❑ Self-talk/cognitions	FH-3.2.9
❑ Unrealistic nutrition-related goals	FH-3.2.10
❑ Unscientific beliefs/attitudes	FH-3.2.11

Behavior (4)

Patient/client activities and actions, which influence achievement of nutrition-related goals.

Adherence (4.1)

❑ Self-reported adherence score	FH-4.1.1
❑ Nutrition visit attendance	FH-4.1.2
❑ Ability to recall nutrition goals	FH-4.1.3
❑ Self-monitoring at agreed upon rate	FH-4.1.4
❑ Self-management as agreed upon	FH-4.1.5

Avoidance behavior (4.2)

❑ Avoidance	FH-4.2.1
❑ Restrictive eating	FH-4.2.2
❑ Cause of avoidance behavior	FH-4.2.3

Bingeing and purging behavior (4.3)

❑ Binge eating behavior	FH-4.3.1
❑ Purging behavior	FH-4.3.2

Mealtime behavior (4.4)

❑ Meal duration	FH-4.4.1
❑ Percent of meal time spent eating	FH-4.4.2
❑ Preference to drink rather than eat	FH-4.4.3
❑ Refusal to eat/chew	FH-4.4.4
❑ Spitting food out	FH-4.4.5
❑ Rumination	FH-4.4.6
❑ Patient/client/caregiver fatigue during feeding process resulting in inadequate intake	FH-4.4.7
❑ Willingness to try new foods	FH-4.4.8
❑ Limited number of accepted foods	FH-4.4.9
❑ Rigid sensory preferences	FH-4.4.10

Social network (4.5)

❑ Ability to build and utilize social network	FH-4.5.1

Edition: 2009

ssessment

Factors Affecting Access to Food and Food/Nutrition-Related Supplies (5)

Factors that affect intake and availability of a sufficient quantity of safe, healthful food as well as food/nutrition-related supplies.

Food/nutrition program participation (5.1)

❑ Eligibility for government programs	FH-5.1.1
❑ Participation in government programs	FH-5.1.2
❑ Eligibility for community programs	FH-5.1.3
❑ Participation in community programs	FH-5.1.4

Safe food/meal availability (5.2)

❑ Availability of shopping facilities	FH-5.2.1
❑ Procurement, identification of safe food	FH-5.2.2
❑ Appropriate meal preparation facilities	FH-5.2.3
❑ Availability of safe food storage	FH-5.2.4
❑ Appropriate storage technique	FH-5.2.5

Safe water availability (5.3)

❑ Availability of potable water	FH-5.3.1
❑ Appropriate water decontamination	FH-5.3.2

Food and nutrition-related supplies availability (5.4)

❑ Access to food and nutrition-related supplies	FH-5.4.1
❑ Access to assistive eating devices	FH-5.4.2
❑ Access to assistive food preparation devices	FH 5.4.3

Physical Activity and Function (6)

Physical activity, cognitive and physical ability to engage in specific tasks, e.g., breastfeeding, self-feeding.

Breastfeeding (6.1)

❑ Initiation of breastfeeding	FH-6.1.1
❑ Duration of breastfeeding	FH-6.1.2
❑ Exclusive breastfeeding	FH-6.1.3
❑ Breastfeeding problems	FH-6.1.4

Nutrition-related ADLs and IADLs (6.2)

❑ Physical ability to complete tasks for meal preparation	FH-6.2.1
❑ Physical ability to self-feed	FH-6.2.2
❑ Ability to position self in relation to plate	FH-6.2.3
❑ Receives assistance with intake	FH 6.2.4
❑ Ability to use adaptive eating devices	FH 6.2.5
❑ Cognitive ability to complete tasks for meal preparation	FH-6.2.6
❑ Remembers to eat, recalls eating	FH-6.2.7
❑ Mini Mental State Examination Score	FH-6.2.8
❑ Nutrition-related activities of daily living (ADL) score	FH-6.2.9
❑ Nutrition-related instrumental activities of daily living (IADL) score	FH-6.2.10

Physical activity (6.3)

❑ Physical activity history	FH-6.3.1
❑ Consistency	FH-6.3.2
❑ Frequency	FH-6.3.3
❑ Duration	FH-6.3.4
❑ Intensity	FH-6.3.5
❑ Type of physical activity	FH-6.3.6
❑ Strength	FH-6.3.7
❑ TV/screen time	FH-6.3.8
❑ Other sedentary activity time	FH-6.3.9
❑ Involuntary physical movement	FH-6.3.10

Nutrition-Related Patient/Client-Centered Measures (7)

Patient/client's perception of his/her nutrition intervention and its impact on life.

Nutrition quality of life (7.1)

❑ Nutrition quality of life responses	FH-7.1.1

ANTHROPOMETRIC MEASUREMENTS   (AD)

Height, weight, body mass index (BMI), growth pattern indices/percentile ranks, and weight history.

Body composition/growth/weight history (1.1)

❑ Height/length	AD-1.1.1
❑ Weight	AD-1.1.2
❑ Frame size	AD-1.1.3
❑ Weight change	AD-1.1.4
❑ Body mass index	AD-1.1.5
❑ Growth pattern indices/percentile ranks	AD-1.1.6
❑ Body compartment estimates	AD-1.1.7

BIOCHEMICAL DATA, MEDICAL TESTS AND PROCEDURES   (BD)

Laboratory data, (e.g., electrolytes, glucose, and lipid panel) and tests (e.g., gastric emptying time, resting metabolic rate).

Acid-base balance (1.1)

❑ Arterial pH	BD-1.1.1
❑ Arterial bicarbonate	BD-1.1.2
❑ Partial pressure of carbon dioxide in arterial blood, $PaCO_2$	BD-1.1.3
❑ Partial pressure of oxygen in arterial blood, PaO_2	BD-1.1.4
❑ Venous pH	BD-1.1.5
❑ Venous bicarbonate	BD-1.1.6

Electrolyte and renal profile (1.2)

❑ BUN	BD-1.2.1
❑ Creatinine	BD-1.2.2
❑ BUN:creatinine ratio	BD-1.2.3
❑ Glomerular filtration rate	BD-1.2.4
❑ Sodium	BD-1.2.5
❑ Chloride	BD-1.2.6
❑ Potassium	BD-1.2.7
❑ Magnesium	BD-1.2.8
❑ Calcium, serum	BD-1.2.9
❑ Calcium, ionized	BD-1.2.10
❑ Phosphorus	BD-1.2.11
❑ Serum osmolality	BD-1.2.12
❑ Parathyroid hormone	BD-1.2.13

Essential fatty acid profile (1.3)

❑ Triene:Tetraene ratio	BD-1.3.1

Gastrointestinal profile (1.4)

❑ Alkaline phophatase	BD-1.4.1
❑ Alanine aminotransferase, ALT	BD-1.4.2
❑ Aspartate aminotransferase, AST	BD-1.4.3
❑ Gamma glutamyl transferase, GGT	BD-1.4.4
❑ Gastric residual volume	BD-1.4.5
❑ Bilirubin, total	BD-1.4.6
❑ Ammonia, serum	BD-1.4.7
❑ Toxicology report, including alcohol	BD-1.4.8
❑ Prothrombin time, PT	BD-1.4.9
❑ Partial thromboplastin time, PTT	BD-1.4.10
❑ INR (ratio)	BD-1.4.11
❑ Fecal fat	BD-1.4.12
❑ Amylase	BD-1.4.13
❑ Lipase	BD-1.4.14

Gastrointestinal profile, cont'd (1.4)

❑ Other digestive enzymes (*specify*)	BD-1.4.15
❑ D-xylose	BD-1.4.16
❑ Hydrogen breath test	BD-1.4.17
❑ Intestinal biopsy	BD-1.4.18
❑ Stool culture	BD-1.4.19
❑ Gastric emptying time	BD-1.4.20
❑ Small bowel transit time	BD-1.4.21
❑ Abdominal films	BD-1.4.22
❑ Swallow study	BD-1.4.23

Glucose/endocrine profile (1.5)

❑ Glucose, fasting	BD-1.5.1
❑ Glucose, casual	BD-1.5.2
❑ HgbA1c	BD-1.5.3
❑ Preprandial capillary plasma glucose	BD-1.5.4
❑ Peak postprandial capillary plasma glucose	BD-1.5.5
❑ Glucose tolerance test	BD-1.5.6
❑ Cortisol level	BD-1.5.7
❑ IGF-binding protein	BD-1.5.8
❑ Thyroid function tests (TSH, T4, T3)	BD-1.5.9

Inflammatory profile (1.6)

❑ C-reactive protein	BD-1.6.1

Lipid profile (1.7)

❑ Cholesterol, serum	BD-1.7.1
❑ Cholesterol, HDL	BD-1.7.2
❑ Cholesterol, LDL	BD-1.7.3
❑ Cholesterol, non-HDL	BD-1.7.4
❑ Total cholesterol:HDL cholesterol	BD-1.7.5
❑ LDL:HDL	BD-1.7.6
❑ Triglycerides, serum	BD-1.7.7

Metabolic rate profile (1.8)

❑ Resting metabolic rate, measured	BD-1.8.1
❑ RQ	BD-1.8.2

Mineral profile (1.9)

❑ Copper, serum or plasma	BD-1.9.1
❑ Iodine, urinary excretion	BD-1.9.2
❑ Zinc, serum or plasma	BD-1.9.3
❑ Other	BD-1.9.4

Nutritional anemia profile (1.10)

❑ Hemoglobin	BD-1.10.1
❑ Hematocrit	BD-1.10.2
❑ Mean corpuscular volume	BD-1.10.3
❑ Red blood cell folate	BD-1.10.4
❑ Red cell distribution width	BD-1.10.5
❑ B12, serum	BD-1.10.6
❑ Methylmalonic acid, serum	BD-1.10.7
❑ Folate, serum	BD-1.10.8
❑ Homocysteine, serum	BD-1.10.9
❑ Ferritin, serum	BD-1.10.10
❑ Iron, serum	BD-1.10.11
❑ Total iron-binding capacity	BD-1.10.12
❑ Transferrin saturation	BD-1.10.13

Protein profile (1.11)

❑ Albumin	BD-1.11.1
❑ Prealbumin	BD-1.11.2
❑ Transferrin	BD-1.11.3
❑ Phenylalanine, plasma	BD-1.11.4
❑ Tyrosine, plasma	BD-1.11.5
❑ Amino acid, other, specify	BD-1.11.6

Urine profile (1.12)

❑ Urine color	BD-1.12.1
❑ Urine osmolality	BD-1.12.2
❑ Urine specific gravity	BD-1.12.3
❑ Urine test, specify	BD-1.12.4
❑ Urine volume	BD-1.12.5

Vitamin profile (1.13)

❑ Vitamin A, serum or plasma retinol	BD-1.13.1
❑ Vitamin C, plasma or serum	BD-1.13.2
❑ Vitamin D, 25-hydroxy	BD-1.13.3
❑ Vitamin E, plasma alpha-tocopherol	BD-1.13.4
❑ Thiamin, activity coefficient for erythrocyte transketolase activity	BD-1.13.5
❑ Riboflavin, activity coefficient for erythrocyte glutathione reductase activity	BD-1.13.6
❑ Niacin, urinary N'methyl-nicotinamide concentration	BD-1.13.7
❑ Vitamin B6, plasma or serum pyridoxal 5'phosphate concentration	BD-1.13.8
❑ Other	BD-1.13.9

NUTRITION-FOCUSED PHYSICAL FINDINGS (PD)

Findings from an evaluation of body systems, muscle and subcutaneous fat wasting, oral health, suck/swallow/breathe ability, appetite, and affect.

Nutrition-focused physical findings (1.1)

❑ Overall appearance (specify) _____	PD-1.1.1
❑ Body language (specify) _____	PD-1.1.2
❑ Cardiovascular-pulmonary (specify) _____	PD-1.1.3
❑ Extremities, muscles and bones (specify) _____	PD-1.1.4
❑ Digestive system (mouth to rectum) (specify) _____	PD-1.1.5
❑ Head and eyes (specify) _____	PD-1.1.6
❑ Nerves and cognition (specify) _____	PD-1.1.7
❑ Skin (specify) _____	PD-1.1.8
❑ Vital signs (specify) _____	PD-1.1.9

CLIENT HISTORY (CH)

Current and past information related to personal, medical, family, and social history.

Personal History (1)

General patient/client information such as age, gender, race/ethnicity, language, education, and role in family.

Personal data (1.1)

❑ Age	CH-1.1.1
❑ Gender	CH-1.1.2
❑ Race/Ethnicity	CH-1.1.3
❑ Language	CH-1.1.4
❑ Literacy factors	CH-1.1.5
❑ Education	CH-1.1.6
❑ Role in family	CH-1.1.7
❑ Tobacco use	CH-1.1.8
❑ Physical disability	CH-1.1.9
❑ Mobility	CH-1.1.10

Patient/Client/Family Medical/Health History (2)

Patient/client or family disease states, conditions, and illnesses that may have nutritional impact.

Patient/client OR family nutrition-oriented medical/health history (2.1)

Specify issue(s) and whether it is patient/client history (P) or family history (F)

❑ Patient/client chief nutrition complaint (specify) _____	CH-2.1.1 P or F
❑ Cardiovascular (specify) _____	CH-2.1.2 P or F
❑ Endocrine/metabolism (specify) _____	CH-2.1.3 P or F
❑ Excretory (specify) _____	CH-2.1.4 P or F
❑ Gastrointestinal (specify) _____	CH-2.1.5 P or F
❑ Gynecological (specify) _____	CH-2.1.6 P or F
❑ Hematology/oncology (specify) _____	CH-2.1.7 P or F
❑ Immune (e.g., food allergies) (specify) _____	CH-2.1.8 P or F
❑ Integumentary (specify) _____	CH-2.1.9 P or F
❑ Musculo-skeletal (specify) _____	CH-2.1.10 P or F
❑ Neurological (specify) _____	CH-2.1.11 P or F
❑ Psychological (specify) _____	CH-2.1.12 P or F
❑ Respiratory (specify) _____	CH-2.1.13 P or F

Treatments/therapy/alternative medicine (2.2)

Documented medical or surgical treatments, complementary and alternative medicine that may impact nutritional status of the patient

❑ Medical treatment/therapy (specify) _____	CH-2.2.1
❑ Surgical treatment (specify) _____	CH-2.2.2
❑ Complementary/alternative medicine (specify) _____	CH-2.2.3

Social History (3)

Patient/client socioeconomic status, housing situation, medical care support and involvement in social groups.

Social history (3.1)

❑ Socioeconomic factors (specify) _____	CH-3.1.1
❑ Living/housing situation (specify) _____	CH-3.1.2
❑ Domestic issues (specify) _____	CH-3.1.3
❑ Social and medical support (specify) _____	CH-3.1.4
❑ Geographic location of home (specify) _____	CH-3.1.5
❑ Occupation (specify) _____	CH-3.1.6
❑ Religion (specify) _____	CH-3.1.7
❑ History of recent crisis (specify) _____	CH-3.1.8
❑ Daily stress level	CH-3.1.9

COMPARATIVE STANDARDS (CS)

Energy Needs (1)

Estimated energy needs (1.1)

❑ Total energy estimated needs	CS-1.1.1
❑ Method for estimating needs	CS-1.1.2

Macronutrient Needs (2)

Estimated fat needs (2.1)

❑ Total fat estimated needs	CS-2.1.1
❑ Type of fat needed	CS-2.1.2
❑ Method for estimating needs	CS-2.1.3

Estimated protein needs (2.2)

❑ Total protein estimated needs	CS-2.2.1
❑ Type of protein needed	CS-2.2.2
❑ Method for estimating needs	CS-2.2.3

Estimated carbohydrate needs (2.3)

❑ Total carbohydrate estimated needs	CS-2.3.1
❑ Type of carbohydrate needed	CS-2.3.2
❑ Method for estimating needs	CS-2.3.3

Estimated fiber needs (2.4)

❑ Total fiber estimated needs	CS-2.4.1
❑ Type of fiber needed	CS-2.4.2
❑ Method for estimating needs	CS-2.4.3

Fluid Needs (3)

Estimated fluid needs (3.1)

❑ Total fluid estimated needs	CS-3.1.1
❑ Method for estimating needs	CS-3.1.2

Micronutrient Needs (4)

Estimated vitamin needs (4.1)

❑ A (1)	❑ Riboflavin (7)
❑ C (2)	❑ Niacin (8)
❑ D (3)	❑ Folate (9)
❑ E (4)	❑ B6 (10)
❑ K (5)	❑ B12 (11)
❑ Thiamin (6)	
❑ Other (specify) (12)	
❑ Method for estimating needs (13)	

Estimated mineral needs (4.2)

❑ Calcium (1)	❑ Potassium (5)
❑ Chloride (2)	❑ Phosphorus (6)
❑ Iron (3)	❑ Sodium (7)
❑ Magnesium (4)	❑ Zinc (8)
❑ Other (specify) (9)	
❑ Method for estimating needs (10)	

Weight and Growth Recommendation (5)

Recommended body weight/body mass index/growth (5.1)

❑ Ideal/reference body weight (IBW)	CS-5.1.1
❑ Recommended body mass index (BMI)	CS-5.1.2
❑ Desired growth pattern	CS-5.1.3

Edition: 2009

Dietary Reference Intakes (DRIs) Interpretation

Purpose

To provide guidance on how to appropriately use the Dietary Reference Intakes (DRIs). Since all DRIs are for healthy individuals in a particular life stage and gender group, they may not be applicable reference standards for all clinical scenarios (1).

Application in the Nutrition Care Process

DRIs can be used to evaluate a "healthy" individual's "usual" intake. Usual intake should reflect long-term average intake over many days; if intake is reported for a small number of days, then the probability of adequacy should be interpreted with caution (1). However assessment in the context of the Nutrition Care Process often involves an individual patient/client whose intake is not "usual" and/or who is not "healthy."

Therefore, when assessing adequacy of intake for a patient/client, the registered dietitian will need to use clinical judgment to determine adequacy with special consideration for the following two factors:

- Intake may not be "usual" and/or
- Patient may not be "healthy"

Intake may not be usual

The ability and appropriateness of assessing "usual" intake will vary depending on the specific circumstances and may be independent of the care setting.

For example, in an acute care setting, it may be necessary to assess current intake (e.g., nutrition support for a trauma patient) or "usual" intake prior to admission in order to evaluate current nutritional status (e.g., cystic fibrosis patient/client). Assessing "usual" intake may be appropriate and achievable for the long-term care resident. Additionally, in the ambulatory care setting, while "usual" intake will generally be used, it may be more appropriate to assess intake since the beginning of an event, such as a new-onset disease diagnosis.

If a patient/client's estimated intake is less than normally recommended for a healthy individual, then the determination of suboptimal nutrient intake(s) based on a comparison with the DRI will need to be carefully evaluated given the specific circumstances.

Patient/client may not be "healthy"

The DRIs are based on recommendations for apparently healthy individuals. However, when a patient/client has an illness, injury, disease, or other medical condition, he/she may no longer be considered "healthy." Therefore, the DRIs may not be the most appropriate reference standard to assess intake adequacy for individuals with altered nutrient requirements due to one or more medical condition. However, if no other reference standard exists, it may be safe to assume in most situations that a patient/client's intake goal/nutrition prescription should not be below the appropriate DRI (RDA or AI) considering the potential for altered nutrient requirements.

In summary, although intake data and recommendations are estimates, assessing intake is still worthwhile and may identify nutrients either under- or over-consumed by individuals. To increase dietary assessment accuracy, ensure that dietary data are as complete as possible, portions are correctly specified, and food composition data are accurate. Whenever possible, nutrient intake data should be considered in combination with clinical, biochemical, anthropometric information, medical diagnosis, clinical status and/or other factors as well as diet to provide a valid assessment of nutritional status based on a totality of the evidence.

What are the DRIs?

They are four categories of reference values set when adequate evidence-based information is available about nutrients or food components (1).

- **Estimated Average Requirement (EAR)**—Mean requirement for a nutrient or the average daily nutrient intake level estimated to meet the requirement of half of the healthy individuals in a particular life stage and gender group.

- **Recommended Dietary Allowance (RDA)**—Recommended intake or the average daily nutrient intake level sufficient to meet the nutrient requirement of 97 to 98 percent of individuals in a particular life stage and gender group.

- **Adequate Intake (AI)**—*Recommended intake* – a recommended intake level based on observed or experimentally determined approximations or estimates of nutrient intake by a group (or groups) of healthy people that are assumed to be adequate – used when an RDA cannot be determined.

- **Tolerable Upper Intake Level (UL)**—the highest average daily nutrient intake level likely to pose no risk of adverse health effects to almost all individuals in the general population. As intake increases above the UL, the risk of adverse effects increases.

When the DRIs are determined to be appropriate reference standards for assessing intake adequacy, the following must be considered:

DRI	Assessing the intake of healthy individuals in a specific life stage and gender category (2)
RDA	For nutrients with a RDA, estimated usual intakes at or above the RDA have a high probability of adequacy.
EAR	For nutrients with an EAR, estimated usual intakes below the EAR very likely need to be improved (because the probability of adequacy is 50% or less); those between the EAR and the RDA probably need to be improved (because the probability of adequacy is less than 97% to 98%).
AI	For nutrients with an AI, estimated usual intakes at or above the AI can be considered adequate. Although the adequacy of intakes below the AI cannot be determined, they should be improved to meet the AI.
UL	For nutrients with a UL, estimated usual intakes below the UL can be considered to be not at risk for toxicity.
DRI	**Assessing the intake of a group (3).**
RDA	Do not use to assess intakes of groups.
EAR	For nutrients with an EAR, use the EAR to assess the prevalence of inadequate intakes or the proportion of a population that has estimated usual intakes below median requirements. Choose between two methods- the probability approach or the EAR cut-point method.
AI	For nutrients with an AI, estimated mean intakes at or above this level implies a low prevalence of inadequate intakes. However, when estimated mean intakes of groups are below the AI, it is not possible to make any assumptions about the prevalence of inadequacy.
UL	For nutrients with a UL, estimated usual intakes above the UL are used to estimate the percentage of the population at risk of adverse effects from excessive nutrient intake.

NOTE: For statistical calculation methods, see reference 1.

References

1. Institute of Medicine, National Academy of Sciences. *Dietary Reference Intakes: Applications in Dietary Assessment*. Washington, DC: National Academies Press; 2000.

2. Barr SI, Murphy SP, Poos MI. Interpreting and using the dietary reference intakes in dietary assessment of individuals and groups. *J Am Diet Assoc*. 2002; 102:780-788.

3. Murphy SP, Poos MI. Dietary Reference Intakes: Summary of applications in dietary assessment. *Public Health Nutr*. 2002;5:843-849.

Assessment

Edition: 2009

Nutrition Assessment and/or Nutrition Monitoring and Evaluation Terms and Definitions

Nutrition Assessment and/or Monitoring and Evaluation Term	Term Number	Definition	Reference Sheet Page Numbers
DOMAIN: FOOD/NUTRITION-RELATED HISTORY	FH	Food and nutrient intake, medication/herbal supplement intake, knowledge/beliefs/attitudes and behavior, food and supply availability, physical activity, and nutrition quality of life	
Class: Food and Nutrient Intake (1)		Composition and adequacy of food and nutrient intake, meal and snack patterns, current and previous diets and/or food modifications, and eating environment	
Subclass: Diet History (1.1)		Description of food and drink regularly provided or consumed, past diets followed or prescribed and counseling received, and the eating environment.	
Diet order	FH-1.1.1	A general or modified diet prescribed and documented in a patient/client medical record by a credentialed provider as part of a medical treatment plan	47-48
Diet experience	FH-1.1.2	Previous nutrition/diet orders, diet education/counseling, and diet characteristics that influence patient's/client's dietary intake	49-50
Eating environment	FH-1.1.3	The aggregate of surrounding things, conditions or influences that affect food intake	51-53
Subclass: Energy Intake (1.2)		Total energy intake from all sources including food, beverages, breast milk/formula, supplements, and via enteral and parenteral routes	
Energy intake	FH-1.2.1	Amount of energy intake from all sources, e.g., food, beverages, supplements, and via enteral and parenteral routes	54-55
Subclass: Food and Beverage Intake (1.3)		Type, amount, and pattern of intake of foods and food groups, indices of diet quality, intake of fluids, breast milk and infant formula	
Fluid/beverage intake	FH-1.3.1	Amount and type of fluid/beverage intake consumed orally	56-58
Food intake	FH-1.3.2	Amount, type and pattern of food consumed and quality of diet	59-61
Breast milk/infant formula intake	FH-1.3.3	Amount of breast milk, and/or the amount, type, and concentration on infant formula consumed orally	62-64

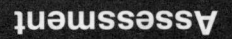

Nutrition Assessment and/or Nutrition Monitoring and Evaluation Terms and Definitions

Nutrition Assessment and/or Monitoring and Evaluation Term	Term Number	Definition	Reference Sheet Page Numbers
Subclass: Enteral and Parenteral Intake (1.4)		Specialized nutrition support intake from all sources including enteral and parenteral routes	
Enteral/parenteral nutrition intake	FH-1.4.1	Amount or type of enteral and/or parenteral nutrition intake provided via a tube or intravenously	65-67
Subclass: Bioactive Substances Intake (1.5)		Alcohol, plant stanol and sterol esters, soy protein, psyllium and β-glucan, and caffeine intake from all sources including food, beverages, supplements and via enteral and parenteral routes	
Alcohol intake	FH-1.5.1	Amount and pattern of alcohol consumption	68-69
Bioactive substance intake	FH-1.5.2	Amount and type of bioactive substances consumed	70-71
Caffeine intake	FH-1.5.3	Amount of caffeine intake from all sources, e.g., food, beverages, supplements, medications, and via enteral and parenteral routes	72-73
Subclass: Macronutrient Intake (1.6)		Fat and cholesterol, protein, carbohydrate, and fiber intake from all sources including food, beverages, supplements, and via enteral and parenteral routes	
Fat and cholesterol intake	FH-1.6.1	Fat and cholesterol consumption from all sources, e.g., food, beverages, supplements, and via enteral and parenteral routes	74-76
Protein intake	FH-1.6.2	Protein intake from all sources, e.g., food, beverages, supplements, and via enteral and parenteral routes	77-79
Carbohydrate intake	FH-1.6.3	Carbohydrate consumption from all sources, e.g., food, beverages, supplements, and via enteral and parenteral routes	80-82
Fiber intake	FH-1.6.4	Amount and/or type of plant source matter consumed that is not completely digested, but may be at least partially fermented in the distal bowel, and is derived from all sources (e.g., food, beverages, supplements, and via enteral routes)	83-84

Nutrition Assessment and/or Nutrition Monitoring and Evaluation Terms and Definitions

Nutrition Assessment and/or Monitoring and Evaluation Term	Term Number	Definition	Reference Sheet Page Numbers
Subclass: Micronutrient Intake (1.7)		Vitamin and mineral intake from all sources, e.g., foods, beverages, supplements, and enteral and/or parenteral routes	
Vitamin intake	FH-1.7.1	Vitamin intake from all sources, including food, beverages, supplements, and via enteral and parenteral routes	85-87
Mineral/element intake	FH-1.7.2	Mineral/element intake from all sources, e.g., food, beverages, supplements, and via enteral and parenteral routes	88-90
Class: Medication and Herbal Supplement Use (2)		Prescription and over-the counter medications, including herbal preparations and complementary medicine products used	
Medication and herbal supplements	FH-2.1	Prescription and over-the-counter medications, including herbal preparations and complementary medicine products that may impact nutritional status	91-93
Class: Knowledge/ Beliefs/Attitudes (3)		Understanding of nutrition-related concepts and conviction of the truth and feelings/emotions toward some nutrition-related statement or phenomenon, along with readiness to change nutrition-related behaviors	
Food and nutrition knowledge	FH-3.1	Content areas and level of understanding about food, nutrition and health, or nutrition-related information and guidelines relevant to patient/client needs	94-96
Beliefs and attitudes	FH-3.2	Conviction of the truth of some nutrition-related statement or phenomenon, and feelings or emotions toward that truth or phenomenon, along with a patient's/client's readiness to change food, nutrition, or nutrition-related behaviors	97-99

Assessment

Nutrition Assessment and/or Nutrition Monitoring and Evaluation Terms and Definitions

Nutrition Assessment and/or Monitoring and Evaluation Term	Term Number	Definition	Reference Sheet Page Numbers
Class: Behavior (4)		Patient/client activities and actions which influence achievement of nutrition-related goals	
Adherence	FH-4.1	Level of compliance or adherence with nutrition-related recommendations or behavioral changes agreed upon by patient/client to achieve nutrition-related goals	100-102
Avoidance behavior	FH-4.2	Keeping away from something or someone to postpone an outcome or perceived consequence	103-105
Bingeing and purging behavior	FH-4.3	Eating a larger amount of food than normal for the individual during a short period of time (within any two hour period) accompanied by a lack of control over eating during the binge episode (i.e., the feeling that one cannot stop eating). This may be followed by compensatory behavior to make up for the excessive eating, referred to as purging.	106-108
Mealtime behavior	FH-4.4	Manner of acting, participating or behaving at mealtime which influences patient/client's food and beverage intake	109-110
Social network	FH-4.5	Ability to build and utilize a network of family, friends, colleagues, health professionals, and community resources for encouragement, emotional support and to enhance one's environment to support behavior change	111-112

Nutrition Assessment and/or Nutrition Monitoring and Evaluation Terms and Definitions

Nutrition Assessment and/or Monitoring and Evaluation Term	Term Number	Definition	Reference Sheet Page Numbers
Class: Factors Affecting Access to Food and Food/Nutrition-Related Supplies (5)		Factors that affect intake and availability of a sufficient quantity of safe, healthful food as well as food/nutrition-related supplies.	
Nutrition program participation	FH-5.1	Patient/client eligibility for and participation in food assistance programs	113-114
Safe food/meal availability	FH-5.2	Availability of enough healthful, safe food	115-116
Safe water availability	FH-5.3	Availability of potable water	117-118
Food/nutrition-related supplies availability	FH-5.4	Access to necessary food/nutrition-related supplies	119-120
Class: Physical Activity and Function (6)		Physical activity, cognitive and physical ability to engage in specific tasks, e.g., breastfeeding and self-feeding	
Breastfeeding	FH-6.1	Degree to which breastfeeding plans and experience meet nutritional and other needs of the infant and mother	121-122
Nutrition-related ADLs (*activities of daily living*) and IADLs (*instrumental activities of daily living*)	FH-6.2	Level of cognitive and physical ability to perform nutrition-related activities of daily living and instrumental activities of daily living by older and/or disabled persons	123-125
Physical activity	FH-6.3	Level of physical activity and/or amount of exercise performed	126-128
Class: Nutrition-Related Patient/Client Centered Measures (7)		Patient/client's perception of his/her nutrition intervention and its impact on life	
Nutrition quality of life	FH-7.1	Extent to which the Nutrition Care Process impacts a patient/client's physical, mental and social well-being related to food and nutrition	129-130
Satisfaction		To be added	

Assessment

Nutrition Assessment and/or Nutrition Monitoring and Evaluation Terms and Definitions

Nutrition Assessment and/or Monitoring and Evaluation Term	Term Number	Definition	Reference Sheet Page Numbers
DOMAIN: ANTHROPOMETRIC MEASUREMENTS (1)	AD	Height, weight, body mass index (BMI), growth pattern indices/percentile ranks, and weight history.	
Body composition/Growth/Weight history	AD-1.1	Measures of the body, including fat, muscle, and bone components and growth	130-134
DOMAIN: BIOCHEMICAL DATA, MEDICAL TESTS AND PROCEDURES (1)	BD	Laboratory data, (e.g., electrolytes, glucose, and lipid panel) and tests (e.g., gastric emptying time, resting metabolic rate).	
Acid-base balance	BD-1.1	Balance between acids and bases in the body fluids. The pH (hydrogen ion concentration) of the arterial blood provides an index for the total body acid-base balance.	135-136
Electrolyte and renal profile	BD-1.2	Laboratory measures associated with electrolyte balance and kidney function	137-138
Essential fatty acid profile	BD-1.3	Laboratory measures of essential fatty acids	139-140
Gastrointestinal profile	BD-1.4	Laboratory measures and medical tests associated with function of the gastrointestinal tract and related organs	141-142
Glucose/endocrine profile	BD-1.5	Laboratory measures associated with glycemic control and endocrine findings	143-144
Inflammatory profile	BD-1.6	Laboratory measures of inflammatory proteins	145-146
Lipid profile	BD-1.7	Laboratory measures associated with lipid disorders	147-149
Metabolic rate profile	BD-1.8	Measures associated with or having implications for assessing metabolic rate	150-151
Mineral profile	BD-1.9	Laboratory measures associated with body mineral status	152-153

Nutrition Assessment and/or Nutrition Monitoring and Evaluation Terms and Definitions

Nutrition Assessment and/or Monitoring and Evaluation Term	Term Number	Definition	Reference Sheet Page Numbers
DOMAIN: BIOCHEMICAL DATA, MEDICAL TESTS AND PROCEDURES (1), cont'd	BD	Laboratory data, (e.g., electrolytes, glucose, lipid panel and gastric emptying time) and tests (e.g., gastric emptying time, resting metabolic rate).	
Nutritional anemia profile	BD-1.10	Laboratory measures associated with nutritional anemias	154-155
Protein profile	BD-1.11	Laboratory measures associated with hepatic and circulating proteins	156-157
Urine profile	BD-1.12	Physical and/or chemical properties of urine	158-159
Vitamin profile	BD-1.13	Laboratory measures associated with body vitamin status	160-162
DOMAIN: NUTRITION-FOCUSED PHYSICAL FINDINGS	PD	Findings from an evaluation of body systems, muscle and subcutaneous fat wasting, oral health, suck/swallow/breathe ability, appetite, and affect.	
Nutrition-focused physical findings	PD-1.1	Nutrition-related physical characteristics associated with pathophysiological states derived from a nutrition-focused physical exam, interview, or the medical record	163-166

Assessment

Nutrition Assessment and/or Nutrition Monitoring and Evaluation Terms and Definitions

Nutrition Assessment and/or Monitoring and Evaluation Term	Term Number	Definition	Reference Sheet Page Numbers
DOMAIN: CLIENT HISTORY *Note: This Domain is used for nutrition assessment only.*	CH	Current and past information related to personal, medical, family, and social history.	
Class: Personal History (1)		General patient/client information such as age, gender, race/ethnicity, language, education, and role in family	
Personal data	CH-1.1	General patient/client information such as age, gender race/ethnicity, occupation, tobacco use and physical disability	167-168
Class: Patient/Client/Family Medical/Health History (2)		Patient/client or family disease states, conditions, and illnesses that may have a nutritional impact	
Patient/client OR family nutrition-oriented medical/health history	CH-2.1	Patient/client or family member disease states, conditions, and illnesses that may impact nutritional status	169-171
Treatments/therapy/complementary/ alternative medicine	CH-2.2	Documented medical or surgical treatments, complementary and alternative medicine that may impact nutritional status of the patient	172-173
Class: Social History(3)		Patient/client socioeconomic factors, housing situation, medical care support and involvement in social groups	
Social history	CH-3.1	Patient/client information such as socioeconomic factors, housing situation, medical support, occupation, religion, history of recent crisis and involvement in social groups	174-176

Diet Order (FH-1.1.1)

Definition
A general or modified diet prescribed and documented in a patient/client medical record by a credentialed provider as part of a medical treatment plan

Nutrition Assessment
Indicators

General, healthful diet ***

Modified diet, specify, e.g., type, amount of energy and/or nutrients/day, distribution, texture***

Enteral nutrition order, specify, e.g., formula, rate/schedule, access***

Parenteral nutrition order, specify, e.g., solution, access, rate ***

Examples of the measurement methods or data sources for these indicators: Medical record, referring health care provider or agency, resident/client history

Typically used with the following domains of nutrition interventions: Food and/or nutrient delivery, nutrition education, nutrition counseling, coordination of nutrition care, resident/client history

Typically used with the following nutrition diagnoses: Inadequate or excess energy, macronutrient or micronutrient intake, inadequate or excess oral food intake, swallowing difficulty

Clinical judgment must be used to select indicators and determine the appropriate measurement techniques and reference standards for a given patient population and setting. Once identified, these indicators, measurement techniques, and reference standards should be identified in policies and procedures or other documents for use in patient/client records, quality or performance improvement, or in formal research projects.

Evaluation

Criteria for evaluation
Comparison to Goal or Reference Standard:
1) Goal (tailored to patient/client needs)
   OR
2) Reference standard

*** *Denotes indicator is used for nutrition assessment only. Other indicators are used for both nutrition assessment and nutrition monitoring and evaluation.*

Assessment

Food/Nutrition-Related History Domain – Diet History

Diet Order (FH-1.1.1)

Patient/Client Example(s)

Example(s) of one or two of the Nutrition Care Indicators (includes sample initial assessment documentation for one of the indicators)

Indicator(s) selected

Modified diet

Criteria for evaluation

Comparison to Goal or Reference Standard:

    1) Goal: Not generally used

       OR

    2) Reference standard: No validated standard exists

Sample nutrition assessment documentation

Initial nutrition assessment with patient/client	Patient/client prescribed a 2400-calorie diabetic diet.

References

The following are some suggested references for indicators, measurement techniques, and reference standards; other references may be appropriate.

1. Hager, M. Hospital Therapeutic Diet Orders and the Centers for Medicare & Medicaid Services: Steering through Regulations to Provide Quality Nutrition Care and Avoid Survey Citations. *J Am Diet Assoc*. 2006; 106 (2):198-204.

2. *ADA Nutrition Care Manual*. 2006. Available at: www.nutritioncaremanual.org. Accessed December 14, 2006.

3. Hager, M. Therapeutic Diet Order Writing: Current Issues and Considerations: Future of clinical dietetic practice. *Topics in Clinical Nutrition*. 2007;22(1):28-36.

4. Niedert KC. Position of the American Dietetic Association: Liberalization of the Diet Prescription Improves Quality of Life for Older Adults in Long-Term Care. *J Am Diet Assoc*. 2005;105(12):1955-1965.

*** Denotes indicator is used for nutrition assessment only. Other indicators are used for both nutrition assessment and nutrition monitoring and evaluation.

Diet Experience (FH-1.1.2)

Definition
Previous nutrition/diet orders, diet education/counseling, and diet characteristics that influence patient's/client's dietary intake

Nutrition Assessment
Indicators
Previously prescribed diets***
- Previous modified diet (specify, e.g., type, amount of energy and/or nutrients/day, distribution, texture)***
- Enteral nutrition order (specify)***
- Parenteral nutrition order (specify)***

Previous diet/nutrition education/counseling (specify, e.g., type, year)***

Self-selected diets followed (specify, e.g., commercial diets, diet books, culturally directed)***

Dieting attempts ***
- Number of past diet attempts (number)***
- Results (specify, e.g., successful/unsuccessful, pounds lost)***
- Successful strategies (specify, e.g., no snacking, self-monitoring)***

Examples of the measurement methods or data sources for these indicators: Patient/client report, medical record, resident/client history, food and nutrition delivery coordination of care

Typically used with the following domains of nutrition interventions: Nutrition education, nutrition counseling

Typically used with the following nutrition diagnoses: Disordered eating pattern, not ready for diet/lifestyle change, excessive oral food/beverage intake, food- and nutrition-related knowledge deficit, harmful beliefs/attitudes about food- or nutrition-related topics, undesirable food choices, swallowing difficulty, intake of unsafe food

Clinical judgment must be used to select indicators and determine the appropriate measurement techniques and reference standards for a given patient population and setting. Once identified, these indicators, measurement techniques, and reference standards should be identified in policies and procedures or other documents for use in patient/client records, quality or performance improvement, or in formal research projects.

*** *Denotes indicator is used for nutrition assessment only. Other indicators are used for both nutrition assessment and nutrition monitoring and evaluation.*

Assessment

Diet Experience (FH-1.1.2)

Evaluation

Criteria for evaluation
Comparison to Goal or Reference Standard:
- 1) Goal (tailored to patient/client needs)
  - OR
- 2) Reference standard

Patient/Client Example(s)
Example(s) of one or two of the Nutrition Care Indicators (includes sample initial assessment documentation for one of the indicators)

Indicator(s) selected
Previous diet/nutrition education/counseling

Criteria for evaluation
Comparison to Goal or Reference Standard:
- 1) Goal: Not generally used
  - OR
- 2) Reference standard: No validated standard exists

Sample nutrition assessment documentation

Initial nutrition assessment with patient/client	Patient/client completed a 6-week diabetic education class in 2004.

References
The following are some suggested references for indicators, measurement techniques, and reference standards; other references may be appropriate.

1. Hager, M. Hospital Therapeutic Diet Orders and the Centers for Medicare & Medicaid Services: Steering through Regulations to Provide Quality Nutrition Care and Avoid Survey Citations. *J Am Diet Assoc.* 2006; 106 (2):198-204.
2. *ADA Nutrition Care Manual.* 2006. Available at: www.nutritioncaremanual.org. Accessed December 14, 2006.
3. Hager, M. Therapeutic Diet Order Writing: Current Issues and Considerations: Future of clinical dietetic practice. *Topics in Clinical Nutrition.* 2007;22(1):28-36.

*** Denotes indicator is used for nutrition assessment only. Other indicators are used for both nutrition assessment and nutrition monitoring and evaluation.

Eating Environment (FH-1.1.3)

Definition
The aggregate of surrounding things, conditions or influences that affect food intake

Nutrition Assessment and Monitoring and Evaluation
Indicators

Location (specify, e.g., home, school, day care, restaurant, nursing home, senior center)

Atmosphere
- Acceptable noise level (yes/no)
- Appropriate lighting (yes/no)
- Appropriate room temperature (yes/no)
- Appropriate table height (yes/no)
- Appropriate table/meal service/set-up (yes/no)
- Eats at designated eating location (does not wander) (yes/no)
- Eats without distractions (e.g., watching TV/reading) (yes/no)
- No unpleasant odors (yes/no)

Caregiver/companion
- Allowed to select foods (often, sometimes, never)
- Caregiver influences/controls what client eats (e.g. encourages, forces) (yes/no)
- Caregiver models expected eating behavior (yes/no)
- Caretaker presence (present/not present)
- Favorite food is offered or withheld to influence behavior (reward/punishment) (yes/no)
- Has companionship while eating (another or others present) (yes/no)
- Meal/snacks offered at consistent times ("grazing" discouraged) (yes/no)

Appropriate breastfeeding accommodations/facility (yes/no)

Examples of the measurement methods or data sources for these indicators: Patient/client report, medical record, referring health care provider or agency, observation

Typically used with the following domains of nutrition interventions: Food and/or Nutrient Delivery, nutrition education, nutrition counseling, coordination of nutrition care

*** *Denotes indicator is used for nutrition assessment only. Other indicators are used for both nutrition assessment and nutrition monitoring and evaluation.*

Assessment

Eating Environment (FH-1.1.3)

Typically used to determine and to monitor and evaluate change in the following nutrition diagnoses: Inadequate oral food/beverage intake, self-feeding difficulty, poor nutrition quality of life, limited access to food

Clinical judgment must be used to select indicators and determine the appropriate measurement techniques and reference standards for a given patient population and setting. Once identified, these indicators, measurement techniques, and reference standards should be identified in policies and procedures or other documents for use in patient/client records, quality or performance improvement, or in formal research projects.

Evaluation

Criteria for evaluation
Comparison to Goal or Reference Standard:
 1) Goal (tailored to patient/client needs)
  OR
 2) Reference standard

Patient/Client Example(s)

Example(s) of one or two of the Nutrition Care Indicators (includes sample initial and reassessment documentation for one of the indicators)

Indicator(s) selected
Eats at designated eating location

Criteria for evaluation
Comparison to Goal or Reference Standard:
 1) Goal: Two-year-old child with inadequate intake of calories/nutrients. Goal is to improve intake through modifications in feeding environment and meal pattern.
  OR
 2) Reference standard: No validated standard exists

*** *Denotes indicator is used for nutrition assessment only. Other indicators are used for both nutrition assessment and nutrition monitoring and evaluation.*

Eating Environment (FH-1.1.3)

Sample nutrition assessment and monitoring and evaluation documentation

Initial nutrition assessment with patient/client	Caregiver completed 3-day food record indicating multiple (10) feeding opportunities throughout the day. Child consumes mostly juice, dry cereal and chips. Prefers foods that can be consumed from bottle or finger foods. Child does not sit at the table to eat, but wanders the house and is allowed to request and receive snacks ad lib. Energy and nutrient intake is less than 75% of standard. Referral to behavioral specialist offered.
Reassessment after nutrition intervention	Caregiver completed follow-up 3-day food record indicating reduced number of feeding opportunities throughout the day (6-7). States child resisted at first, but now eats at table at regular meal/snack times. Caregiver is continuing to work with behavior specialist for both mealtime and other behavior issues. Energy and nutrient intake have improved to 85-90% of standard.

References

The following are some suggested references for indicators, measurement techniques, and reference standards; other references may be appropriate.

1. Spruijt-Metz D, Lindquist CH, Birch LL, Fisher JO, Goran MI. Relation between mothers' child-feeding practices and children's adiposity. *Am J Clin Nutr*. 2002; 75:581-586.
2. Boutelle KN, Birnbaum AS, Lytle LA, Murray DM, Story M. Associations between perceived family meal environment and parent intake of fruit, vegetables and fat. *J Nutri Ed Behav*. 2003; 35: 24-29.
3. Birch LL, Fisher, JO. Development of eating behaviors among children and adolescents. *Pediatrics*. 1998;101: 539-549.
4. O'Dea JA. Why do kids eat healthful food? Perceived benefits of and barriers to healthful eating and physical activity among children and adolescents. *J Am Diet Assoc*. 2003; 103(4): 497-501.
5. Birch LL, Fisher, JO. Mothers' child-feeding practices influence daughters' eating and weight. *Am J Clin Nutr*. 2000; 71: 1054-1061.
6. Birch LL. Development of food preferences. *Ann Rev Nutr*. 1999; 19:41-62.
7. Campbell K, Crawford, D. Family food environments as determinants of preschool-aged children's eating behaviours: implications for obesity prevention policy. *Aust J Nutr Diet*. 2005; 58:19-25.
8. Hurtsi, UK. Factors influencing children's food choice. *Ann Med*. 1999; 31 (Suppl 1): 26-32.
9. Birch LL, Fisher JO, Davison, KK. Learning to overeat: Maternal use of restrictive feeding practices promotes girls' eating in the absence of hunger. 2003. *Am J Clin Nutr*. 78: 215-220.
10. Wansink, B, Cheney, MM. Super bowls: serving bowl size and food consumption. *JAMA*. (2005); 293:1727-1728
11. Wansink, B. Environmental factors that increase the food intake and consumption volume of unknowing consumers. *Ann Rev Nutr*. 2004;24:455-479
12. Rozin, P, Kabnick, K, Pete, E, Fischler, C, Shields, C. The ecology of eating: smaller portion sizes in France than in the United States help explain the French paradox *Psychol Sci*. 2003; 14:450-454
13. Rozin, P. The meaning of food in our lives: a cross-cultural perspective on eating and well-being *J Nutr Educ Behav*. 2005;37(suppl):107-112.
14. Birch LL, Davison KK. Family environmental factors influencing the developing behavioral controls of food intake and childhood overweight. *Pediatr Clin North Am*. 2001;48(4):893-907.
15. Hetherington MM. Cues to overeat: psychological factors influencing overconsumption. *Proc Nutr Soc*. 2007;66(1):113-23.

*** Denotes indicator is used for nutrition assessment only. Other indicators are used for both nutrition assessment and nutrition monitoring and evaluation.

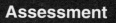

Assessment

Energy Intake (FH-1.2.1)

Definition
Amount of energy intake from all sources, e.g., food, beverages, breast milk/formula, supplements, and via enteral and parenteral routes

Note: Whenever possible, nutrient intake data should be considered in combination with clinical, biochemical, anthropometric information, medical diagnosis, clinical status, and/or other factors as well as diet to provide a valid assessment of nutritional status based on a totality of the evidence. (Dietary Reference Intakes. Applications in Dietary Assessment. Institute of Medicine. Washington, D.C.: National Academy Press; 2000.)

Nutrition Assessment and Monitoring and Evaluation
Indicators
Total energy intake (specify, e.g., calories/day, calories/kg/day)

Note: Weight and weight change can be found on the body composition/growth/weight history reference sheet.

Examples of the measurement methods or data sources for these indicators: Food intake records, 24-hour recall, 3-5 day food diary, food frequency questionnaire, caretaker intake records, menu analysis, intake and output records

Typically used with the following domains of nutrition interventions: Food and/or nutrient delivery, nutrition education, nutrition counseling, coordination of nutrition care

Typically used to determine and to monitor and evaluate change in the following nutrition diagnoses: Inadequate energy intake, excessive energy intake, evident protein-calorie malnutrition, inadequate protein-energy intake, underweight, involuntary weight loss, overweight/obesity, involuntary weight gain, swallowing difficulty, breastfeeding difficulty, altered GI function, limited adherence to nutrition-related recommendations

Clinical judgment must be used to select indicators and determine the appropriate measurement techniques and reference standards for a given patient population and setting. Once identified, these indicators, measurement techniques, and reference standards should be identified in policies and procedures or other documents for use in patient/client records, quality or performance improvement, or in formal research projects.

Evaluation
Criteria for evaluation
Comparison to Goal or Reference Standard:
1) Goal (tailored to individual's needs)
   OR
2) Reference standard (estimated or measured energy requirement)

Patient/Client Example
Indicator(s) selected
Total energy intake

*** Denotes indicator is used for nutrition assessment only. Other indicators are used for both nutrition assessment and nutrition monitoring and evaluation.

Energy Intake (FH-1.2.1)

Criteria for evaluation

Comparison to Goal or Reference Standard:

1) Goal: Food diary indicates patient/client consumes approximately 2600 kcal/day. Patient/client's target calorie intake level is 1800 kcal/day.

OR

2) Reference standard: Patient/client's I & O indicates patient/client's intake at approximately 2000 kcal/day, 80% of goal based on an estimated energy requirement of 2500 kcal/day.

Sample nutrition assessment and monitoring and evaluation documentation

Initial encounter with patient/client	Based on patient/client food diary, patient/client consuming approximately 2600 kcal/day, 144% of recommended level of 1800 kcal. Will evaluate calorie intake at next encounter in two weeks.
Reassessment after nutrition intervention	Significant progress toward meeting goal. Based on patient/client food diary, patient/client consuming approximately 2100 kcal/day, 117% of recommended level of 1800 kcal. Will evaluate calorie intake at next encounter in two weeks.

References

The following are some suggested references for indicators, measurement techniques, and reference standards for the outcome; other references may be appropriate.

1. Institute of Medicine, Food and Nutrition Board. Dietary Reference Intakes for Energy, Carbohydrate, Fiber, Fat, Fatty Acids, Cholesterol, Protein and Amino Acids. Food and Nutrition Board. National Academy of Sciences. Washington, DC: National Academy Press; 2002. Available at: www.iom.edu/Object.File/Master/21/372/DRI%20Tables%20after%20electrolytes%20plus%20micro-macroEAR_2.pdf

2. Frankenfield D, Roth-Yousey L, Compher C. Comparison of predictive equations for resting metabolic rate in healthy nonobese adults: A systematic review. *J Amer Diet Assoc.* 2005;105:775-789.

3. American Dietetic Association. Pamela Charney, Ainsley Malone, eds. *ADA Pocket Guide to Nutrition Assessment.*

4. Compher C. Frankenfield D, Keim N, Roth-Yousey L. Best practice methods to apply to measurement of resting metabolic rate in adults: A systematic review. *J Amer Diet Assoc.* 2006;106:881-903.

5. © 2006 ADA Evidence Analysis Library. Accessed on: 10/28/2006 from http://ada.portalxm.com/eal/template.cfm? key=1309&cms_preview=1

6. American Society for Parenteral and Enteral Nutrition Board of Directors and The Clinical Guidelines Task Force. Guidelines for the use of parenteral and enteral nutrition in adult and pediatric patients: Life cycle and metabolic conditions. *J Parenter Enteral Nutr.* 2002;26(Suppl):S45-S60.

7. American Society for Parenteral and Enteral Nutrition Board of Directors and The Clinical Guidelines Task Force. Guidelines for the use of parenteral and enteral nutrition in adult and pediatric patients: Specific guidelines for disease - adults. *J Parenter Enteral Nutr.* 2002;26(Suppl):S61-S96.

8. American Society for Parenteral and Enteral Nutrition Board of Directors and The Clinical Guidelines Task Force. Guidelines for the use of parenteral and enteral nutrition in adult and pediatric patients: Specific guidelines for disease - pediatrics. *J Parenter Enteral Nutr.* 2002;26(Suppl):S111-S138.

9. US Departments of Agriculture and Health and Human Services. *Dietary Guidelines for Americans 2005.* Available at: www.healthierus.gov/dietaryguidelines.

10. ADA Nutritional Care Manual. 2006. Available at: www.nutritioncaremanual.org. Accessed January 30, 2008.

11. ADA Evidence Analysis Library. Accessed on: January 30, 2008 from http://www.ada.portalxm.com/eal/topic.cfm?cat=2883 and http://www.ada.portalxm.com/eal/topic.cfm?cat=2954

*** Denotes indicator is used for nutrition assessment only. Other indicators are used for both nutrition assessment and nutrition monitoring and evaluation.

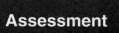

Assessment

Food/Nutrition-Related History Domain – Food and Beverage Intake

Fluid/Beverage Intake (FH-1.3.1)

Definition
Amount and type of fluid/beverage intake consumed orally

> *Note: Whenever possible, nutrient intake data should be considered in combination with clinical, biochemical, anthropometric information, medical diagnosis, clinical status, and/or other factors as well as diet to provide a valid assessment of nutritional status based on a totality of the evidence. (*Dietary Reference Intakes. Applications in Dietary Assessment. *Institute of Medicine. Washington, D.C.: National Academy Press; 2000.)*

Nutrition Assessment and Monitoring and Evaluation
Indicators

Oral fluid amounts (specify, e.g., oz or mL or cups/day)
- Water
- Coffee and tea
- Juice
- Milk
- Soda (specify regular or artificially sweetened)

Food-derived fluids (e.g., 3 oz fluid in 4 oz apple sauce) (mL/day)

Liquid meal replacement or supplement (oz or mL/day)

> *Note: Biochemical measures of hydration status are found on the Electrolyte and Renal Profile and the Urine Profile reference sheets.*

Examples of the measurement methods or data sources for these indicators: Food intake records, 24-hour recall, food frequency questionnaire, intake and output data, observation

Typically used with the following domains of nutrition interventions: Food and/or nutrient delivery, nutrition education, nutrition counseling, coordination of nutrition care

Typically used to determine and to monitor and evaluate change in the following nutrition diagnoses: Excessive or inadequate oral food/beverage intake, food-medication interaction, underweight, overweight/obesity, involuntary weight loss, involuntary weight gain, disordered eating pattern, undesirable food choices, limited adherence to nutrition related recommendations, inability or lack of desire to manage self-care, swallowing difficulty, breastfeeding difficulty, altered GI function

Clinical judgment must be used to select indicators and determine the appropriate measurement techniques and reference standards for a given patient population and setting. Once identified, these indicators, measurement techniques, and reference standards should be identified in policies and procedures or other documents for use in patient/client records, quality or performance improvement, or in formal research projects.

*** Denotes indicator is used for nutrition assessment only. Other indicators are used for both nutrition assessment and nutrition monitoring and evaluation.

Fluid/Beverage Intake (FH-1.3.1)

Evaluation

Criteria for evaluation

Comparison to Goal or Reference Standard:

    1) Goal (tailored to patient/client's needs)

        OR

    2) Reference standard

Patient/Client Example(s)

Example(s) of one or two of the Nutrition Care Indicators (includes sample initial and reassessment documentation for one of the indicators)

Indicator(s) selected

Oral fluid amounts

Criteria for evaluation

Comparison to Goal or Reference Standard:

    1) Goal: Patient/client currently drinks 12 oz of fluid per day and has a personal goal of consuming 64 oz of fluid per day.

        OR

    2) Reference standard: No validated standard exists.

Sample nutrition assessment and monitoring and evaluation documentation

Initial nutrition assessment with patient/client	Based on patient/client food diary, patient/client consuming approximately 1000 mL fluid per day. Goal is to consume approximately 3000 mL/day. Will monitor fluid intake at next encounter.
Reassessment after nutrition intervention	Significant progress toward recommended fluid intake. Based upon fluid intake records, patient/client increased consumption of fluids from 1000 mL to 2600 mL per day.

References

The following are some suggested references for indicators, measurement techniques, and reference standards for the outcome; other references may be appropriate.

    1. Institute of Medicine, Food and Nutrition Board. Dietary Reference Intakes for Energy, Carbohydrate, Fiber, Fat, Fatty Acids, Cholesterol, Protein and Amino Acids. Washington, DC: National Academy Press; 2002. Available at: www.iom.edu/report.asp?id=4340.

    2. American Society for Parenteral and Enteral Nutrition Board of Directors and The Clinical Guidelines Task Force. Guidelines for the use of parenteral and enteral nutrition in adult and pediatric patients: Specific guidelines for disease—adults. *J Parenter Enteral Nutr*. 2002;26(Suppl):S61-S96.

*** Denotes indicator is used for nutrition assessment only. Other indicators are used for both nutrition assessment and nutrition monitoring and evaluation.

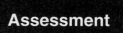

Assessment

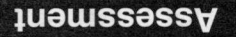

Food/Nutrition-Related History Domain – Food and Beverage Intake

Fluid/Beverage Intake (FH-1.3.1)

References, cont'd

3. Queen PM, Lang CE. *Handbook of Pediatric Nutrition*. Gaitherburg, MD: Aspen Press; 1993.

4. American Society for Parenteral and Enteral Nutrition Board of Directors and The Clinical Guidelines Task Force. Guidelines for the use of parenteral and enteral nutrition in adult and pediatric patients: Specific guidelines for disease—pediatrics. *J Parenter Enteral Nutr*. 2002;26(Suppl):S111-S138.

5. Fluid needs in nephrolithiasis. *ADA Nutritional Care Manual*. 2006. Available at: http://nutritioncaremanual.org.

6. American College of Sports Medicine website. Available at: http://www.acsm.org.

7. United States Department of Agriculture. USDA National Nutrient Database for Standard Reference. Available at: http://www.nal.usda.gov/fnic/foodcomp/search/ Accessed on: February 13, 2008

8. American Dietetic Association. *Nutrition care of the older adult* (2nd ed.). Chicago, IL. 2004.

9. Consultant Dietititians in Health Care Facilities Dietetic Practice Group. *Nutrition management and restorative dining for older adults*. (2001). Chicago, IL:American Dietetic Association.

*** *Denotes indicator is used for nutrition assessment only. Other indicators are used for both nutrition assessment and nutrition monitoring and evaluation.*

Food Intake (FH-1.3.2)

Definition

Amount, type, and pattern of food consumed and quality of diet

> *Note: Whenever possible, nutrient intake data should be considered in combination with clinical, biochemical, anthropometric information, medical diagnosis, clinical status, and/or other factors as well as diet to provide a valid assessment of nutritional status based on a totality of the evidence.* (Dietary Reference Intakes. Applications in Dietary Assessment. *Institute of Medicine. Washington, D.C.: National Academy Press; 2000.)*

Nutrition Assessment and Monitoring and Evaluation
Indicators

Amount of food

- Grains (servings, cups, or ounces)
- Fruits (servings or cups)
- Vegetables (servings or cups)
- Fruit and vegetable (servings or cups)
- Milk/milk products (servings or cups)
- Meat, poultry, fish, eggs, beans, nut products (servings or ounces)
- Fat and oils (servings or teaspoons)
- Concentrated sweets (servings)
- Percent total meal eaten (percent)

Types of food/meals

- Foods liked (specify foods)
- Foods disliked (specify foods)
- Fortified/enriched foods (specify, e.g., amount or servings calcium fortified orange juice)
- Ready to eat food selections (e.g., type and number/day or week)
- Convenience frozen meals (e.g., type and number/day or week)
- Self-prepared foods/snacks (specify type e.g., low or high in sodium, fat, fiber)

Note: Liquid meal replacements/supplements are found on the Fluid Intake reference sheet.

* Snack is defined as a light, quick meal eaten between, or instead of, a main meal.

Meal/snack* pattern

- Number of meals (number/day)
- Number of snack(s) (number/day)

Diet Quality Index

- Healthy Eating Index (HEI)
- Children's Diet Quality Index (C-DQI)
- Revised Children's Diet Quality Index (RC-DQI)
- Other (specify)

Food variety (present/absent)

*** Denotes indicator is used for nutrition assessment only. Other indicators are used for both nutrition assessment and nutrition monitoring and evaluation.

Assessment

Food/Nutrition-Related History Domain – Food and Beverage Intake

Food Intake (FH-1.3.2)

Examples of the measurement methods or data sources for these indicators: Food intake records, 24-hour recall, food frequency questionnaire, menu analysis, MyPyramid Tracker, Healthy Eating Index, C-DQI, RC-DQI

Typically used with the following domains of nutrition interventions: Food and/or nutrient delivery, nutrition education, nutrition counseling, coordination of nutrition care

Typically used to determine and to monitor and evaluate change in the following nutrition diagnoses: Excessive or inadequate oral food/beverage intake, food-medication interaction, underweight, overweight/obesity, disordered eating pattern, involuntary weight gain, involuntary weight loss, undesirable food choices, limited adherence to nutrition related recommendations, inability or lack of desire to manage self-care, limited access to food, intake of unsafe food, inadequate or excessive energy, macronutrient or micronutrient intake

Clinical judgment must be used to select indicators and determine the appropriate measurement techniques and reference standards for a given patient population and setting. Once identified, these indicators, measurement techniques, and reference standards should be identified in policies and procedures or other documents for use in patient/client records, quality or performance improvement, or in formal research projects.

Evaluation

Criteria for evaluation
Comparison to Goal or Reference Standard:
1) Goal (tailored to patient/client needs)
   OR
2) Reference standard

Patient/Client Example(s)

Example(s) of one or two of the Nutrition Care Indicators (includes sample initial and reassessment documentation for one of the indicators)

Indicator(s) selected
Amount of food

Criteria for evaluation
Comparison to Goal or Reference Standard:
1) Goal: Patient/client currently eats approximately 1-2 fruit and vegetable servings per day. Goal is to increase fruit and vegetable intake to 5 servings per day.
   OR
2) Reference standard: Patient/client's current intake of 1-2 servings of fruit and vegetable per day is below the DASH Eating Plan recommendation of 9 servings of fruits and vegetables per day.

*** *Denotes indicator is used for nutrition assessment only. Other indicators are used for both nutrition assessment and nutrition monitoring and evaluation.*

Food Intake (FH-1.3.2)

Sample nutrition assessment and monitoring and evaluation documentation

Initial nutrition assessment with patient/client	Based on patient/client recall, patient/client consuming approximately 1-2 servings of fruits and vegetables per day. Will monitor fruit and vegetable intake at next encounter.
Reassessment after nutrition intervention	Some progress toward goal of 9 servings of fruits and vegetables per day. Based upon food records, patient/client increased consumption of fruits and vegetables from approximately 1 to 4 servings per day.

References

The following are some suggested references for indicators, measurement techniques, and reference standards for the outcome; other references may be appropriate.

1. US Departments of Agriculture and Health and Human Services. Dietary Guidelines for Americans 2005. Available at: www.healthierus.gov/dietaryguidelines.

2. US Department of Agriculture Center for Nutrition Policy and Promotion. *The Food Guide Pyramid for Young Children 2 to 6 Years Old*. Bethesda, MD: US Department of Agriculture; Center for Nutrition Policy and Promotion; 1998.

3. United States Department of Agriculture Human Nutrition Information Service. My Pyramid. 2005. Available at: http://www.mypyramid.gov. Accessed January 9, 2007.

4. *ADA Nutrition Care Manual*. 2006. Available at: www.nutritioncaremanual.org. Accessed December 11, 2006.

5. Ledikwe JH, Blanck HM, Khan LK, Serdula MK, Seymour JD, Tohill BC, Rolls BJ. Low-energy-density diets are associated with high diet quality in adults in the United States. *J Am Diet Assoc*. 2006;106:1172-1180.

6. Rolls B. *The Volumetrics Eating Plan*. New York, NY: HarperCollins Publishers, Inc; 2005.

7. American Academy of Pediatrics Committee on Nutrition. *Pediatric Nutrition Handbook*. 5th ed. Elk Grove Village, IL: American Academy of Pediatrics; 2004.

8. Kranz S, Hartman T, Siega-Riz AM, Herring AH. A diet quality index for American preschoolers based on current dietary intake recommendations and an indicator of energy balance. *J Am Diet Assoc*. 2006;106:1594-1604.

9. McCollough ML, Feskanich D, Stampfer MJ Giovannucci EL, Rimm EB, Hu FB, Spiegelman D, Hunter DJ, Colditz GA, Willett WC. Diet Quality and major chronic disease risk in men and women: Moving toward improved dietary guidance. *Am J Clin Nutr*. 2002;76:1261-1271.

10. Kennedy ET, Ohls J, Carlson S, Fleming K. The Health Eating Index: Design and applications. *J Am Diet Assoc*. 1995;95:1103-1108.

11. Fogli-Cawley JJ, Dwyer JT, Saltzman E, McCullough ML, Troy LM, Jacques PF. The 2005 Dietary Guidelines for Americans Adherence Index: development and application. *J Nutr*. 2006 Nov;136(11):2908-15.

12. McCullough ML, Willett WC. Evaluating adherence to recommended diets in adults: the Alternate Healthy Eating Index. *Public Health Nutr*. 2006;9:152-157.

13. Feskanich D, Rockett HR, Colditz GA. Modifying the Healthy Eating Index to assess diet quality in children and adolescents. *J Am Diet Assoc*. 2004 Sep;104(9):1375-83.

14. Position of the American Dietetic Association: Dietary Guidance for Healthy Children Ages 2 to 11 Years. *J Am Diet Assoc*. 2004 ;104(4): 660-677.

15. Dwyer M, Picciano MF, Raiten DJ. Collection of food and dietary supplement intake data: What we eat in America-NHANES. *J Nutr*. 2003;133:590S-600S

16. Kant AK, Ballard-Barbash R, Schatzkin A. Evening eating and its relation to self-reported body weight and nutrient intake in women, CFSII 1985-1986. *J Am Coll Nutr*. 1995. 14:358-363.

17. Willett WC. *Nutritional Epidemiology*. Oxford, UK: Oxford University Press; 1990.

*** *Denotes indicator is used for nutrition assessment only. Other indicators are used for both nutrition assessment and nutrition monitoring and evaluation.*

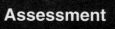

Assessment

Food/Nutrition-Related History Domain – Food and Beverage Intake

Breast Milk/Infant Formula Intake (FH-1.3.3)

Definition
Amount of breast milk, and/or the amount, type, and concentration on infant formula consumed orally

Nutrition Assessment and Monitoring and Evaluation
Indicators
Breast milk intake (adequacy or ounces or mL/day)
- Number of feedings (feedings/24-hour period)
- Duration of feedings (number of minutes)
- Modifier/supplement (specify, e.g., thickener, lipid, formula, protein)

Infant formula intake (ounces or mL/day)
- Type (specify, e.g., brand, cow's milk-based, soy-based, preterm formula, or other specialty with or without DHA and ARA)
- Concentration (specify, e.g., kcal/oz or kcal/mL)
- Number of feedings (number/day)
- Volume of formula per feeding (oz or mL; amount prepared – amount left in bottle)
- Number and volume or weight of cans of formula used per week (powder, liquid concentrate or ready to feed)
- Modifier/supplement (specify, e.g., thickener, lipid, formula, protein)

Note: Initiation, duration, exclusivity of breastfeeding and breastfeeding problems can be found on the Breastfeeding reference sheet.

Weight change is found on the Body Composition/Growth/Weight History reference sheet.

Number of wet diapers per day is found on the Urine Profile reference sheet.

Number/consistency of bowel movements is found on the Nutrition-focused Physical Exam reference sheet.

If provided via tube use the Enteral and Parenteral Nutrition Intake reference sheet.

Examples of the measurement methods or data sources for these indicators: Intake records, 24-hour recall, usual intake recall, observation of feeding (bottle or breast).

Typically used with the following domains of nutrition interventions: Food and/or nutrient delivery, nutrition education, nutrition counseling, coordination of nutrition care

*** Denotes indicator is used for nutrition assessment only. Other indicators are used for both nutrition assessment and nutrition monitoring and evaluation.

Breast Milk/Infant Formula Intake (FH-1.3.3)

Typically used to determine and to monitor and evaluate change in the following nutrition diagnoses: Underweight, overweight, involuntary weight gain, involuntary weight loss, limited adherence to nutrition related recommendations, inadequate or excessive energy intake, inadequate or excessive food/beverage or fluid intake

Clinical judgment must be used to select indicators and determine the appropriate measurement techniques and reference standards for a given patient population and setting. Once identified, these indicators, measurement techniques, and reference standards should be identified in policies and procedures or other documents for use in patient/client records, quality or performance improvement, or in formal research projects.

Evaluation
Criteria for evaluation
Comparison to Goal or Reference Standard:
1) Goal (tailored to patient/client needs)
   OR
2) Reference standard

Patient/Client Example(s)

Example(s) of one or two of the Nutrition Care Indicators (includes sample initial and reassessment documentation for one of the indicators)

Indicator(s) selected
Infant formula intake

Criteria for evaluation
Comparison to Goal or Reference Standard:
1) Goal: Patient/client currently consumes approximately 100 mL/kg body weight infant formula per day. Goal is to increase intake to 150 mL/kg per day.
   OR
2) Reference standard: Patient/client's current intake of 100 mL/kg/day day is below the recommended intake of 150 mL/kg/day to support adequate growth.

Sample nutrition assessment and monitoring and evaluation documentation

Initial nutrition assessment with patient/client	Based on mother's recall, patient/client consuming approximately 100 mL/kg/day of infant formula per day, 33% below the recommended level of 150 mL per day. Will monitor formula intake at next encounter.
Reassessment after nutrition intervention	Significant progress toward goal of consuming 150 mL/kg per day. Based upon mother's records, patient/client increased consumption of infant formula to approximately 140 mL/kg per day over the past 7 days.

*** Denotes indicator is used for nutrition assessment only. Other indicators are used for both nutrition assessment and nutrition monitoring and evaluation.

Assessment

Food/Nutrition-Related History Domain – Food and Beverage Intake

Breast Milk/Infant Formula Intake (FH-1.3.3)

References
The following are some suggested references for indicators, measurement techniques, and reference standards for the outcome; other references may be appropriate.

1. US Department Health and Human Services, Public Health Service, Health Resources and Services Administration, Maternal and Child Health Bureau. Gaining & Growing: Assuring Nutritional Care of Preterm Infants. Available at: http://depts.washington.edu/growing/Nourish/index~4.htm. Accessed on: January 17, 2008

2. Lawrence, RA & Lawrence RM Breastfeeding: *A Guide for the Medical Profession* 6th Edition, Mosby, 2005

3. Kurtz D; Measuring breastmilk intake. *Neonatal Intensive Care*, March/April, pp22-25, 1995

4. Riordan J, Gilt-Hopple K, Angeron J: Indicators of effective breastfeeding and estimates of breast milk intake. *J Human Lactation*. 21(4):406-12, Nov 2005

5. Brenner MG. You can provide efficient, effective and reimbursable breastfeeding support—here's how. Contemporary *Pediatrics*. Sept 28, 2005

6. Gartner LM, et al, American Academy of Pediatrics Section on Breastfeeding; Breastfeeding and the use of human milk. *Pediatrics*. 115(2):496-506, Feb 2005

7. Kent JC, et al; Volume and frequency of breastfeedings and fat content of breastmilk throughout the day. *Pediatrics*. 117(3):e387-395, March 2006

8. Dewey KG, Heinig MJ, Nommsen LA, Lonnerdal B. Maternal versus infant factors related to breast milk intake and residual milk volume: the DARLING study. *Pediatrics*. 1991 Jun;87(6):829-37.

9. Neville MC, et al. Studies in human lactation: milk volumes in lactating women during the onset of lactation and full lactation. *Am J Clin Nutr*. 1988 Dec;48(6):1375-86.

10. Dewey KG, Finley DA, Lonnerdal B. Breast milk volume and composition during late lactation (7-20 months). *J Pediatr Gastroenterol Nutr*. 1984 Nov;3(5):713-20.

11. Butte NF, Garza C, Smith EO, Nichols BL. Human milk intake and growth in exclusively breast-fed infants. *J Pediatr*. 1984 Feb;104(2):187-95.

12. Dewey KG, Lonnerdal B. Milk and nutrient intake of breast-fed infants from 1 to 6 months: relation to growth and fatness. *J Pediatr Gastroenterol Nutr*. 1983;2(3):497-506.

13. www.abbottnutrition.com (formerly www.ross.com)

14. Nestle Good Start. Available at: http://www.verybestbaby.com/GoodStart/NutritionInfo.aspx?ProductId=108F6251-3DFA-4BF2-9C48-79D2C7E451EA#chart1 Accessed on: January 17, 2008.

15. Mead Johnson Nutritionals. Available at: www.meadjohnson.com Accessed on: January 17, 2008.

16. Bright Beginnings Milk Formulas with DHA. Available at: http://www.brightbeginnings.com/products/baby-formula.asp Accessed on: January 17, 2008

17. Nutricia North America: Specialized Clinical Nutrition. Available at: www.shsna.com Accessed on: January 17, 2008.

18. Fomon SJ and Ziegler EE. Renal solute load and potential renal solute load in infancy. *Journal of Pediatrics*, 134:11-14 January, 1999

19. Morale SE, et al. Duration of long-chain polyunsaturated fatty acids availability in the diet and visual acuity. *Early Human Development*, 81:197-203, 2005

20. Birch EE, et al; Visual maturation of term infants fed long-chain polyunsaturated fatty acid-supplemented or control formula for 12 mo. *Am J Clin Nutr*. 81:871-9, 2005

21. Clandinin MT, Van Aerde JE, Merkel KL, Harris CL, Springer MA, Hansen JW, Diersen-Schade DA. Growth and development of preterm infants fed infant formulas containing docosahexaenoic acid and arachidonic acid. *J Pediatrics*. 146(4):461-468, April 2005

22. Vanderhoof JA, et al; Efficacy of a pre-thickened infant formula: A multicenter, double-blind, randomized placebo-controlled parallel group trial in 104 infants with symptomatic gastroesophageal reflux. *Clinical Pediatrics*. 42:483-495, 2003

23. The Pediatric Nutrition Practice Group American Dietetic Association. *Pediatric Manual of Clinical Dietetics*, 2nd edition, updated 2008; chapters 4, 10 and 11.

24. Otten JJ, Pitzi Hellwig J, and Meyers LD (editors). *Dietary Reference Intakes: The Essential Guide to Nutrient Requirements*. The National Academies Press, Washington DC, 2006

*** *Denotes indicator is used for nutrition assessment only. Other indicators are used for both nutrition assessment and nutrition monitoring and evaluation.*

Enteral and Parenteral Nutrition Intake (FH-1.4.1)

Definition

Amount or type of enteral and/or parenteral nutrition provided via a tube or intravenously.

> *Note: Whenever possible, nutrient intake data should be considered in combination with clinical, biochemical, anthropometric information, medical diagnosis, clinical status, and/or other factors as well as diet to provide a valid assessment of nutritional status based on a totality of the evidence. (*Dietary Reference Intakes. Applications in Dietary Assessment. *Institute of Medicine. Washington, D.C.: National Academy Press; 2000.)*

Nutrition Assessment and Monitoring and Evaluation
Indicators

Access (specify)

- Enteral nutrition e.g., nasocentric, oroenteric, percutaneous, or surgical access with gastric, duodenal or jejunal placement
- Parenteral nutrition e.g., peripheral, central, and/or type of catheter

Formula/solution (specify)

- Enteral nutrition e.g., formula name, calories/mL, special additive/supplemental fat, carbohydrate or protein
- Parenteral nutrition e.g., solution composition

Discontinuation (specify)

Initiation (specify)

Rate/schedule (mL/hour × number of hours; specify intermittent schedule of mL × number of feedings or time schedule)

> *Note: Enteral/parenteral nutrition tolerance can be accomplished with the Physical Exam Reference Sheet and/or the pertinent biochemical/sign or symptom reference sheet.*

Examples of the measurement methods or data sources for these indicators: Patient/client report/recall, patient/client record, home evaluation, intake and output record

Typically used with the following domains of nutrition interventions: Food and/or nutrient delivery, nutrition education, coordination of nutrition care

Typically used to determine and to monitor and evaluate change in the following nutrition diagnoses: Inadequate or excess intake of enteral or parenteral nutrition, inadequate fluid intake, food-medication interaction, involuntary weight loss or gain

Clinical judgment must be used to select indicators and determine the appropriate measurement techniques and reference standards for a given patient population and setting. Once identified, these indicators, measurement techniques, and reference standards should be identified in policies and procedures or other documents for use in patient/client records, quality or performance improvement, or in formal research projects.

*** Denotes indicator is used for nutrition assessment only. Other indicators are used for both nutrition assessment and nutrition monitoring and evaluation.

Assessment

Food/Nutrition-Related History Domain – Enteral/Parenteral Nutrition

Enteral and Parenteral Nutrition Intake (FH-1.4.1)

Evaluation

Criteria for evaluation
Comparison to Goal or Reference Standard:
1) Goal (tailored to patient/client needs)
   OR
2) Reference standard

Patient/Client Example

Example(s) of one or two of the Nutrition Care Indicators (includes sample initial and reassessment documentation for one of the indicators)

Indicator (s) selected
Rate/schedule (mL/hour × number of hours)

Criteria for evaluation
Comparison to Goal or Reference Standard:
1) Goal: Patient/client's enteral nutrition is at a rate of 50 mL per hour × 24 hours of 1 calorie per mL formula compared to the nutrition prescription of 80 mL/hour × 24 hours to meet estimated nutrition requirements.
   OR
2) Reference standard: There is no reference standard for this outcome as the provision of EN/PN is individualized.

Sample nutrition assessment and monitoring and evaluation documentation

Initial nutrition assessment with patient/client	Enteral nutrition rate of 25 mL per hour × 24 hours of 1 calorie per mL formula compared to the nutrition prescription of 80 mL/hour to meet estimated nutrition requirements. Monitor enteral nutrition initiation and rate advancement.
Reassessment after nutrition intervention	Enteral nutrition at 70 mL per hour × 24 hours. Significant progress toward nutrition prescription of 1 calorie per mL formula at 80 mL per hour × 24 hours.

References

The following are some suggested references for indicators, measurement techniques, and reference standards; other references may be appropriate.

1. American Dietetic Association. Pamela Charney, Ainsley Malone, eds. *ADA Pocket Guide to Nutrition Assessment*. Chicago, IL: American Dietetic Association; 2004.

2. ADA Nutrition Care Manual. 2004. Available at: www.nutritioncaremanual.org. Accessed November 29, 2006.

3. Cavicchi M, Philippe Beau P, Crenn P, Degott C, Messing B. Prevalence of liver disease and contributing factors in patients receiving home parenteral nutrition for permanent intestinal failure. *Intern Med.* 2000;132:525-532.

*** *Denotes indicator is used for nutrition assessment only. Other indicators are used for both nutrition assessment and nutrition monitoring and evaluation.*

Edition: 2009

Enteral and Parenteral Nutrition Intake (FH-1.4.1)

References, cont'd

4. Centers for Medicare and Medicaid Services. National coverage determination (NCD) for enteral and parenteral nutrition therapy. Available at: http://www.cms.hhs.gov/mcd/viewncd.asp?ncd_id=180.2&ncd_version=1&basket=ncd%3A180%2E2%3A1%3AEnteral+and+Parenteral+Nutritional+Therapy. Accessed December 22, 2006.

5. Compher C, Frankenfield D, Keim N, Roth-Yousey L. Best practice methods to apply to measurement of resting metabolic rate in adults: A systematic review. *J Amer Diet Assoc*. 2006;106:881-903.

6. Guidelines for the use of parenteral and enteral nutrition in adult and pediatric patients: Administration of specialized nutrition support – issues unique to pediatrics. *J Parenter Enteral Nutr*. 2002;26(Suppl):S97-S110.

7. Guidelines for the use of parenteral and enteral nutrition in adult and pediatric patients: Specific guidelines for disease - adults. *J Parenter Enteral Nutr*. 2002;26(Suppl):S61-S96.

8. Guidelines for the use of parenteral and enteral nutrition in adult and pediatric patients: Access for administration of nutrition support. *J Parenter Enteral Nutr*. 2002 Jan-Feb;26(1 Suppl):33SA-41SA.

9. Guidelines for the use of parenteral and enteral nutrition in adult and pediatric patients: Specific guidelines for disease - pediatrics. *J Parenter Enteral Nutr*. 2002;26(Suppl):S111-S138.

10. Guidelines for the use of parenteral and enteral nutrition in adult and pediatric patients: Life cycle and metabolic conditions. *J Parenter Enteral Nutr*. 2002;26(Suppl):S45-S60.

11. Kovacevich DS, Frederick A, Kelly D, Nishikawa R, Young L; American Society for Parenteral and Enteral Nutrition Board of Directors; Standards for Specialized Nutrition Support Task Force. Standards for specialized nutrition support: home care patients. *Nutr Clin Pract*. 2005;20:579-590.

12. Nevin Folino N., ed. *Pediatric Manual of Clinical Dietetics*. American Dietetic Association. Chicago, IL: 2003.

13. Steiger E; HPEN Working Group. Consensus statements regarding optimal management of home parenteral nutrition (HPN) access. *J Parenter Enteral Nutr*. 2006;30(1 Suppl):S94-S95.

*** Denotes indicator is used for nutrition assessment only. Other indicators are used for both nutrition assessment and nutrition monitoring and evaluation.

Assessment

Food/Nutrition-Related History Domain – Bioactive Substances

Alcohol Intake (FH-1.5.1)

Definition
Amount and pattern of alcohol consumption

Nutrition Assessment and Monitoring and Evaluation
Indicators

Drink size/volume (ounces)

Frequency (drinks/day and/or number of drinking days per week)

Pattern of alcohol consumption (number/size of drinks on drinking days)

Note: 1 drink = 5 oz wine, 12 oz beer, 1.5 oz distilled alcohol

Examples of the measurement methods or data sources for these indicators: Patient/client report/recall, self-monitoring log

Typically used with the following domains of nutrition interventions: Nutrition education, nutrition counseling

Typically used to determine and to monitor and evaluate change in the following nutrition diagnoses: Excess intake of alcohol; excess or inadequate intake of energy; altered nutrition-related laboratory values; impaired nutrient utilization; overweight/obesity

Clinical judgment must be used to select indicators and determine the appropriate measurement techniques and reference standards for a given patient population and setting. Once identified, these indicators, measurement techniques, and reference standards should be identified in policies and procedures or other documents for use in patient/client records, quality or performance improvement, or in formal research projects.

Evaluation

Criteria for evaluation
Comparison to Goal or Reference Standard:
1) Goal (tailored to patient/client needs)
   OR
2) Reference standard

*** *Denotes indicator is used for nutrition assessment only. Other indicators are used for both nutrition assessment and nutrition monitoring and evaluation.*

Alcohol Intake (FH-1.5.1)

Patient/Client Example

Example(s) of one or two of the Nutrition Care Indicators (includes sample initial and reassessment documentation for one of the indicators)

Indicator(s) selected

Pattern of alcohol consumption (number/size of drinks on drinking days)

Criteria for evaluation

Comparison to Goal or Reference Standard:

1) Goal: Patient/client's intake of one, 5 ounce glass of wine 2-3 times per week is significantly above and non-compliant with the goal to abstain from alcohol during pregnancy.

   OR

2) Reference standard: Patient/client's intake of three to four, 5 ounce glasses of wine on drinking days is significantly above (above or consistent with) the recommendation of one 5 ounce glass of wine per day for adult females.

Sample nutrition assessment and monitoring and evaluation documentation

Initial nutrition assessment with patient/client	Based upon recall, patient/client consuming three to four, 5 ounce glasses of wine on drinking days, which is above the recommended amount for females. Will monitor change in alcohol intake at next encounter.
Reassessment after nutrition intervention	Progress toward reference standard of up to one, 5 ounce glass of wine per day. Based upon 7-day record, patient/client consuming 3 ounces of wine on drinking days.

References

The following are some suggested references for indicators, measurement techniques, and reference standards; other references may be appropriate.

1. Dietary Guidelines for Americans, 2005. Available at: http://www.health.gov/dietaryguidelines/dga2005/document/html/executivesummary.htm. Accessed October 27, 2006.

2. National Institutes of Health, National Institute on Alcoholism and Alcohol Abuse. Task Force on Recommended Alcohol Questions, National Council on Alcohol Abuse and Alcoholism Recommended Sets of Alcohol Consumption Questions. Available at: http://www.niaaa.nih.gov/Resources/ResearchResources/TaskForce.htm. Accessed October 27, 2006.

3. Sobell SC, Sobell MB. Alcohol Consumption Measures. Available at: http://pubs.niaaa.nih.gov/publications/Assesing%20Alcohol/measures.htm. Accessed February 7, 2008.

*** *Denotes indicator is used for nutrition assessment only. Other indicators are used for both nutrition assessment and nutrition monitoring and evaluation.*

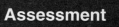

Assessment

Food/Nutrition-Related History Domain – Bioactive Substances

Bioactive Substance Intake (FH-1.5.2)

Definition

Amount and type of bioactive substances consumed

> *Note: Bioactive Substances are not included as part of the Dietary Reference Intakes, and therefore there are no established minimum requirements or Tolerable Upper Intake Levels. However, RDs can assess whether estimated intakes are adequate or excessive using the patient/client goal or nutrition prescription for comparison.*

> *Working definition of bioactive substances—physiologically active components of foods that may offer health benefits beyond traditional macro- or micro-nutrient requirements. There is not scientific consensus about a definition for bioactive substances/components.*

Nutrition Assessment and Monitoring and Evaluation

Indicators

Plant sterol and stanol esters (grams/day)

Soy protein (grams/day)

Psyllium and β-glucan (grams/day)

> *Note: Only bioactive substances with an FDA Health Claim based upon Significant Scientific Agreement (SSA) are included above.*

Examples of the measurement methods or data sources for these indicators: Patient/client report/recall, self-monitoring log

Typically used with the following domains of nutrition interventions: Nutrition education, nutrition counseling

Typically used to determine and to monitor and evaluate change in the following nutrition diagnoses: Inadequate or excess intake of bioactive substances, food-medication interaction

Clinical judgment must be used to select indicators and determine the appropriate measurement techniques and reference standards for a given patient population and setting. Once identified, these indicators, measurement techniques, and reference standards should be identified in policies and procedures or other documents for use in patient/client records, quality or performance improvement, or in formal research projects.

Evaluation

Criteria for evaluation

Comparison to Goal or Reference Standard:

    1) Goal (tailored to patient/client needs)
       OR
    2) Reference standard

*** Denotes indicator is used for nutrition assessment only. Other indicators are used for both nutrition assessment and nutrition monitoring and evaluation.

Bioactive Substance Intake (FH-1.5.2)

Patient/Client Example
Example(s) of one or two of the Nutrition Care Indicators (includes sample initial and reassessment documentation for one of the indicators)

Indicator(s) selected
Plant sterol and stanol esters (grams/day)

Criteria for evaluation
Comparison to Goal or Reference Standard:
1) Goal: The patient/client does not consume plant sterol or stanol esters compared to the goal intake of 2-3 grams per day.
   OR
2) Reference standard: No validated standard exists.

Sample nutrition assessment and monitoring and evaluation documentation

Initial assessment with patient/client	Based upon recall, patient/client not consuming (0 grams) stanol/sterol ester per day, which is below the goal intake of 2-3 grams per day. Will monitor change in stanol/sterol ester intake at next encounter.
Reassessment after nutrition intervention	Good progress toward the goal of 2-3 g/day of stanol/sterol ester. Based upon 7-day diet record, patient/client consuming 2-3 grams stanol/sterol ester per day, 2-3 days per week.

References
The following are some suggested references for indicators, measurement techniques, and reference standards; other references may be appropriate.
1. ADA Disorders of Lipid Metabolism Evidence-Based Nutrition Practice Guideline, 2006. Available at: http://www.adaevidencelibrary.com/topic.cfm?cat=3015. Accessed November 5, 2005.
2. Position of the American Dietetic Association: Functional foods. *J Am Diet Assoc.* 2004;104:814-826.

*** *Denotes indicator is used for nutrition assessment only. Other indicators are used for both nutrition assessment and nutrition monitoring and evaluation.*

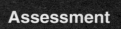

Assessment

Food/Nutrition-Related History Domain – Bioactive Substances

Caffeine Intake (FH-1.5.3)

Definition
Amount of caffeine intake from all sources, e.g., food, beverages, supplements, medications, and via enteral and parenteral routes

Nutrition Assessment and Monitoring and Evaluation
Indicators
Total caffeine intake (mg/day, e.g. naturally occurring caffeine in leaves, seeds, fruits of plants and sources with added caffeine such as water/beverages, medications)

Examples of the measurement methods or data sources for these indicators: Patient/client report/recall, self-monitoring log

Typically used with the following domains of nutrition interventions: Nutrition education, nutrition counseling

Typically used to determine and to monitor and evaluate change in the following nutrition diagnoses: Food and nutrition-related knowledge deficit

Clinical judgment must be used to select indicators and determine the appropriate measurement techniques and reference standards for a given patient population and setting. Once identified, these indicators, measurement techniques, and reference standards should be identified in policies and procedures or other documents for use in patient/client records, quality or performance improvement, or in formal research projects.

Evaluation

Criteria for evaluation
Comparison to Goal or Reference Standard:
1) Goal (tailored to patient/client needs)
   OR
2) Reference standard

Patient/Client Example
Example(s) of one or two of the Nutrition Care Indicators (includes sample initial and reassessment documentation for one of the indicators)

Indicator(s) selected
Total caffeine intake (mg/day)

*** *Denotes indicator is used for nutrition assessment only. Other indicators are used for both nutrition assessment and nutrition monitoring and evaluation.*

Caffeine Intake (FH-1.5.3)

Criteria for evaluation

Comparison to Goal or Reference Standard:

1) Goal: The patient/client's intake is 600 mg of caffeine per day, which is above the goal of < 300 mg caffeine/day.
   OR
2) Reference standard: The patient/client's intake is approximately 600 mg of caffeine/day which is above (above, below or consistent with) of the reference standard of 400 mg caffeine/day.

Sample nutrition assessment and monitoring and evaluation documentation

Initial assessment with patient/client	Based upon recall, patient/client consuming approximately 600 mg caffeine/day, which is above the reference standard of 400 mg/day. Will monitor change in caffeine intake at next encounter.
Reassessment after nutrition intervention	No progress toward the reference standard of 400 mg caffeine /day. Based upon 3-day diet record, patient/client still consuming 600 mg caffeine/day.

References

The following are some suggested references for indicators, measurement techniques, and reference standards; other references may be appropriate.

1. Bech BH, Obel C, Henriksen TB, Olsen J. Effect of reducing caffeine intake on birth weight and length of gestation: randomised controlled trial. *BMJ*. 2007;334:409.
2. Department of Health and Human Services, National Institute of Environmental Health Sciences, National Toxicology Program. Center for the Evaluation of Risks to Human Reproduction (CERHR) Available at: http://cerhr.niehs.nih.gov/common/caffeine.html. Accessed October 31, 2006.
3. Frary CD, Johnson RK, Wang MQ. Food sources and intakes of caffeine in the diets of persons in the United States. *J Am Diet Assoc*. 2005;105:110-113.
4. Higdon JV, Frei B. Coffee and health: a review of recent human research. *Crit Rev Food Sci Nutr*. 2006;46:101-123.
5. Kaiser LL, Allen L. Position of the American Dietetic Association: Nutrition and lifestyle for a healthy pregnancy outcome. *J Amer Diet Assoc*. 2008;108:553-561.
6. McCusker RR, Goldberger BA, Cone EJ. Caffeine content of specialty coffees. *J Anal Toxicol*. 2003;27:520-522.
7. McCusker RR, Goldberger BA, Cone EJ. Caffeine content of energy drinks, carbonated sodas, and other beverages. *J Anal Toxicol*. 2006;30:112-114.
8. Nawrot P, Jordan S, Eastwood J, Rotstein J, Hugenholtz A, Feeley M. Effects of caffeine on human health. *Food Addit Contam*. 2003; 20: 1–30.
9. Nutrient Data Laboratory, USDA National Nutrient Database for Standard Reference. Available at: http://www.nal.usda.gov/fnic/foodcomp/search/. Accessed on October 30, 2006.
10. Organization of Teratology Information Services (OTIS). Caffeine and Pregnancy. Available at: http://www.otispregnancy.org/pdf/caffeine.pdf. Accessed November 11, 2006.
11. Winkelmayer WC, Stampfer MJ, Willett WC, Curhan, GC. Habitual Caffeine Intake and the Risk of Hypertension in Women *JAMA*. 2005;294:2330-2335.

*** *Denotes indicator is used for nutrition assessment only. Other indicators are used for both nutrition assessment and nutrition monitoring and evaluation.*

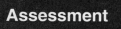
Assessment

Food/Nutrition-Related History Domain – Macronutrient Intake

Fat and Cholesterol Intake (FH-1.6.1)

Definition

Fat and cholesterol consumption from all sources, e.g., food, beverages, supplements, and via enteral and parenteral routes

*Note: Whenever possible, nutrient intake data should be considered in combination with clinical, biochemical, anthropometric information, medical diagnosis, clinical status, and/or other factors as well as diet to provide a valid assessment of nutritional status based on a totality of the evidence. (*Dietary Reference Intakes. Applications in Dietary Assessment. *Institute of Medicine. Washington, D.C.: National Academy Press; 2000.)*

Nutrition Assessment and Monitoring and Evaluation

Indicators

Total fat (specify, e.g., grams/day, grams/kg/day, percent of calories)

Saturated fat (specify, e.g., grams/day or % of calories/day)

Trans fatty acids (specify, e.g., grams/day or % of calories/day)

Polyunsaturated fat (specify, e.g., grams/day or % of calories/day)

Monounsaturated fat (specify, e.g., grams/day or % of calories/day)

Omega-3 fatty acids
- Marine-derived (specify, e.g., grams/day)
- Plant-derived
  - Alpha-linolenic acid (specify, e.g., grams/day or % of calories/day)

Dietary cholesterol (specify, e.g., mg/day)

Essential fatty acids (specify, e.g., grams or ratio)

Note: Plant sterol and stanol esters can be found on the Bioactive Substance Intake Reference Sheet.

Examples of the measurement methods or data sources for these indicators: Food intake records, 24-hour recall, food frequency questionnaires, menu analysis, fat and cholesterol targeted questionnaires and monitoring devices

Typically used with the following domains of nutrition interventions: Food and/or nutrient delivery, nutrition education, nutrition counseling

Typically used to determine and to monitor and evaluate change in the following nutrition diagnoses: Inadequate and excessive fat intake, inappropriate intake of food fats, overweight/obesity, altered nutrition-related lab values, altered food and nutrition-related knowledge deficit

Clinical judgment must be used to select indicators and determine the appropriate measurement techniques and reference standards for a given patient population and setting. Once identified, these indicators, measurement techniques, and reference standards should be identified in policies and procedures or other documents for use in patient/client records, quality or performance improvement, or in formal research projects.

*** Denotes indicator is used for nutrition assessment only. Other indicators are used for both nutrition assessment and nutrition monitoring and evaluation.

Edition: 2009

Fat and Cholesterol Intake (FH-1.6.1)

Evaluation

Criteria for evaluation

Comparison to Goal or Reference Standard:
1) Goal (tailored to patient/client's needs)
   OR
2) Reference standard

Patient/Client Example(s)

Example(s) of one or two of the Nutrition Care Indicators (includes sample initial and reassessment documentation for one of the indicators)

Indicator(s) selected

Total fat (% of calories from fat)

Criteria for evaluation

Comparison to Goal or Reference Standard:
1) Goal: Patient/client currently consumes 40% of calories from fat. Goal is to decrease fat intake to 25-35% of calories.
   OR
2) Reference standard: Patient/client's intake of 350 mg of cholesterol per day is 175% of the Adult Treatment Panel III guidelines of less than 200 mg of dietary cholesterol per day.

Sample nutrition assessment and monitoring and evaluation documentation

Initial nutritional assessment with patient/client	Based upon a three-day food diary, patient/client is consuming approximately 40% of calories from fat. Patient/client goal is to reduce total fat intake to 25-35% of calories. Will monitor fat and calorie intake at next appointment.
Reassessment after nutrition intervention	Significant progress toward the goal intake of 25-35% calories from fat. Based on a three-day food diary patient/client's total fat intake decreased from approximately 40% to 38% calories from fat/day. Will continue to monitor progress at next encounter in 6 weeks.

*** *Denotes indicator is used for nutrition assessment only. Other indicators are used for both nutrition assessment and nutrition monitoring a*

Fat and Cholesterol Intake (FH-1.6.1)

References

The following are some suggested references for indicators, measurement techniques, and reference standards for the outcome; other references may be appropriate.

1. American Heart Association Nutrition Committee: Lichtenstein, A, Appel, L, Brands M, Carnethon M, Daniels S, Franch HA, Franklin B, Kris-Etherton P, Harris WS, Howard B, Karanja N, Lefevre M, Rudel L, Sacks F, Van Horn L, Winston M, Wylie-Rosett J. Diet and lifestyle recommendations revision 2006: a scientific statement from the American Heart Association Nutrition Committee. *Circulation*. 2006;114:82-96.

2. Bantle JP, Wylie-Rosett J, Albright AL, Apovian CM, Clark NG, Franz MJ, Hoogwerf BJ, Lichtenstein AH, Mayer-Davis E, Mooradian AD, Wheeler ML. Nutrition recommendations and interventions for diabetes-2006: a position statement of the American Diabetes Association. *Diabetes Care*. 2006;29:2140-2157.

3. Committee on Nutrient Relationships in Seafood—National Academies. *Seafood choices: Balancing Benefits and Risks*. National Academies Press; 2006.

4. US Departments of Agriculture and Health and Human Services. Dietary Guidelines for Americans 2005. Available at: www.healthierus.gov/dietaryguidelines/.

5. US Department of Health and Human Services. National Institutes of Health. National Heart, Lung and Blood Institute. *Third Report of the Expert Panel on Detection, Evaluation, and Treatment of High Blood Cholesterol in Adults (Adult Treatment Panel III)*. Bethesda, MD: National Institutes of Health; 2001.

6. Institute of Medicine, Food and Nutrition Board. Dietary Reference Intakes for Energy, Carbohydrate, Fiber, Fat, Fatty Acids, Cholesterol, Protein and Amino Acids. Washington, DC: National Academy Press; 2002. Available at: www.iom.edu/report.asp?id=4340.

7. American Society for Parenteral and Enteral Nutrition Board of Directors and The Clinical Guidelines Task Force. Guidelines for the use of parenteral and enteral nutrition in adult and pediatric patients: Specific guidelines for disease—adults. *J Parenter Enteral Nutr*. 2002;26(Suppl):S61-S96.

8. US Departments of Agriculture and Health and Human Services. Dietary Guidelines for Americans 2005. Available at: www.healthierus.gov/dietaryguidelines.

9. ADA Nutrition Care Manual. 2006. Available at: www.nutritioncaremanual.org. Accessed December 11, 2006.

10. ADA Evidence Analysis Library. Accessed on: January 30, 2008 from http://www.ada.portalxm.com/eal/topic.cfm?cat=1447

11. McCoin M, Sikand G, Johnson EQ, Kris-Etherton PM, Burke F, Carson J, Champagne CM, Karmally W, Van Horn L. The effectiveness of medical nutriton therapy delivered by registered dietitians for disorders of lipid metabolism: A call for further research. *J Am Diet Assoc*. 2008; 108(2):233-239.

12. Van Horn L, McCoin M, Kris-Etherton PM, Burke F, Carson J, Champagne CM, Karmally W Sikand G. The evidence for dietary prevention and treatment of cardiovascular disease. *J Am Diet Assoc*. 2008; 108(2):287-331.

*** *Denotes indicator is used for nutrition assessment only. Other indicators are used for both nutrition assessment and nutrition monitoring and evaluation.*

Protein Intake (FH-1.6.2)

Definition
Protein intake from all sources (e.g., food, beverages, supplements, and via enteral and parenteral routes)

Note: Whenever possible, nutrient intake data should be considered in combination with clinical, biochemical, anthropometric information, medical diagnosis, clinical status, and/or other factors as well as diet to provide a valid assessment of nutritional status based on a totality of the evidence. (Dietary Reference Intakes. Applications in Dietary Assessment. Institute of Medicine. Washington, D.C.: National Academy Press; 2000.)

Nutrition Assessment and Monitoring and Evaluation
Indicators

Total protein (specify, e.g., grams/day, grams/kg/day, percent of calories)

High biological value protein (specify, e.g., grams/day, percent of calories)

Casein (specify, e.g., g/day)

Whey (specify, e.g., g/day)

Amino acids (specify, e.g., % crystalline amino acids)

Essential amino acids (specify, e.g., mg/day)

Note: Soy protein can be found on the Bioactive Substance Intake Reference Sheet.

Examples of the measurement methods or data sources for these indicators: Food intake records, 24-hour recall, food frequency questionnaires, protein intake collection tools, nutrition fact labels, other product information, nutrient composition tables

Typically used with the following domains of nutrition interventions: Food and/or nutrient delivery, nutrition education, nutrition counseling, coordination of nutrition care

Typically used to determine and to monitor and evaluate change in the following nutrition diagnoses: Inadequate and excessive protein intake, inappropriate intake of amino acids, evident protein-energy malnutrition, inadequate protein-energy intake, altered GI function, limited adherence to nutrition-related recommendations

Clinical judgment must be used to select indicators and determine the appropriate measurement techniques and reference standards for a given patient population and setting. Once identified, these indicators, measurement techniques, and reference standards should be identified in policies and procedures or other documents for use in patient/client records, quality or performance improvement, or in formal research projects.

*** Denotes indicator is used for nutrition assessment only. Other indicators are used for both nutrition assessment and nutrition monitoring and evaluation.

Assessment

Food/Nutrition-Related History Domain – Macronutrient Intake

Protein Intake (FH-1.6.2)

Evaluation

Criteria for evaluation
Comparison to Goal or Reference Standard:
1) Goal (tailored to patient/client's needs)
   OR
2) Reference standard

Patient/Client Example(s)
Example(s) of one or two of the Nutrition Care Indicators (includes sample initial and reassessment documentation for one of the indicators)

Indicator(s) selected
Total protein

Criteria for evaluation
Comparison to Goal or Reference Standard:
1) Goal: Patient's/client's current intake of 25 g protein per day is below the recommended level of 55–65 g per day.
   OR
2) Reference standard: (Used when patient goal is based on the population standard) Patient's/client's intake of 12 g protein/day is less then the DRI of 53 g/day (0.8 g/kg BW). Patient/client's goal is to increase protein intake to approximately 55 g/day.

Sample nutrition assessment and monitoring and evaluation documentation

Initial nutrition assessment with patient/client	Enteral feeding currently providing 25 g protein/day, well below the recommended level of 55–65 g/day (1-1.2 g/kg BW). Will continue to monitor protein intake daily.
Reassessment after nutrition intervention	Some progress toward goal intake of 55–65 g protein/day. Current intake approximately 30 g protein/day, 25 g protein below desired level. Will continue to monitor protein intake daily.

*** *Denotes indicator is used for nutrition assessment only. Other indicators are used for both nutrition assessment and nutrition monitoring and evaluation.*

Protein Intake (FH-1.6.2)

References

The following are some suggested references for indicators, measurement techniques, and reference standards for the outcome; other references may be appropriate.

1. Institute of Medicine, Food and Nutrition Board. Dietary Reference Intakes for Energy, Carbohydrate, Fiber, Fat, Fatty Acids, Cholesterol, Protein and Amino Acids. Washington, DC: National Academy Press; 2002. Available at: www.iom.edu/report.asp?id=4340.

2. Young VR, Borgouha S. Adult human amino acid requirements. *Curr Opin Clin Metab Care*. 1999;2:39-45.

3. Charney P, Malone A, eds. ADA Pocket Guide to Nutrition Assessment. Chicago, IL: American Dietetic Association; 2004.

4. American Society for Parenteral and Enteral Nutrition Board of Directors and The Clinical Guidelines Task Force. Guidelines for the use of parenteral and enteral nutrition in adult and pediatric patients: Specific guidelines for disease—adults. *J Parenter Enteral Nutr*. 2002;26(Suppl):S61-S96

5. American Society for Parenteral and Enteral Nutrition Board of Directors and The Clinical Guidelines Task Force. Guidelines for the use of parenteral and enteral nutrition in adult and pediatric patients: Life cycle and metabolic conditions. *J Parenter Enteral Nutr*. 2002;26(Suppl):S45-S60.

6. American Society for Parenteral and Enteral Nutrition Board of Directors and The Clinical Guidelines Task Force. Guidelines for the use of parenteral and enteral nutrition in adult and pediatric patients: Specific guidelines for disease—pediatrics. *J Parenter Enteral Nutr*. 2002;26(Suppl):S111-S138

7. ADA Nutrition Care Manual. 2006. Available at: www.nutritioncaremanual.org. Accessed December 14, 2006.

8. NKF-K/DOQI. Clinical Practice Guidelines for Nutrition in Chronic Renal Failure. *Am J Kidney Dis*. 2001;37(1 Suppl 2):S66-70.

*** Denotes indicator is used for nutrition assessment only. Other indicators are used for both nutrition assessment and nutrition monitoring and evaluation.

Assessment

Food/Nutrition-Related History Domain – Macronutrient Intake

Carbohydrate Intake (FH-1.6.3)

Definition
Carbohydrate consumption from all sources, (e.g., food, beverages, supplements, and via enteral and parenteral routes)

> *Note: Whenever possible, nutrient intake data should be considered in combination with clinical, biochemical, anthropometric information, medical diagnosis, clinical status, and/or other factors as well as diet to provide a valid assessment of nutritional status based on a totality of the evidence. (*Dietary Reference Intakes. Applications in Dietary Assessment. *Institute of Medicine. Washington, D.C.: National Academy Press; 2000.)*

Nutrition Assessment and Monitoring and Evaluation
Indicators
Total carbohydrate (specify, e.g., grams/day, grams/meal, grams/kg/min, percent of calories)

Sugar (specify, e.g., grams/day, percent of calories)

Starch (specify, e.g., grams/day, percent of calories)

Glycemic index (specify)

Glycemic load (specify)

Source of carbohydrate intake (food, beverage, tube feeding, parenteral nutrition, medication)

> *Note: Fiber intake is listed on the Fiber Intake Reference Sheet.*
>> *Psyllium and β-glucan can be found on the Bioactive Substance Intake reference sheet.*

Examples of the measurement methods or data sources for these indicators: Food intake records, 24-hour or typical day's recall, food frequency questionnaires, menu analysis, carbohydrate counting tools, intake/output sheets (for tube feeding or parenteral nutrition)

Typically used with the following domains of nutrition interventions: Food and/or nutrient delivery, nutrition education, nutrition counseling, coordination of nutrition care

Typically used to determine and to monitor and evaluate change in the following nutrition diagnoses: Inadequate and excessive carbohydrate intake, inappropriate intake of types of carbohydrate, inconsistent carbohydrate intake, altered nutrition-related laboratory values, food medication interaction

Clinical judgment must be used to select indicators and determine the appropriate measurement techniques and reference standards for a given patient population and setting. Once identified, these indicators, measurement techniques, and reference standards should be identified in policies and procedures or other documents for use in patient/client records, quality or performance improvement, or in formal research projects.

*** *Denotes indicator is used for nutrition assessment only. Other indicators are used for both nutrition assessment and nutrition monitoring and evaluation.*

Carbohydrate Intake (FH-1.6.3)

Evaluation

Criteria for evaluation
Comparison to Goal or Reference Standard:
1) Goal (tailored to patient/client's needs)
    OR
2) Reference standard

Patient/Client Example(s)

Example(s) of one or two of the Nutrition Care Indicators (includes sample initial and reassessment documentation for one of the indicators)

Indicator(s) selected
Total carbohydrate (distribution by meal)

Criteria for evaluation
Comparison to Goal or Reference Standard:
1) Goal: Patient's/client's current carbohydrate intake in the morning ranges from 0 to 95 grams. The goal is that the patient/client will consume approximately 30 g carbohydrate at breakfast six days per week.
    OR
2) Reference standard: No validated standard exists.

Sample nutrition assessment and monitoring and evaluation documentation

Initial nutrition assessment with patient/client	Based upon carbohydrate counting tools, patient/client consumed 30 g carbohydrate at breakfast 2 days/week. Goal is to consume 30 g carbohydrate for breakfast 6 days per week.
Reassessment after nutrition intervention	Some progress made toward goal. Based upon carbohydrate counting tools, patient/client consumed 30 g carbohydrate at breakfast 2 days/week. Will monitor breakfast carbohydrate intake at next encounter.

*** *Denotes indicator is used for nutrition assessment only. Other indicators are used for both nutrition assessment and nutrition monitoring and evaluation.*

Edition: 2009

Assessment

Food/Nutrition-Related History Domain – Macronutrient Intake

Carbohydrate Intake (FH-1.6.3)

References

The following are some suggested references for indicators, measurement techniques, and reference standards for the outcome; other references may be appropriate.

1. Institute of Medicine, Food and Nutrition Board. Dietary Reference Intakes for Energy, Carbohydrate, Fiber, Fat, Fatty Acids, Cholesterol, Protein and Amino Acids. Washington, DC: National Academy Press; 2002. Available at: www.iom.edu/report.asp?id=4340.

2. American Society for Parenteral and Enteral Nutrition Board of Directors and The Clinical Guidelines Task Force. Guidelines for the use of parenteral and enteral nutrition in adult and pediatric patients: Specific guidelines for disease—adults. *J Parenter Enteral Nutr*. 2002;26(Suppl):S61-S96.

3. ADA Nutrition Care Manual. 2009. Available at: www.nutritioncaremanual.org. Accessed December 14, 2006.

4. The American Diabetes Association. Standards of Medical Care in Diabetes (Position Statement)–2008. *Diabetes Care*. 2008;31:S12-S54..

5. US Departments of Agriculture and Health and Human Services. Dietary Guidelines for Americans 2005. Available at: www.healthierus.gov/dietaryguidelines.

*** *Denotes indicator is used for nutrition assessment only. Other indicators are used for both nutrition assessment and nutrition monitoring and evaluation.*

Fiber Intake (FH-1.6.4)

Definition

Amount and/or type of plant source matter consumed that is not completely digested, but may be at least partially fermented in the distal bowel, and is derived from all sources (e.g., food, beverages, supplements, and via enteral routes)

*Note: Whenever possible, nutrient intake data should be considered in combination with clinical, biochemical, anthropometric information, medical diagnosis, clinical status, and/or other factors as well as diet to provide a valid assessment of nutritional status based on a totality of the evidence. (*Dietary Reference Intakes. Applications in Dietary Assessment. *Institute of Medicine. Washington, D.C.: National Academy Press; 2000.)*

Nutrition Assessment and Monitoring and Evaluation

Indicators

Total fiber (g/day)

Soluble fiber (g/day)

Insoluble fiber (g/day)

- Fructooligosaccharides (g/day)

Note: Psyllium and β-glucan can be found on the Bioactive Substance Intake reference sheet

Examples of the measurement methods or data sources for these indicators: Food intake records, 24-hour recall, food frequency questionnaires, menu analysis, fiber counting tools, nutrition fact labels, other product information, nutrient composition tables

Typically used with the following domains of nutrition interventions: Food and/or nutrient delivery, nutrition education, nutrition counseling, coordination of nutrition care

Typically used to determine and to monitor and evaluate change in the following nutrition diagnoses: Inadequate and excessive fiber intake, altered GI function, disordered eating pattern, inadequate bioactive substance intake

Clinical judgment must be used to select indicators and determine the appropriate measurement techniques and reference standards for a given patient population and setting. Once identified, these indicators, measurement techniques, and reference standards should be identified in policies and procedures or other documents for use in patient/client records, quality or performance improvement, or in formal research projects.

Evaluation

Criteria for evaluation

Comparison to Goal or Reference Standard:

1) Goal (tailored to patient/client's needs)

OR

2) Reference standard

*** Denotes indicator is used for nutrition assessment only. Other indicators are used for both nutrition assessment and nutrition monitoring and evaluation.

Assessment

Food/Nutrition-Related History Domain – Food and Nutrition Intake

Fiber Intake (FH-1.6.4)

Patient/Client Example(s)
Example(s) of one or two of the Nutrition Care Indicators (includes sample initial and reassessment documentation for one of the indicators)

Indicator(s) selected
Total dietary fiber intake including those from foods and dietary fiber supplements.

Criteria for evaluation
Comparison to Goal or Reference Standard:
1) Goal: Patient/client with current fiber intake of 15 g per day. Goal is to increase fiber intake to approximately 25 g per day.
   OR
2) Reference standard: Patient/client's current intake of 15 g of dietary fiber per day is below the DRI of 25 g/day for a 40-year-old woman.

Sample nutrition assessment and monitoring and evaluation documentation

Initial nutrition assessment with patient/client	Based upon patient/client's food diary, patient/client is consuming approximately 15 g of fiber/day. Will monitor fiber intake at next encounter in three weeks.
Reassessment after nutrition intervention	Goal achieved. Patient/client's intake of 27 g fiber exceeded goal intake of 25 g/day. Will continue to monitor to ensure success is sustained.

References
The following are some suggested references for indicators, measurement techniques, and reference standards for the outcome; other references may be appropriate.

1. Institute of Medicine, Food and Nutrition Board. *Dietary Reference Intakes for Energy, Carbohydrate, Fiber, Fat, Fatty Acids, Cholesterol, Protein and Amino Acids*. Washington, DC: National Academy Press; 2002. Available at: www.iom.edu/report.asp?id=4340.
2. Marlett JA, McBurney MI, Slavin JL. Position of the American Dietetic Association: Health implications of dietary fiber. *J Am Diet Assoc*. 2002;102:993-1000.
3. Institute of Food Science and Technology. Information statement: Dietary fiber. Available at: http://www.ifst.org/uploadedfiles/cms/store/ATTACHMENTS/dietaryfibre.pdf Accessed on January 29, 2008.
4. US Department of Health and Human Services. National Institutes of Health. National Heart, Lung and Blood Institute. *Third Report of the Expert Panel on Detection, Evaluation, and Treatment of High Blood Cholesterol in Adults (Adult Treatment Panel III)*. Bethesda, MD: National Institutes of Health; 2001
5. ADA Nutrition Care Manual. 2006. Available at: www.nutritioncaremanual.org. Accessed December 14, 2006.
6. Thomson CA. Practice Paper of the American Dietetic Association: Dietary Supplements. *J Am Diet Assoc*. 2005;105(3):460-470.

*** Denotes indicator is used for nutrition assessment only. Other indicators are used for both nutrition assessment and nutrition monitoring and evaluation.

Vitamin Intake (FH-1.7.1)

Definition

Vitamin intake from all sources, e.g., food, beverages, supplements, and via enteral and parenteral routes

*Note: Whenever possible, nutrient intake data should be considered in combination with clinical, biochemical, anthropometric information, medical diagnosis, clinical status, and/or other factors as well as diet to provide a valid assessment of nutritional status based on a totality of the evidence. (*Dietary Reference Intakes. Applications in Dietary Assessment. *Institute of Medicine. Washington, D.C.: National Academy Press; 2000.)*

Nutrition Assessment and Monitoring and Evaluation

Indicators

Vitamin A (µg/day)

Vitamin C (mg/day)

Vitamin D (µg/day)

Vitamin E (mg/day)

Vitamin K (µg/day)

Thiamin (mg/day)

Riboflavin (mg/day)

Multivitamin (yes/no)

Niacin (mg/day)

Vitamin B6 (mg/day)

Folate (µg/day)

Vitamin B12 (µg/day)

Pantothenic acid (mg/day)

Biotin (µg/day)

Note: Laboratory measures associated with body vitamin status can be found on the Vitamin Profile Reference Sheet.

Examples of the measurement methods or data sources for these indicators: Patient/client report or recall, food frequency, home evaluation, supplement use questionnaire

Typically used with the following domains of nutrition interventions: Food and/or nutrient delivery, nutrition education, nutrition counseling, coordination of nutrition care

Typically used to determine and to monitor and evaluate change in the following nutrition diagnoses: Excess or inadequate intake of vitamins, parenteral, or enteral nutrition

Clinical judgment must be used to select indicators and determine the appropriate measurement techniques and reference standards for a given patient population and setting. Once identified, these indicators, measurement techniques, and reference standards should be identified in policies and procedures or other documents for use in patient/client records, quality or performance improvement, or in formal research projects.

*** *Denotes indicator is used for nutrition assessment only. Other indicators are used for both nutrition assessment and nutrition monitoring and evaluation.*

Assessment

Food/Nutrition-Related History Domain – Micronutrient Intake

Vitamin Intake (FH-1.7.1)

Evaluation

Criteria for evaluation

Comparison to Goal or Reference Standard:

    1) Nutrition prescription or goal (tailored to patient/client needs)

       OR

    2) Reference standard

Patient/Client Example

Example(s) of one or two of the Nutrition Care Indicators (includes sample initial and reassessment documentation for one of the indicators)

Indicator(s) selected

Vitamin D (µg/day)

Criteria for evaluation

Comparison to Goal or Reference Standard:

    1) Nutrition prescription or goal: Use if patient/client's nutrition prescription/goal is different from the reference standard.

       OR

    2) Reference standard: The patient/client's intake of 4 µg of Vitamin D is below (above, below, consistent with) the Adequate Intake (AI) for males, age 14-18.

Sample nutrition assessment and monitoring and evaluation documentation

Initial nutrition assessment with patient/client	Based upon recall, patient/client with cystic fibrosis consuming approximately 4 µg for Vitamin D, which is below the Adequate Intake (AI) of 5 µg per day for Vitamin D for a 15 year old male. Patient/client has also discontinued fat-soluble vitamin supplement. Will monitor Vitamin D intake at next encounter, intake of fat-soluble vitamin supplement, and request 25-Hydroxy, Vitamin D level (Vitamin Profile Reference Sheet).
Reassessment after nutrition intervention	25-Hydroxy, Vitamin D level below expected range (from Vitamin Profile). Significant progress toward the Adequate Intake of 5 µg for Vitamin D. Based upon 3-day diet record, patient/client has increased consumption of Vitamin D from food sources to 5-7µg for Vitamin D which is consistent with the Adequate Intake for healthy individuals, and is taking fat-soluble vitamin supplement on average 5 days per week. Despite meeting Adequate Intake, since patient/client has cystic fibrosis, will need to continue fat-soluble vitamin supplementation in addition to food sources. Repeat lab in 3 months.

*** *Denotes indicator is used for nutrition assessment only. Other indicators are used for both nutrition assessment and nutrition monitoring and evaluation.*

Vitamin Intake (FH-1.7.1)

References

The following are some suggested references for indicators, measurement techniques, and reference standards; other references may be appropriate.

1. ADA Nutrition Care Manual. 2004. Available at: www.nutritioncaremanual.org. Accessed December 11, 2006.

2. Gartner LM, Greer FR, American Academy of Pediatrics Committee on Nutrition. Prevention of rickets and vitamin D deficiency: new guidelines for vitamin D Intake. *Pediatrics* 2003:111:908-10.

3. Guidelines for the use of parenteral and enteral nutrition in adult and pediatric patients: Normal requirements - adults. *J Parenter Enteral Nutr.* 2002;26(Suppl):S22-S24.

4. Guidelines for the use of parenteral and enteral nutrition in adult and pediatric patients: Normal requirements - pediatrics. *J Parenter Enteral Nutr.* 2002;26(Suppl):S25-S32.

5. National Academy of Sciences, Institute of Medicine. *Dietary Reference Intakes for Calcium, Phosphorus, Magnesium, Vitamin D, and Fluoride.* Washington, DC: National Academy Press; 1997.

6. National Academy of Sciences, Institute of Medicine. *Dietary Reference Intakes: Thiamin, riboflavin, niacin, vitamin B6, folate, vitamin B12, pantothenic acid, biotin, and choline.* National Academy Press. Washington, DC, 1998.

7. National Academy of Sciences, Institute of Medicine. *Dietary Reference Intakes for Vitamin A, Vitamin K, Arsenic, Boron, Chromium, Copper, Iodine, Iron, Manganese, Molybdenum, Nickel, Silicon, Vanadium, and Zinc.* National Academy Press, Washington, DC, 2001.

8. National Academy of Sciences, Institute of Medicine. *Dietary Reference Intakes: Vitamin C, Vitamin E, Selenium, and Carotenoids.* National Academy Press, Washington, DC, 2000.

9. Nevin Folino N., ed. *Pediatric Manual of Clinical Dietetics.* American Dietetic Association. Chicago, IL: 2003.

*** *Denotes indicator is used for nutrition assessment only. Other indicators are used for both nutrition assessment and nutrition monitoring and evaluation.*

87

Assessment

Mineral/Element Intake (FH-1.7.2)

Definition
Mineral/element intake from all sources, e.g., food, beverages, supplements, and via enteral and parenteral routes

> *Note: Whenever possible, nutrient intake data should be considered in combination with clinical, biochemical, anthropometric information, medical diagnosis, clinical status, and/or other factors as well as diet to provide a valid assessment of nutritional status based on a totality of the evidence. (Dietary Reference Intakes. Applications in Dietary Assessment. Institute of Medicine. Washington, D.C.: National Academy Press; 2000.)*

Nutrition Assessment and Monitoring and Evaluation
Indicators

Calcium (mg/day)	Selenium (µg/day)
Copper (µg/day)	Zinc (mg/day)
Fluoride (mg/day)	Potassium (g/day)
Iodine (µg/day)	Sodium (mg/day)
Iron (mg/day)	Chloride (mg/day)
Magnesium (mg/day)	Chromium (µg/day)
Phosphorus (mg/day)	
Multi-mineral (yes/no)	
Multi-trace element (yes/no)	

Examples of the measurement methods or data sources for these indicators: Patient/client report or recall, food frequency, home evaluation, home care or pharmacy report, supplement use questionnaire

Typically used with the following domains of nutrition interventions: Food and/or nutrient delivery, nutrition education, nutrition counseling, coordination of nutrition care

Typically used to determine and to monitor and evaluate change in the following nutrition diagnoses: Excess or inadequate intake of minerals, food-medication interaction, altered nutrition-related laboratory values, impaired nutrient utilization, undesirable food choices, limited adherence to nutrition-related recommendations

Clinical judgment must be used to select indicators and determine the appropriate measurement techniques and reference standards for a given patient population and setting. Once identified, these indicators, measurement techniques, and reference standards should be identified in policies and procedures or other documents for use in patient/client records, quality or performance improvement, or in formal research projects.

*** Denotes indicator is used for nutrition assessment only. Other indicators are used for both nutrition assessment and nutrition monitoring and evaluation.

Mineral/Element Intake (FH-1.7.2)

Evaluation

Criteria for evaluation

Comparison to Goal or Reference Standard:
1) Nutrition prescription or goal (tailored to individual's needs)
   OR
2) Reference standard

Patient/Client Example

Example(s) of one or two of the Nutrition Care Indicators (includes sample initial and reassessment documentation for one of the indicators)

Indicator(s) selected

Sodium (mg/day)
Calcium (mg/day)

Criteria for evaluation

Comparison to Goal or Reference Standard:
1) Nutrition prescription or goal: The patient/client's intake of sodium is approximately 6000 mg per day, which is above the nutrition prescription of 4000 mg per day.
   OR
2) Reference standard: The patient/client's intake of calcium is 500 mg per day which is 50% of the Adequate Intake (AI) for adult females, 31-50 years of age.

Sample nutrition assessment and monitoring and evaluation documentation

Initial nutrition assessment with patient/client	Based upon recall, patient/client consuming approximately 500 mg/day, which is below the adequate intake for calcium per day for females 31-50 years of age. Will monitor calcium intake at next encounter.
Reassessment after nutrition intervention	Significant progress toward the adequate intake of 1000 mg of calcium per day. Based upon 3-day diet record, patient/client has increased consumption from 500 mg/day to 750 mg/day of the adequate daily intake for calcium.

*** Denotes indicator is used for nutrition assessment only. Other indicators are used for both nutrition assessment and nutrition monitoring and evaluation.*

Assessment

Mineral/Element Intake (FH-1.7.2)

References

The following are some suggested references for indicators, measurement techniques, and reference standards; other references may be appropriate.

1. ADA Adult Weight Management Evidence-Based Guideline, 2006. Available at: http://www.adaevidencelibrary.com/topic.cfm?cat=2798. Accessed October 30, 2006.

2. ADA Nutrition Care Manual. 2004. Available at: www.nutritioncaremanual.org. Accessed December 12, 2006.

3. Appel LJ, Moore TJ, Obarzanek E, Vollmer WM, Svetkey LP, Sacks FM, Bray GA, Vogt TM, Cutler JA, Windhauser MM, Lin P, Karanja N, Simons-Morton D, McCullough M, Swain J, Steele P, Evans MA, Miller ER, Harsha DW. A clinical trial of the effects of dietary patterns on blood pressure. *NEJM*. 1997;336:1117-1124.

4. Dietary Guidelines for Americans, 2005. Available at: http://www.health.gov/dietaryguidelines/dga2005/document/html/executivesummary.htm. Accessed October 27, 2006.

5. Guidelines for the use of parenteral and enteral nutrition in adult and pediatric patients: Normal requirements - adults. *J Parenter Enteral Nutr*. 2002;26(Suppl):S22-S24.

6. Guidelines for the use of parenteral and enteral nutrition in adult and pediatric patients: Normal requirements - pediatrics. *J Parenter Enteral Nutr*. 2002;26(Suppl):S25-S32.

7. National Academy of Sciences, Institute of Medicine. *Dietary Reference Intakes for Calcium, Phosphorus, Magnesium, Vitamin D, and Fluoride*. Washington, DC: National Academy Press; 1997.

8. National Academy of Sciences, Institute of Medicine. *Dietary Reference Intakes for Vitamin A, Vitamin K, Arsenic, Boron, Chromium, Copper, Iodine, Iron, Manganese, Molybdenum, Nickel, Silicon, Vanadium, Zinc*. Washington, DC: National Academy Press; 2001.

9. National Academy of Sciences, Institute of Medicine. *Dietary Reference Intakes for Vitamin C, Vitamin E, Selenium, and Carotenoids*. Washington, DC: National Academy Press; 2000.

10. National Academy of Sciences, Institute of Medicine. *Dietary Reference Intakes for Water, Potassium, Sodium, Chloride, and Sulfate*, Washington DC: National Academy Press; 2004.

11. Nevin Folino N., ed. *Pediatric Manual of Clinical Dietetics*. American Dietetic Association. Chicago, IL: 2003.

12. Your Guide to Lowering Your Blood Pressure. Available at: http://www.nhlbi.nih.gov/hbp/prevent/h_eating/h_eating.htm. Accessed November 16, 2006.

*** *Denotes indicator is used for nutrition assessment only. Other indicators are used for both nutrition assessment and nutrition monitoring and evaluation.*

Medication and Herbal Supplements (FH-2.1)

Definition

Prescription and over-the-counter medications, including herbal preparations and complementary medicine products that may impact nutritional status

Nutrition Assessment and Monitoring and Evaluation

Indicators

Medications

- Prescription medication
  - Current prescriptions with nutrient/food-medication interactions, specify
  - Insulin or insulin secretagogues, specify
  - Medication, alter blood pressure, specify
  - Medication, alter breast milk production, specify
  - Medication, lipid lowering, specify
  - Medications, alter glucose levels, specify
  - Other, specify
- Over-the-counter (OTC) medications
  - Current OTC products with nutrient/food-medication implications, specify
  - Medication, alter blood pressure, specify
  - Medication, alter breast milk production, specify
  - Medication, lipid lowering, specify
  - Medications, alter glucose levels, specify
  - Other, specify

Herbal/complementary medicine products (e.g., gingko, St John's Wart, elderberry, garlic, ephedra), specify

Misuse of medications (e.g., accidental overdose, illegal drugs, laxatives, diuretics, drug use during pregnancy), specify

Note: Vitamin and mineral supplements can be found on the vitamin and mineral intake reference sheets. Alcohol is found on the alcohol intake reference sheet

Examples of the measurement methods or data sources for these indicators: Patient/client report, medical record, referring health care provider or agency

Typically used with following domains of nutrition interventions: Food and/or nutrient delivery, nutrition education, nutrition counseling, coordination of nutrition care

*** *Denotes indicator is used for nutrition assessment only. Other indicators are used for both nutrition assessment and nutrition monitoring and evaluation.*

Assessment

Food/Nutrition-Related History Domain – Medication and Herbal Supplement Use

Medication and Herbal Supplements (FH-2.1)

Typically used to determine the following nutrition diagnoses: Food-medication interaction, increased energy expenditure, evident protein-energy malnutrition, inadequate or excessive energy, food/beverage, fluid, carbohydrate, protein, fat, vitamin and mineral intake, involuntary weight gain or loss, overweight/obesity, underweight, intake of unsafe foods, disordered eating pattern

Clinical judgment must be used to select indicators and determine the appropriate measurement techniques and reference standards for a given patient population and setting. Once identified, these indicators, measurement techniques, and reference standards should be identified in policies and procedures or other documents for use in patient/client records, quality or performance improvement, or in formal research projects.

Evaluation

Criteria for evaluation
Comparison to Goal or Reference Standard:
  1) Goal (tailored to patient/client's needs)
     OR
  2) Reference standard

Patient/Client Example(s)

Example(s) of one or two of the Nutrition Care Indicators (includes sample initial and reassessment documentation for one of the indicators)

Indicator(s) selected
Current prescription medication with nutrient/food-medication interactions – Prednisone

Criteria for evaluation
Comparison to Goal or Reference Standard:
  1) Goal: Patient/client with prescription for 50 mg/d prednisone and concerned about concurrent weight gain caused by increased appetite and fluid retention. Goal is to minimize weight gain and maintain good nutritional status during prednisone therapy.
     OR
  2) Reference standard: Not applicable

*** *Denotes indicator is used for nutrition assessment only. Other indicators are used for both nutrition assessment and nutrition monitoring and evaluation.*

Medication and Herbal Supplements (FH-2.1)

Sample nutrition assessment and monitoring and evaluation documentation

Initial nutrition assessment with patient/client	Patient/client prescribed 50 mg/d prednisone for rheumatoid arthritis. Current weight 182 lbs. Long-term therapy may result in a need for protein, calcium, potassium, phosphorus, folate and vitamin A, C and D supplementation. Patient/client currently taking a vitamin/mineral supplement and concerned about weight gain caused by increased appetite and fluid retention.
Reassessment after nutrition intervention	Patient/client prednisone dose reduced to 25 mg/d. Currently taking a one-a-day multivitamin/multimineral and snacking on raw vegetables between meals. Weight stable.

References

The following are some suggested references for indicators, measurement techniques, and reference standards; other references may be appropriate.

1. Charney P, Malone A eds. ADA *Pocket Guide to Nutrition Assessment*. Chicago, IL, The Amercian Dietetic Association; 2004.
2. Position of the American Dietetic Association: Integration of nutrition and pharmacotherapy. *J Am Diet Assoc*. 2003;103:1363-1370.
3. Pronksy ZM. *Food-Medication Interactions Handbook*, 15th ed. Birchrunville, PA: Food-Medication Interactions; 2008.
4. ADA Nutrition Care Manual. 2006. Available at: www.nutritioncaremanual.org. Accessed December 14, 2006.
5. Thomson CA. Practice Paper of the American Dietetic Association: Dietary Supplements. *J Am Diet Assoc*. 2005;105(3):460-470.
6. ADA Evidence Analysis Library. Accessed on: 10/28/2006 from http://www.ada.portalxm.com/eal/category.cfm?cid=5&cat=0
7. U.S. National Library of Medicine, National Institutes of Health, Medline Plus. Accessed on: 12/18/2007 from http://www.nlm.nih.gov/medlineplus/canceralternativetherapies.html
8. National Institutes of Health and the National Center for Complementary and Alternative Medicine. Accessed on: 11/ 29/2007 from http://nccam.nih.gov/health/.

*** Denotes indicator is used for nutrition assessment only. Other indicators are used for both nutrition assessment and nutrition monitoring and evaluation.

Assessment

Food and Nutrition Knowledge (FH-3.1)

Definition
Content areas and level of understanding about food, nutrition and health, or nutrition-related information and guidelines relevant to patient/client needs

Nutrition Assessment and Monitoring and Evaluation
Indicators

> Use the following terms to specify *level of knowledge* by each area of concern:
> - *Inadequate*
> - *Basic* (survival, identify facts, little application)
> - *Moderate* (some application of knowledge in typical situations)
> - *Comprehensive* (synthesize and evaulate knowledge for application in new situations)

Area(s) and level of knowledge
- Breastfeeding (e.g., signs of infant satiety)
  - Consequences of food behavior
  - Disease/condition
  - Goal setting techniques
  - Food label
  - Food products
  - Food/nutrient requirements
  - Health knowledge gap (e.g., understanding of health or health guidance versus true health)
  - Healthcare literacy
  - Laboratory results compared to desirable
  - Level of physical conditioning
  - Nutrition recommendations
  - Physiological functions
  - Self-management parameters
  - Control food portions
  - Food preparation/cooking
  - Manage behavior in response to stimuli (e.g., identify triggers/cues, develop a plan, modify environment or behavior)
  - Plan meals/snacks
  - Select healthful foods/meals
  - Self-monitor
  - Other (specify topic and level of knowledge)
- Diagnosis specific or global nutrition-related knowledge score (specify instrument used e.g., Type 2 Diabetes BASICS Pre/Post Knowledge Test and score)

*** *Denotes indicator is used for nutrition assessment only. Other indicators are used for both nutrition assessment and nutrition monitoring and evaluation.*

Food and Nutrition Knowledge (FH-3.1)

Examples of the measurement methods or data sources for this indicator: Pre- and/or post-tests administered orally, on paper or by computer, scenario discussions, patient/client restates key information, review of food records, practical demonstration/test, survey, nutrition quotient, nutrition questionnaire, nutrition assessment inventory

Typically used to determine and monitor and evaluate change in the following domains of nutrition interventions: Nutrition education, nutrition counseling

Typically used to determine and to monitor and evaluate change in the following nutrition diagnoses: Food- and nutrition-related knowledge deficit, limited adherence to nutrition-related recommendations, undesirable food choices, breastfeeding difficulty, overweight/obesity, intake domain

Clinical judgment must be used to select indicators and determine the appropriate measurement techniques and reference standards for a given patient population and setting. Once identified, these indicators, measurement techniques, and reference standards should be identified in policies and procedures or other documents for use in patient/client records, quality or performance improvement, or in formal research projects.

Evaluation

Criteria for evaluation
Comparison to Goal or Reference Standard:
1) Goal (tailored to individual's needs)
   OR
2) Reference standard

Patient/Client Example(s)

Example(s) of one or two of the Nutrition Care Indicators (includes sample initial and reassessment documentation for one of the indicators)

Indicator(s) selected
Area and level of knowledge (carbohydrate counting)

Criteria for evaluation
Comparison to Goal or Reference Standard:
1) Goal: Patient/client will be able to accurately read a food label and identify the total number of grams of carbohydrate per serving.
   OR
2) Reference standard: No validated standard exists.

*** Denotes indicator is used for nutrition assessment only. Other indicators are used for both nutrition assessment and nutrition monitoring and evaluation.

Edition: 2009

Assessment

Food/Nutrition-Related History Domain – Food and Nutrition Knowledge

Food and Nutrition Knowledge (FH-3.1)

Sample nutrition assessment and monitoring and evaluation documentation

Initial nutrition assessment with patient/client	Patient/client with newly diagnosed diabetes with inadequate knowledge regarding carbohydrate counting.
Reassessment after nutrition intervention	Patient/client with basic knowledge regarding carbohydrate counting. Able to apply knowledge to common scenarios, but not consistently able to apply knowledge to own diet. Will continue to monitor at next encounter in one week.

References

The following are some suggested references for indicators, measurement techniques, and reference standards for the outcome; other references may be appropriate.

1. Bloom B. S. *Taxonomy of Educational Objectives, Handbook I: The Cognitive Domain.* New York: David McKay Co Inc. 1956.
2. Krathwohl, D. R., Bloom, B. S., & Masia, B. B. *Taxonomy of Educational Objectives, the Classification of Educational Goals. Handbook II: Affective Domain.* New York: David McKay Co., Inc. 1973.
3. Snetselaar LG. *Nutrition Counseling Skills for Medical Nutrition Therapy.* Gaithersburg, MD; 1997:133,209.
4. ADA Evidence Analysis Library. Available at: www.adaevidencelibrary.com. Accessed 11/3/2006.
5. Kessler H, Wunderlich SM. Relationship between use of food labels and nutrition knowledge of people with diabetes. *Diabetes Educ.* 1999; 25.
6. Chapman-Novakofski K, Karduck J. Improvement in knowledge, social cognitive theory variables, and movement through stages of change after a community-based diabetes education program. *J Am Diet Assoc.* 2005; 105:1613-1616.
7. International Diabetes Center. *Type 2 Diabetes BASICS Pre/Post Knowledge Test.* 2nd ed. Minneapolis, MN: International Diabetes Center, 2004.
8. Powers MA, Carstensen K, Colon K, Rickheim P, Bergenstal RM. Diabetes BASICS: Education, innovation, revolution. Diabetes Spectrum. 2006;19:90-98.
9. Obayashi S, Bianchi LJ, Song WO. Reliability and validity of nutrition knowledge, social-psychological factors, and food label use scales from the 1995 Diet and Health Knowledge Survey. *J Nutr Educ Behav.* 2003;35:83-92.
10. Kunkel ME, Bell LB, Luccia BHD. Peer Nutrition Education Program To Improve Nutrition Knowledge Of Female Collegiate Athletes. *J Nutr Educ Behav.* 2001; 33:114-115.
11. Shilts MK, Horowitz M, Townsend MS. Goal Setting as a Strategy for Dietary and Physical Activity Behavior Change: A Review of the Literature. *Am J Health Promot.* 2004 Nov-Dec;19(2):81-93
12. ADA Evidence Analysis Library. Available at: http://www.adaevidencelibrary.com/default.cfm?home=1&auth=1. Accessed on: March 14, 2008.
13. Wansink B. Position of the American Dietetic Association: Food and Nutrition Misinformation. *J Am Diet Assoc.*2006;106(4):601-607.
14. Thomson CA. Practice Paper of the American Dietetic Association: Dietary Supplements. *J Am Diet Assoc.* 2005;105(3):460-470.
15. Rothman RL, Malone R, Bryant B, Wolfe C, Padgett P, DeWalt DA, Weinberger M, Pignone M. The spoken knowledge in low literacy in diabetes scale: A diabetes knowledge scale. The Diabetes Educator.2005; 31: 215-224
16. Powell CK, Hill EG, Clancy DE. The relationship between health literacy and diabetes knowledge and readiness to take health actions. *The Diabetes Educator.* 2007;33:144-151.
17. Kay BF, Lund MM, Taylor PN, Herbold NH. Assessment of firefighters' cardiovascular disease-related knowledge and behaviors. *J Am Diet Assoc.* 2001;101(7):807-9.

*** Denotes indicator is used for nutrition assessment only. Other indicators are used for both nutrition assessment and nutrition monitoring and evaluation.

Beliefs and Attitudes (FH-3.2)

Definition
Conviction of the truth of some nutrition-related statement or phenomenon, and feelings or emotions toward that truth or phenomenon, along with a patient's/client's readiness to change food, nutrition, or nutrition-related behaviors

Nutrition Assessment and Monitoring and Evaluation
Indicators

Conflict with personal/family value system (specify)

Distorted body image (yes/no)

End-of-life decisions (specify)

Motivation
- Perceived susceptibility to nutrition-related health problems (e.g., patient/client believes he/she is diabetic or at high-risk for developing diabetes) (yes/no)
- Understanding of severity of risk to health/lifestyle (Perceived severity) (yes/no)
- Belief that benefits of diet change outweigh barriers (benefits are worth the sacrifice and effort) (yes/no)
- Verbalizes desire to change diet and nutrition-related behaviors (yes/no)

Preoccupation with food (yes/no)

Preoccupation with weight (yes/no)

Readiness to change nutrition-related behaviors
- Precontemplation (yes/no)
- Contemplation (yes/no)
- Preparation (yes/no)
- Action (yes/no)
- Maintenance (yes/no)

Self-efficacy
- Breastfeeding self-efficacy (specify, e.g., high, low)
- Eating self-efficacy (specify, e.g., high, low)
- Weight loss self-efficacy (specify, e.g., high, low)
- Other (specify)

Self-talk/cognitions (Documented cognitions related to food/nutrition activity) (positive/negative)

Unrealistic nutrition-related goals (specify, e.g., current weight loss goal of 20 lbs/month is unrealistic)

Unscientific beliefs/attitudes (specify, e.g., specific food with unsubstantiated curative power)

*** Denotes indicator is used for nutrition assessment only. Other indicators are used for both nutrition assessment and nutrition monitoring and evaluation.

Assessment

Beliefs and Attitudes (FH-3.2)

Examples of the measurement methods or data sources for these outcome indicators: Patient/client self-report, patient/client assessment questionnaire or interview, medical record, referring health care provider or agency

Typically used to monitor and evaluate change in the following domains of nutrition interventions: Nutrition education, nutrition counseling

Typically used to determine and to monitor and evaluate change in the following nutrition diagnoses: Harmful beliefs/attitudes about food- or nutrition-related topics; not ready for diet/lifestyle change; inability to manage self-care; self-monitoring deficit, excess or inadequate oral food/beverage, energy, macronutrient, micronutrient or bioactive substance intake; imbalance of nutrients; inappropriate fat foods; inappropriate intake of amino acids; underweight; overweight/obesity; disordered eating pattern; physical inactivity; excess exercise; limited access to food

Clinical judgment must be used to select indicators and determine the appropriate measurement techniques and reference standards for a given patient population and setting. Once identified, these indicators, measurement techniques, and reference standards should be identified in policies and procedures or other documents for use in patient/client records, quality or performance improvement, or in formal research projects.

Evaluation

Criteria for evaluation
Comparison to Goal or Reference Standard:
  1) Goal (tailored to individual's needs)
     OR
  2) Reference standard

Patient/Client Example(s)

Example(s) of one or two of the Nutrition Care Indicators (includes sample initial and reassessment documentation for one of the indicators)

Indicator(s) selected
Readiness to change nutrition-related behaviors

Criteria for evaluation
Comparison to Goal or Reference Standard:
  1) Goal: Patient/client is currently in the precontemplation stage of change. Patient/client goal is to move to the preparation stage of change within 3 months.
     OR
  2) Reference standard: No validated standard exists.

*** *Denotes indicator is used for nutrition assessment only. Other indicators are used for both nutrition assessment and nutrition monitoring and evaluation.*

Beliefs and Attitudes (FH-3.2)

Sample nutrition assessment and monitoring and evaluation documentation

Initial nutrition assessment with patient/client	Assessment results indicate patient/client is currently in the precontemplation stage of change related to need for DASH diet adherence. Will initiate motivational interviewing and reassess in two weeks.
Reassessment after nutrition intervention	Significant progress toward goal. Reassessment indicates that patient/client has moved from the precontemplation stage to the contemplation stage related to need for DASH diet adherence. Will reassess in two weeks.

References

The following are some suggested references for indicators, measurement techniques, and reference standards for the outcome; other references may be appropriate.

1. Glanz K. Current theoretical basis for nutrition intervention and their uses. In Coulston AM, Rock CL, Monsen E. *Nutrition in the Prevention and Treatment of Disease.* San Diego, Ca: Academy Press: 2001:83-93.
2. U.S. Department of Health and Human Services, National Institutes of Health, National Cancer Institute. Theory at a Glance: A Guide for Health Promotion Practice, Spring 2005. Available at: http://www.cancer.gov/PDF/481f5d53-63df-41bc-bfaf-5aa48ee1da4d/TAAG3.pdf, Accessed on February 18, 2008.
3. ADA Evidence Analysis Library. Available at: http://www.adaevidencelibrary.com/topic.cfm?cat=3151. Accessed on: March 14, 2008.
4. Greene GW, Rossi SR. Stages of change for reducing dietary fat intake over 18 months. *J Am Diet Assoc.* 1998; 98:529-534.
5. Krummel DA, Semmens E, Boury J, Gordon PM, Larkin KT. Stages of change for weight management in postpartum women. *J Am Diet Assoc.* 2004; 104(7):1102-1108.
6. Nothwehr F, Snetselaar L, Yang J and Wu H. Stage of Change for Healthful Eating and Use of Behavioral Strategies. *J Am Diet Assoc.* 2006;106: 1035-1041.
7. Jones H, Edwards L, Vallis T, Ruggiero L, Rossi S, Rossi J, Greene G, Prochaska J, Zinman B. Changes in diabetes self-care behaviors make a difference in glycemic control: the Diabetes Stages of Change (DiSC) study. *Diabetes Care.* 2003;26(3):732-7.
8. Clark MM, Abrams DB, Niaura RS. Self-efficacy in weight management. *J Consult Clin Psychol.* 1991;59:739-744.
9. Irwin C, Guyton R. Eating self-efficacy among college students in a behavioral-based weight control program. *Am J Health Studies.* 1997;13:141-151.
10. Kitsantas, A. The role of self-regulation strategies and self-efficacy perceptions in successful weight loss maintenance. *Psychol Health.* 2000;15:811-820.
11. Sutton K, Logue E, Jarjoura D, Baughman K, Smucker W, Capers C. Assessing dietary and exercise stage of change to optimize weight loss interventions. *Obes Res* 2003;11:641-652.
12. Kristal AR, Glanz K, Curry SJ, Patterson RE. How can stages of change be best used in dietary interventions? *J Am Diet Assoc.* 1999; 99: 679-684.
13. Watson K, Baranowski T, Thompson D. Item response modeling: an evaluation of the children's fruit and vegetable self-efficacy questionnaire. *Health Educ Res.* 2006;21 Suppl 1:i47-i57
14. Perri MG, Corsica JA. Improving the maintenance of weight lost in behavioral treatment of obesity. In: Wadden TA, Stunkard AJ (eds). *Handbook of Obesity Treatment.* New York, NY: Guilford Press; 2002:357-379.
15. Miller WR, Rollnick S. *Motivational Interviewing* (2nd ed). New York, NY: Guilford Press; 2002.
16. Dennis C. The breastfeeding self-efficacy scale: psychometric assessment of the short form. *J Obstet Gynecol Neonatal Nurs.* 2003; 32:734-744.

*** Denotes indicator is used for nutrition assessment only. Other indicators are used for both nutrition assessment and nutrition monitoring and evaluation.

Assessment

Food/Nutrition-Related History Domain – Behavior

Adherence (FH-4.1)

Definition
Level of compliance or adherence with nutrition-related recommendations or behavioral changes agreed upon by patient/client to achieve nutrition-related goals

Nutrition Assessment and Monitoring and Evaluation
Indicators

Self-reported adherence score (Rated on scale of 1 to 10, 1 = Not adherent, 10 = Completely adherent)

Nutrition visit attendance (ratio number attended/total)

Ability to recall nutrition goals (full, partial, none)

Self-monitoring at agreed upon rate (Rated on scale of 1 to 10, 1 = Not adherent, 10 = Completely adherent)

Self-management based upon details agreed upon (within the nutrition plan) (Rated on scale of 1 to 10, 1 = Not adherent, 10 = Completely adherent)

Note: Use in conjunction with appropriate Food and Nutrition Intake, Anthropometric Data and Biochemical Data reference sheets.
May be useful in relapse prevention treatment (analyze and control factors that caused the lapse).

Examples of the measurement methods or data sources for these indicators: Nutrition visit attendance, self-monitoring records (e.g., to evaluate fat, sodium, calories, diet quality), patient/client self-report, adherence tools or questionnaires, provider assessment

Typically used with the following domains of nutrition interventions: Food and/or nutrient delivery, nutrition education, nutrition counseling

Typically used to determine and to monitor and evaluate change in the following nutrition diagnosis: Limited adherence to nutrition-related recommendations

Clinical judgment must be used to select indicators and determine the appropriate measurement techniques and reference standards for a given patient population and setting. Once identified, these indicators, measurement techniques, and reference standards should be identified in policies and procedures or other documents for use in patient/client records, quality or performance improvement, or in formal research projects.

Evaluation

Criteria for evaluation
Comparison to Goal or Reference Standard:
1) Goal (tailored to individual's needs)
   OR
2) Reference standard

*** Denotes indicator is used for nutrition assessment only. Other indicators are used for both nutrition assessment and nutrition monitoring and evaluation.*

Adherence (FH-4.1)

Patient/Client Example(s)

Example(s) of one or two of the Nutrition Care Indicators (includes sample initial and reassessment documentation for one of the indicators)

Indicator(s) selected

Self-reported adherence score

Criteria for evaluation

Comparison to Goal or Reference Standard:

1) Goal: Patient/client rates herself a 4 on a scale of 1 to 10 (1 = Not adherent, 10 = Completely adherent) on her level of adherence to nutrition-related goals. Patient/client desires to move to a rating of 8.

   OR

2) Reference standard: No validated standard exists.

Sample nutrition assessment monitoring and evaluation documentation

Initial nutrition assessment with patient/client	Patient/client rates herself a 1 on a scale of 1-10 on her ability to adhere to her meal plan. Patient/client set a goal to adhere to her meal plan 5 days per week. Will evaluate adherence at the next encounter.
Reassessment after nutrition intervention	Some progress toward goal. Patient/client rated herself a 6 on a scale of 1-10 on her ability to meet her adherence goal of following her meal plan 5 days per week. Is doing well on weekdays, but states she must improve on weekends. Discussed ways to improve adherence to meal plan on the weekends. Will monitor at next encounter in two weeks.

References

The following are some suggested references for indicators, measurement techniques, and reference standards for the outcome; other references may be appropriate.

1. Bosworth H, Oddone EZ, Weinberger M. (eds). *Patient Treatment Adherence: Concepts, Interventions, and Measurement*. Psychology Press, 2005.

2. Haynes RB. Improving patient adherence: State of the art, with a special focus on medication taking for cardiovascular disorders. In: Burke LE, Ockene IS (eds). *Compliance in Healthcare and Research*. Armonk, NY: Futura Publishing Company, Inc.; 2001:3-21.

3. Milas N, Nowalk MP, Akpele L, Castoldo L, Coyne T, Doroshenko L, Kigawa L, Korzec-Ramirez D, Scherch LK, Snetselaar L. Factors Associated with Adherence to the Dietary Protein Intervention in the Modification of Diet in Renal Disease Study. *J Am Diet Assoc*. 1995; 95:1295-1300.

4. Snetselaar LG. *Nutrition Counseling Skills for Medical Nutrition Therapy*, 2nd ed. Gaithersburg, MD: Aspen Press; 2007.

5. Schlundt DG, Rea MR, Kline SS, Pichert JW. Situational obstacles to dietary adherence for adults with diabetes. *J Am Diet Assoc*. 1994;94:874-876.

6. DiMatteo MR, Giordani PJ, Lepper HS, Croghan TW. Patient adherence and medical treatment outcomes: a meta-analysis. *Med Care*. 2002;40:794-811.

*** *Denotes indicator is used for nutrition assessment only. Other indicators are used for both nutrition assessment and nutrition monitoring and evaluation.*

Assessment

Food/Nutrition-Related History Domain – Behavior

Adherence (FH-4.1)

References, cont'd

7. Rushe H, McGee HM. Assessing adherence to dietary recommendations for hemodialysis patients: the Renal Adherence Attitudes Questionnaire (RAAQ) and the Renal Adherence Behaviour Questionnaire (RABQ). *J Psychosom Res*. 1998;45:149-157.

8. Sharma S, Murphy SP, Wilkens LR, Shen L, Hankin JH, Henderson B, Kolonel LN. Adherence to the Food Guide Pyramid recommendations among Japanese Americans, Native Hawaiians, and whites: Results from the Multiethnic Cohort Study. *J Am Diet Assoc*. 2003;103:1195-1198.

9. Tinker LF, Perri MG, Patterson RE, Bowen DJ, McIntosh M, Parker LM, Sevick MA, Wodarski LA. The effects of physical and emotional status on adherence to a low-fat dietary pattern in the Women's Health Initiative. *J Am Diet Assoc*. 2002;102:789-800.

*** *Denotes indicator is used for nutrition assessment only. Other indicators are used for both nutrition assessment and nutrition monitoring and evaluation.*

Avoidance Behavior (FH-4.2)

Definition

Keeping away from something or someone to postpone an outcome or perceived consequence

Nutrition Assessment and Monitoring and Evaluation

Indicators

Avoidance

- Specific foods (specify, e.g., grapefruit, seeds)
- Food groups (specify, e.g., milk/milk products)
- Fluids (specify)
- Textures (specify)
- Social situations (specify)
- Other (specify)

Restrictive eating (yes/no)

Cause of avoidance behavior *** (e.g., personal choice, prescribed dietary restriction, GI distress, suspected allergy, eating disorder, cancer treatment side effects, medications, mental illness, Parkinson's disease)

Examples of the measurement methods or data sources for these indicators: Self-monitoring records, patient/client interview

Typically used with the following domains of nutrition interventions: Nutrition counseling

Typically used to determine and to monitor and evaluate change in the following nutrition diagnoses: Disordered eating pattern, overweight/obesity, underweight, GI disorders

Clinical judgment must be used to select indicators and determine the appropriate measurement techniques and reference standards for a given patient population and setting. Once identified, these indicators, measurement techniques, and reference standards should be identified in policies and procedures or other documents for use in patient/client records, quality or performance improvement, or in formal research projects.

*** *Denotes indicator is used for nutrition assessment only. Other indicators are used for both nutrition assessment and nutrition monitoring and evaluation.*

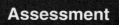

Assessment

Food/Nutrition-Related History Domain – Behavior

Avoidance Behavior (FH-4.2)

Evaluation

Criteria for evaluation
Comparison to Goal or Reference Standard:
    1) Goal (tailored to patient/client needs)
       OR
    2) Reference standard

Patient/Client Example(s)
Example(s) of one or two of the Nutrition Care Indicators (includes sample initial and reassessment documentation for one of the indicators)

Indicator(s) selected
Avoidance of social situations

Criteria for evaluation
Comparison to Goal or Reference Standard:
    1) Goal: Patient/client avoiding social situations in an effort to avoid overeating. Goal is to learn strategies to control eating in social situations.
       OR
    2) Reference standard: No validated standard exists

Sample nutrition assessment and monitoring and evaluation documentation

Initial nutrition assessment with patient/client	Patient/client avoids social situations because she is afraid she will overeat. Reviewed client's food diary and client brainstormed strategies which may help her control eating in social situations. Patient/client will preplan food intake on days she has social engagements, will have a piece of fruit before going to help curb her appetite and will maintain a food diary.
Reassessment after nutrition intervention	Patient/client made some progress toward goal. Attended 2 of 4 social engagements where food was served, and successfully controlled food intake both times. Patient/client will continue to use strategies. Will reevaluate avoidance behavior at next encounter.

*** *Denotes indicator is used for nutrition assessment only. Other indicators are used for both nutrition assessment and nutrition monitoring and evaluation.*

Avoidance Behavior (FH-4.2)

References

The following are some suggested references for indicators, measurement techniques, and reference standards for the outcome; other references may be appropriate.

1. Susan H. Barriers to effective nutritional care for older adults. *Nursing Standard* [serial online]. 2006;21:50-4.

2. Susan H. Nutrition matters for older adults. *Journal of Community Nursing* [serial online]. February 2006;20:24,26,28-30.

3. Zutavern A, Brockow I, Schaaf B, Bolte G, von Berg A, Diez U, Borte M, Herbarth O, Wichmann HE, Heinrich J, LISA Study Group. Timing of solid food introduction in relation to atopic dermatitis and atopic sensitization: Results from a prospective birth cohort study. *Pediatrics* [serial online]. 2006;117:401-411.

4. Ogden J, Karim L, Choudry A, Brown K. Understanding successful behaviour change: the role of intentions, attitudes to the target and motivations and the example of diet. *Health Education Research* [serial online]. 2007;22:397-405.

5. Watson L, Leslie W, Hankey C. Under-nutrition in old age: diagnosis and management. *Reviews in Clinical Gerontology* [serial online]. 2006;16:23-34.

6. Brisbois TD, Hutton JL, Baracos VE, Wismer WV. Taste and smell abnormalities as an independent cause of failure of food intake in patients With advanced cancer-an argument for the application of sensory science. *Journal of Palliative Care* [serial online]. 2006;22:111-4.

7. Cassens, Digna, Johnson, Elenore, Keelan, Stephanie. Enhancing taste, texture, appearance, and presentation of pureed food improved resident quality of life and weight status. *Nutrition Reviews* [serial online]. 1996;54:S51. 2.

8. Reed PS, Zimmerman S, Sloane PD, Williams CS, Boustani M. Characteristics associated with low food and fluid intake in long-term care residents with dementia. *The Gerontologist.* [serial online]. 2005;45:74-80.

9. Joo SH, Wood RA. The impact of childhood food allergy on quality of life. *Pediatrics: Synopsis Book: Best Articles Relevant to Pediatric Allergy* [serial online]. 2003;112:459. 2.

10. Fält B; Granérus A; Unosson M. Avoidance of solid food in weight losing older patients with Parkinson's disease. *Journal of Clinical Nursing.* 2006 Nov; 15 (11):1404-12.

11. Nowak-Wegrzyn A; Sampson HA. Adverse reactions to foods. *Medical Clinics of North America.* 2006 Jan; 90 (1):97-127.

12. Meyer C; Serpell L; Waller G; Murphy F; Treasure J; Leung N. Cognitive avoidance in the strategic processing of ego threats among eating-disordered patients. *International Journal of Eating Disorders.* 2005 Jul; 38 (1):30-6.

13. Talley NJ. Irritable bowel syndrome. *Gastroenterology Clinics of North America.* 2005 Jun; 34 (2): xi-xii, 173-354

14. Sverker A; Hensing G; Hallert C. Controlled by food— lived experiences of coeliac disease. *Journal of Human Nutrition & Dietetics.* 2005 Jun; 18 (3): 171-80

15. Smith CM; Kagan SH. Prevention of systemic mycoses by reducing exposure to fungal pathogens in hospitalized and ambulatory neutropenic patients. *Oncology Nursing Forum.* 2005 May; 32 (3): 565-79.

16. Millson DS; Tepper SJ. Migraine treatment. Headache. *Journal of Head & Face Pain.* 2004 Nov-Dec; 44 (10): 1059-61.

17. Brown AC; Hairfield M; Richards DG; McMillin DL; Mein EA; Nelson CD. Medical nutrition therapy as a potential complementary treatment for psoriasis—five case reports. *Alternative Medicine Review.* 2004 Sep; 9 (3): 297-307.

18. Biddle J; Anderson J. Report on a 12-month trial of food exclusion methods in a primary care setting. *Journal of Nutritional & Environmental Medicine.* 2002 Mar; 12 (1): 11-17.

*** *Denotes indicator is used for nutrition assessment only. Other indicators are used for both nutrition assessment and nutrition monitoring and evaluation.*

Assessment

Food/Nutrition-Related History Domain – Behavior

Bingeing and Purging Behavior (FH-4.3)

Definition
Eating a larger amount of food than normal for the individual during a short period of time (within any two-hour period) accompanied by a lack of control over eating during the binge episode (i.e., the feeling that one cannot stop eating). This may be followed by compensatory behavior to make up for the excessive eating, referred to as purging.

Nutrition Assessment and Monitoring and Evaluation
Indicators

Binge eating behavior (present/absent)
- Number of binge episodes (e.g., number/day, number/ week, number/month)

Purging behavior (present/absent)
- Self-induced vomiting (number/day, number/week, number/month)
- Fasting (yes/no)
- Other (specify)

Note: Misuse of laxatives, diuretics or other drugs is found on the Medication and Herbal Supplements reference sheet.

Amount and type of physical activity is found on the Physical Activity reference sheet.

Examples of the measurement methods or data sources for these indicators: Patient/client interview, medical record, referring health care provider or agency, self-monitoring records

Typically used with following domains of nutrition interventions: Nutrition counseling

Typically used to determine and to monitor and evaluate change in the following nutrition diagnoses: Excessive oral food/beverage intake, disordered eating pattern, overweight/obesity

Clinical judgment must be used to select indicators and determine the appropriate measurement techniques and reference standards for a given patient population and setting. Once identified, these indicators, measurement techniques, and reference standards should be identified in policies and procedures or other documents for use in patient/client records, quality or performance improvement, or in formal research projects.

*** Denotes indicator is used for nutrition assessment only. Other indicators are used for both nutrition assessment and nutrition monitoring and evaluation.*

Bingeing and Purging Behavior (FH-4.3)

Evaluation

Criteria for evaluation

Comparison to Goal or Reference Standard:
1) Goal (tailored to patient/client needs)
   OR
2) Reference standard

Patient/Client Example(s)

Example(s) of one or two of the Nutrition Care Indicators (includes sample initial and reassessment documentation for one of the indicators)

Indicator(s) selected

Number of binge episodes

Criteria for evaluation

Comparison to Goal or Reference Standard:
1) Goal: Patient/client reports 3 binge eating episodes per week. Goal is to reduce binge eating to one episode per week.
   OR
2) Reference standard: No validated standard exists.

Sample nutrition assessment and monitoring and evaluation documentation

Initial encounter with patient/client	Patient/client reports 3 binge-eating episodes this week.
Reassessment after nutrition intervention	Some progress toward goal. Patient/client reported 2 binge eating episodes this week. Will continue to monitor at next encounter.

References

The following are some suggested references for indicators, measurement techniques, and reference standards for the outcome; other references may be appropriate.

1. Fairburn CG. Wilson GT. *Binge Eating:Nature, Assessment and Treatment*. Guillford Press, New York, 1993.
2. Snetselaar LG. *Nutrition Counseling Skills for Medical Nutrition Therapy*, 2nd ed. Gaithersburg, MD: Aspen Press; 2007.
3. Kellogg M. *Counseling Tips for Nutrition Therapists: Practice Workbook*. Philadelphia, PA: Kg Press; 2006.
4. Wonderlich SA, de Zwaan M, Mitchell JE, Peterson C, Crow S. Psychological and dietary treatments of binge eating disorder: conceptual implications. *Int J Eat Disord*. 2003;34 Suppl:S58-73.
5. Telch CF, Agras WS, Linehan MM. Dialectical behavior therapy for binge eating disorder. *J Consult Clin Psychol*. 2001 Dec;69(6):1061-5.
6. Safer DL, Lively TJ, Telch CF, Agras WS. Predictors of relapse following successful dialectical behavior therapy for binge eating disorder. *Int J Eat Disord*. 2002 Sep;32(2):155-63.

*** Denotes indicator is used for nutrition assessment only. Other indicators are used for both nutrition assessment and nutrition monitoring and evaluation.

Edition: 2009

Assessment

Bingeing and Purging Behavior (FH-4.3)

References, cont'd

7. Devlin MJ, Goldfein JA, Petkova E, Liu L, Walsh BT. Cognitive behavioral therapy and fluoxetine for binge eating disorder: two-year follow-up. *Obesity.* 2007;15(7):1702-9.

8. Peterson CB, Mitchell JE, Engbloom S, Nugent S, Mussell MP, Miller JP. Group cognitive-behavioral treatment of binge eating disorder: a comparison of therapist-led versus self-help formats. *Int J Eat Disord.* 1998 Sep;24(2):125-36.

9. Gorin AA, Le Grange D, Stone AA. Effectiveness of spouse involvement in cognitive behavioral therapy for binge eating disorder. *Int J Eat Disord.* 2003 May;33(4):421-33.

10. Ljotsson B, Lundin C, Mitsell K, Carlbring P, Ramklint M, Ghaderi A. Remote treatment of bulimia nervosa and binge eating disorder: a randomized trial of Internet-assisted cognitive behavioural therapy. *Behav Res Ther.* 2007;45(4):649-61. Epub 2006.

11. Celio AA, Wilfley DE, Crow SJ, Mitchell J, Walsh BT. A comparison of the binge eating scale, questionnaire of eating and weight patterns-revised, and eating disorder examination with instructions with the eating disorder examination in the assessment of binge eating disorder and its symptoms. *Int J Eat Disord.* 2004;36:434-444.

12. Henry BW, Ozier AD. Position of the American Dietetic Association: Nutrition Intervention in the Treatment of Anorexia Nervosa, Bulimia Nervosa, and Other Eating Disorders. *J Am Diet Assoc.* 2006;106(12):2073-2082.

*** *Denotes indicator is used for nutrition assessment only. Other indicators are used for both nutrition assessment and nutrition monitoring and evaluation.*

Mealtime Behavior (FH-4.4)

Definition
Manner of acting, participating or behaving at mealtime which influences patient/client's food and beverage intake

Nutrition Assessment and Monitoring and Evaluation
Indicators

Meal duration (minutes)

Percent of meal time spent eating (percent)

Preference to drink rather than eat (yes/no)

Refusal to eat/chew (specify, e.g., meal, food type)

Spitting food out (specify, e.g., food type, frequency)

Rumination (yes/no)

Patient/client/caregiver fatigue during feeding process, resulting in inadequate intake (yes/no)

Willingness to try new foods (yes/no)

Limited number of accepted foods (specify)

Rigid sensory preferences (flavor, temperature, texture)

Examples of the measurement methods or data sources for these indicators: Observation, medical record, referring health care provider or agency, caregiver observation, patient/client interview

Typically used with following domains of nutrition interventions: Food and/or nutrient delivery, coordination of nutrition care

Typically used to determine and to monitor and evaluate change in the following nutrition diagnoses: Self-feeding difficulty, inadequate and excessive oral food/beverage intake

Clinical judgment must be used to select indicators and determine the appropriate measurement techniques and reference standards for a given patient population and setting. Once identified, these indicators, measurement techniques, and reference standards should be identified in policies and procedures or other documents for use in patient/client records, quality or performance improvement, or in formal research projects.

Evaluation

Criteria for evaluation
Comparison to Goal or Reference Standard:
  1) Goal (tailored to patient/client needs)
     OR
  2) Reference standard

*** *Denotes indicator is used for nutrition assessment only. Other indicators are used for both nutrition assessment and nutrition monitoring and evaluation.*

Assessment

Mealtime Behavior (FH-4.4)

Patient/Client Example(s)

Example(s) of one or two of the Nutrition Care Indicators (includes sample initial and reassessment documentation for one of the indicators)

Indicator(s) selected

Percent of meal spent eating (percentage)

Criteria for evaluation

Comparison to Goal or Reference Standard:

1) Goal: Four-year-old patient/client with inadequate food/beverage intake. Lunch meal observation revealed less than 10% of mealtime was spent eating. Goal is to reduce environmental distractions and increase percent of meal spent eating to 55%.

   OR

2) Reference standard: No validated standard exists

Sample nutrition assessment and monitoring and evaluation documentation

Initial nutrition assessment with patient/client	Lunch meal observation revealed that patient/client is highly distracted and spends less than 10% of the mealtime eating.
Reassessment after nutrition intervention	Significant progress toward goal. Environmental distractions were minimized and caregiver eats meals with patient/client. Observation reveals that approximately 40% of mealtime is spent eating. Will monitor at next encounter.

References

The following are some suggested references for indicators, measurement techniques, and reference standards; other references may be appropriate.

1. Powers SW, Patton SR, Byars KC, Mitchell MJ, Jelalian E, Mulvihill MM, Hovell MF, Stark LJ. Caloric intake and eating behavior in infants and toddlers with cystic fibrosis. *Diabetes Care.* 2002;109(5):e75

2. Wardle J, Guthrie CA, Sanderson, S, Rapoport, L. Development of the Children's Eating Behaviour Questionnaire. 2001. *J Child Psychol Psychiat.* 42(7): 963-970.

3. Chial HJ, Camilleri M, Williams DE, Litzinger K, Perrault J. Rumination Syndrome in Children and Adolescents: Diagnosis, Treatment and Prognosis. *Pediatrics.* 2003; 111:158-162.

4. Fung EB, Samson-Fang L, Stallings VA, Conaway M, Liptak G, Henderson RC, Worley G, O'Donnell, M, Calvert B, Rosenbaum P, Chumlea W, Stevenson RD. Feeding dysfunction is associated with poor growth and health status in children with cerebral palsy. *J Am Diet Assoc.* 2002; 102:361-368,373.

5. Lucas B, Pechstein S, Ogata B. Nutrition concerns of children with autism spectrum disorders. *Nutrition Focus.* 2002;17:1-8, Jan-Feb issue.

6. Adams RA, Gordon C, Spangler AA. Maternal stress in caring for children with feeding disabilities: Implications for health care providers. *J Am Diet Assoc.* 1999;99:962-966.

7. Ramsay M, Gisel EG, Boutry M. Non-Organic Failure to Thrive: Growth Failure Secondary to Feeding-Skills Disorder. *Developmental Medicine and Child Neurology.* 1993;35:285-297.

*** *Denotes indicator is used for nutrition assessment only. Other indicators are used for both nutrition assessment and nutrition monitoring and evaluation.*

Social Network (FH-4.5)

Definition
Ability to build and utilize a network of family, friends, colleagues, health professionals, and community resources for encouragement, emotional support and to enhance one's environment to support behavior change

Nutrition Assessment and Monitoring and Evaluation
Indicators

Ability to build and utilize social networks (e.g., may include perceived social support, social integration, and assertiveness)

Examples of the measurement methods used or data sources for these indicators: Self-monitoring records, client/patient self-report, goal tracking tools

Typically used with the following domains of nutrition interventions: Nutrition counseling

Typically used to determine and to monitor and evaluate change in the following nutrition diagnoses: Intake domain, underweight, overweight/obesity, disordered eating pattern, undesirable food choices, inability or lack of desire to manage self-care, breastfeeding difficulty, not ready for diet/lifestyle change, limited adherence to nutrition-related recommendations

Clinical judgment must be used to select indicators and determine the appropriate measurement techniques and reference standards for a given patient population and setting. Once identified, these indicators, measurement techniques, and reference standards should be identified in policies and procedures or other documents for use in patient/client records, quality or performance improvement, or in formal research projects.

Evaluation

Criteria for evaluation
Comparison to Goal or Reference Standard:
1) Goal (tailored to individual's needs)
    OR
2) Reference standard

Patient/Client Example

Example(s) of one or two of the Nutrition Care Indicators (includes sample initial and reassessment documentation for one of the indicators)

Indicator(s) selected
Ability to build and utilize social support (e.g., may include perceived social support, social integration, and assertiveness)

*** *Denotes indicator is used for nutrition assessment only. Other indicators are used for both nutrition assessment and nutrition monitoring and evaluation.*

Assessment

Food/Nutrition-Related History Domain – Behavior

Social Network (FH-4.5)

Criteria for evaluation

Comparison to Goal or Reference Standard:

1) Goal: Overweight patient/client's wife adds fat to all foods prepared at home. Goal is to reduce the amount of fat in meals prepared at home by asking wife to not dress the salad or add fat seasoning to vegetables before serving.

   OR

2) Reference standard: No validated standard exists.

Sample nutrition assessment and monitoring and evaluation documentation

Initial encounter with patient/client	Patient/client states that he rarely verbalizes his nutrition-related desires/needs in family or social situations and rates his ability to elicit social support a 3 on a scale of 1 to 10. Will evaluate at the next encounter.
Reassessment at a later date	Some progress toward goal. Patient/client rated himself a 5, on a scale of 1-10, on his ability to elicit social support. Has begun to verbalize his needs and plans to research restaurants that meet his needs that others will enjoy. Will monitor at next encounter in two weeks.

References

The following are some suggested references for indicators, measurement techniques, and reference standards for the outcome; other references may be appropriate.

1. Barrera M, Toobert D, Angell K, Glasgow R, Mackinnon D. Social support and social-ecological resources as mediators of lifestyle intervention effects for type 2 diabetes. *J Health Psychol.* 2006;11:483-495.

2. Sherbourne CD, Stewart AI. The MOS Social Support Survey. *Social Sci Med.* 1991;32:706-714.

3. Barrera M Jr, Glasgow RE, McKay HG, Boles SM, Feil E. Do internet-based support interventions change perceptions of social support?: an experimental trial of approaches for supporting diabetes self-management. *Am J Comm Psychol.* 2002; 30:637-654.

4. LaGreca AM, Bearman KJ. The diabetes social support questionnaire-family version: evaluating adolescents' diabetes-specific support from family members. *J Pediatr Psychol.* 2002;27:665-676.

5. Glasgow RE, Strycker LA, Toobert DJ, Eakin E. A social-ecologic approach to assessing support for disease self-management: the Chronic Illness Resources Survey. *J Behav Med.* 2000;23:559-583.

*** *Denotes indicator is used for nutrition assessment only. Other indicators are used for both nutrition assessment and nutrition monitoring and evaluation.*

Food/Nutrition Program Participation (FH-5.1)

Definition
Patient/client eligibility for and participation in food assistance programs

Nutrition Assessment and Monitoring and Evaluation
Indicators

Eligibility for government programs (specify, e.g., qualification for federal programs, such as, WIC, Food Stamp Program [refer to state for title of program], School Breakfast/Lunch program, Food Distribution Program on Indian Reservations; state assistance programs, such as, emergency food assistance programs)

Participation in government programs (specify patient/client or family/caregiver influence)

Eligibility for community programs (specify, e.g., qualification for community programs such as food pantries, meal sites, and meal delivery programs)

Participation in community programs (specify patient/client or family/caregiver influence)

Examples of the measurement methods or data sources for these indicators: Patient/client report of eligibility/participation, referral information, home evaluation

Typically used with the following domains of nutrition interventions: Nutrition education, nutrition counseling, coordination of nutrition care

Typically used to determine and to monitor and evaluate change in the following nutrition diagnoses: Limited access to food, inadequate or excessive energy intake

Clinical judgment must be used to select indicators and determine the appropriate measurement techniques and reference standards for a given patient population and setting. Once identified, these indicators, measurement techniques, and reference standards should be identified in policies and procedures or other documents for use in patient/client records, quality or performance improvement, or in formal research projects.

Evaluation

Criteria for evaluation
Comparison to Goal or Reference Standard:
1) Goal (tailored to patient/client needs)
   OR
2) Reference standard

*** *Denotes indicator is used for nutrition assessment only. Other indicators are used for both nutrition assessment and nutrition monitoring and evaluation.*

Assessment

Food/Nutrition-Related History Domain – Factors Affecting Access to Food and/or Food and Nutrition-Related Supplies

Food/Nutrition Program Participation (FH-5.1)

Patient/Client Example(s)
Example(s) of one or two of the Nutrition Care Indicators (includes sample initial and reassessment documentation for one of the indicators)

Indicator(s) selected
Participation in government programs

Criteria for evaluation
Comparison to Goal or Reference Standard:
1) Goal: Patient/client is not participating in federal School Lunch Program as parent has not completed required forms.
   OR
2) Reference standard: No validated standard exists.

Sample nutrition assessment and monitoring and evaluation documentation

Initial nutrition assessment with patient/client	The patient/client not participating in federal School Lunch Program as the required forms are not complete. Will follow-up with family/guardian and monitor change in school lunch program participation at next appointment.
Reassessment after nutrition intervention	Progress toward goal as patient/client's family/guardian has completed School Lunch Program forms.

References
The following are some suggested references for indicators, measurement techniques, and reference standard; other references may be appropriate.

1. Department of Health and Human Services (HHS) Poverty Guidelines, 2006. Available at: http://aspe.hhs.gov/poverty/06poverty.shtml. Accessed November 14, 2006.
2. Dietary Guidelines for Americans, 2005. Available at: http://www.health.gov/dietaryguidelines/dga2005/document/html/executivesummary.htm. Accessed October 25, 2006.
3. Holben DH. Incorporation of food security learning activities into dietetics curricula. *Top Clin Nutr.* 2005;20:339-350.
4. Holben DH, Myles W. Food Insecurity in the United States: How It Affects Our Patients. *Am Fam Physician.* 2004;69;1058-1063.
5. Position of the American Dietetic Association on Food Insecurity and Hunger in the United States. *J Am Diet Assoc.* 2006;106:446-458.
6. U.S. Department of Agriculture, Economic Research Service. Food security in the United States. Available at: http://www.ers.usda.gov/Briefing/FoodSecurity/. Accessed February 28, 2007.

*** *Denotes indicator is used for nutrition assessment only. Other indicators are used for both nutrition assessment and nutrition monitoring and evaluation.*

Edition: 2009

Safe Food/Meal Availability (FH-5.2)

Definition
Availability of enough healthful, safe food

Nutrition Assessment and Monitoring and Evaluation
Indicators

Availability of shopping facilities (specify, e.g., access to facilities with a wide variety of healthful food choices)

Procurement, identification of safe food (specify, e.g., financial resources for obtaining food, identification of spoilage, expiration dates, community gardens, growing own food, hunting, and fishing, identification of foods containing poisons such as specific berries, mushrooms, etc)

Appropriate meal preparation facilities (specify, e.g., access to cooking apparatus and supplies used in preparation, sanitary conditions and supplies for meal preparation, appropriate temperatures of hot/cold food)

Availability of safe food storage (specify, e.g., refrigerator/freezer, dry storage, designated containers)

Appropriate storage techniques (specify, e.g., appropriate refrigeration/freezer temperatures, canning/preservation, length of storage, sanitary conditions)

Examples of the measurement methods or data sources for these indicators: Patient/client report overall food availability/food consumed during the week, referral information, home evaluation

Typically used with the following domains of nutrition interventions: Nutrition education, nutrition counseling, coordination of nutrition care

Typically used to determine and to monitor and evaluate change in the following nutrition diagnoses: Limited access to food, intake of unsafe food, inadequate or excessive energy intake

Clinical judgment must be used to select indicators and determine the appropriate measurement techniques and reference standards for a given patient population and setting. Once identified, these indicators, measurement techniques, and reference standards should be identified in policies and procedures or other documents for use in patient/client records, quality or performance improvement, or in formal research projects.

Evaluation

Criteria for evaluation
Comparison to Goal or Reference Standard:
1) Goal (tailored to patient/client needs)
   OR
2) Reference standard

*** *Denotes indicator is used for nutrition assessment only. Other indicators are used for both nutrition assessment and nutrition monitoring and evaluation.*

Assessment

Food/Nutrition-Related History Domain – Factors Affecting Access to Food and/or Food and Nutrition-Related Supplies

Safe Food/Meal Availability (FH-5.2)

Patient/Client Example(s)

Example(s) of one or two of the Nutrition Care Indicators (includes sample initial and reassessment documentation for one of the indicators)

Indicator(s) selected

Availability of meal preparation facilities

Criteria for evaluation

Comparison to Goal or Reference Standard:
1. Goal: Patient/client has no access to meal preparation facilities when extensive access to meal preparation facilities is the goal.
    OR
2. Reference standard: No validated standard exists.

Sample nutrition assessment and monitoring and evaluation documentation

Initial nutrition assessment with patient/client	The patient/client has no access to meal preparation facilities. Will monitor change in access at next appointment after coordination of nutrition care with social work.
Reassessment after nutrition intervention	Substantial progress toward goal as patient/client has consistent access to meal preparation facility with repair of stove.

References

The following are some suggested references for indicators, measurement techniques, and reference standard; other references may be appropriate.

1. Bickel, G., M. Nord, C. Price, W.L. Hamilton, and J.T. Cook. 2000. Guide to Measuring Household Food Security, Revised 2000. USDA, Food and Nutrition Service. Available at: www.fns.usda.gov/fsec/fi les/fsguide.pdf. Accessed February 26, 2008.
2. Department of Health and Human Services (HHS) Poverty Guidelines, 2006. Available at: http://aspe.hhs.gov/poverty/06poverty.shtml. Accessed November 14, 2006.
3. Dietary Guidelines for Americans, 2005. Available at: http://www.health.gov/dietaryguidelines/dga2005/document/html/executivesummary.htm. Accessed October 25, 2006.
4. Granger LE, Holben DH. Self-identified food security knowledge and practices of family physicians in Ohio. *Top Clin Nutr*. 2004;19:280-285.
5. Holben DH. Incorporation of food security learning activities into dietetics curricula. *Top Clin Nutr*. 2005;20:339-350.
6. Holben DH, Myles W. Food Insecurity in the United States: How It Affects Our Patients. *Am Fam Physician*. 2004;69;1058-1063.
7. Partnership for Food Safety Education. Available at: http://www.fightbac.org. Accessed October 19, 2006.
8. Position of the American Dietetic Association on Food Insecurity and Hunger in the United States. *J Am Diet Assoc*. 2006;106:446-458.
9. Position of the American Dietetic Association: Addressing world hunger, malnutrition, and food insecurity. *J Am Diet Assoc*. 2003;103:1046-1057.
10. Position of the American Dietetic Association: Food and water safety. *J Am Diet Assoc*. 2003;103:1203-1218.
11. Tscholl E, Holben DH. Knowledge and Practices of Ohio Nurse Practitioners and Its Relationship to Food Access of Patients. *J Am Acad Nusr Pract*. 2006;18:335-342.
12. U.S. Department of Agriculture, Economic Research Service. Food security in the United States. Available at: http://www.ers.usda.gov/Briefing/FoodSecurity/. Accessed February 28, 2007.
13. U.S. Environmental Protection Agency, Ground Water and Drinking Water Frequently Asked Questions. Available at: http://www.epa.gov/safewater/faq/faq.html#safe. Accessed November 14, 2006.

*** *Denotes indicator is used for nutrition assessment only. Other indicators are used for both nutrition assessment and nutrition monitoring and evaluation.*

Safe Water Availablity (FH-5.3)

Definition
Availability of potable water

Nutrition Assessment and Monitoring and Evaluation
Indicators
Availability of potable water (specify, e.g., functioning well, access to treated public water supply)

Appropriate water decontamination (specify, e.g., awareness of and compliance with public health warnings, use of strategies such as boiling, chemical, filtration treatment)

Examples of the measurement methods or data sources for these indicators: Patient/client report of water availability and/or decontamination strategies, referral information, home evaluation

Typically used with the following domains of nutrition interventions: Nutrition education, nutrition counseling, coordination of nutrition care

Typically used to determine and to monitor and evaluate change in the following nutrition diagnoses: Insufficient fluid intake, intake of unsafe food

Clinical judgment must be used to select indicators and determine the appropriate measurement techniques and reference standards for a given patient population and setting. Once identified, these indicators, measurement techniques, and reference standards should be identified in policies and procedures or other documents for use in patient/client records, quality or performance improvement, or in formal research projects.

Evaluation

Criteria for evaluation
Comparison to Goal or Reference Standard:
1) Goal (tailored to patient/client needs)
   OR
2) Reference standard

*** *Denotes indicator is used for nutrition assessment only. Other indicators are used for both nutrition assessment and nutrition monitoring and evaluation.*

Assessment

Food/Nutrition-Related History Domain – Factors Affecting Access to Food and/or Food and Nutrition-Related Supplies

Safe Water Availability (FH-5.3)

Patient/Client Example(s)

Example(s) of one or two of the Nutrition Care Indicators (includes sample initial and reassessment documentation for one of the indicators)

Indicator(s) selected

Appropriate water decontamination

Criteria for evaluation

Comparison to Goal or Reference Standard:
1) Goal: Patient/client has limited awareness and no compliance with water decontamination recommendations when extensive awareness and compliance with the decontamination guidelines is the goal.
   OR
2) Reference standard: No validated standard exists.

Sample nutrition assessment and monitoring and evaluation documentation

Initial nutrition assessment with patient/client	The patient/client has limited awareness and no compliance with water decontamination recommendations (e.g., community has a boil water alert for water used for drinking and cooking) when extensive awareness and compliance with the decontamination guidelines is the goal. Will monitor change in compliance at next appointment.
Reassessment after nutrition intervention	Substantial progress toward goal as patient/client is complying with water decontamination guidelines.

References

The following are some suggested references for indicators, measurement techniques, and reference standard; other references may be appropriate.

1. Position of the American Dietetic Association: Addressing world hunger, malnutrition, and food insecurity. *J Am Diet Assoc.* 2003;103:1046-1057.
2. Position of the American Dietetic Association: Food and water safety. *J Am Diet Assoc.* 2003;103:1203-1218.
3. U.S. Environmental Protection Agency, Ground Water and Drinking Water Frequently Asked Questions. Available at: http://www.epa.gov/safewater/faq/faq.html#safe. Accessed November 14, 2006.

*** *Denotes indicator is used for nutrition assessment only. Other indicators are used for both nutrition assessment and nutrition monitoring and evaluation.*

Food/Nutrition-Related Supplies Availability (FH-5.4)

Definition
Access to necessary food/nutrition-related supplies

Nutrition Assessment and Monitoring and Evaluation
Indicators

Access to food/nutrition-related supplies (specify, e.g., glucose monitor, monitoring strips, lancets, pedometer, PN/EN supplies, thickeners, blood pressure related devices)

Access to assistive eating devices (specify, e.g., modified utensils, plates, bowls, gavage feeding supplies)

Access to assistive food preparation devices (specify, e.g., modified utensils for food preparation, electric can openers, rocking knives, one-handed devices)

Examples of the measurement methods or data sources for these indicators: Patient/client report, referral information, home evaluation

Typically used with the following domains of nutrition interventions: Nutrition education, nutrition counseling, coordination of nutrition care

Typically used to determine and to monitor and evaluate change in the following nutrition diagnoses: Inability or lack of desire to manage self-care, inadequate oral food/beverage intake, self-feeding difficulty, limited adherence to nutrition-related recommendations

Clinical judgment must be used to select indicators and determine the appropriate measurement techniques and reference standards for a given patient population and setting. Once identified, these indicators, measurement techniques, and reference standards should be identified in policies and procedures or other documents for use in patient/client records, quality or performance improvement, or in formal research projects.

Evaluation

Criteria for evaluation
Comparison to Goal or Reference Standard:
1) Goal (tailored to patient/client needs)
    OR
2) Reference standard

*** Denotes indicator is used for nutrition assessment only. Other indicators are used for both nutrition assessment and nutrition monitoring and evaluation.

Assessment

Food/Nutrition-Related Supplies Availability (FH-5.4)

Patient/Client Example(s)

Example(s) of one or two of the Nutrition Care Indicators (includes sample initial and reassessment documentation for one of the indicators)

Indicator(s) selected

Access to food/nutrition-related supplies

Criteria for evaluation

Comparison to Goal or Reference Standard:
1) Goal: Patient/client has limited access to a sufficient quantity of glucose monitoring strips when extensive access is the goal.
   OR
2) Reference standard: No validated standard exists.

Sample nutrition assessment and monitoring and evaluation documentation

Initial nutrition assessment with patient/client	The patient/client has limited access to a sufficient quantity of glucose monitoring strips. Will monitor change in access to glucose monitoring strips at next appointment.
Reassessment after nutrition intervention	Some progress toward goal as patient/client has moderate access to a sufficient supply of glucose monitoring strips.

References

The following are some suggested references for indicators, measurement techniques, and reference standard; other references may be appropriate.

1. Department of Health and Human Services (HHS) Poverty Guidelines, 2006. Available at: http://aspe.hhs.gov/poverty/06poverty.shtml. Accessed November 14, 2006.
2. Holben DH, Myles W. Food Insecurity in the United States: How It Affects Our Patients. *Am Fam Physician*. 2004;69;1058-1063.
3. Position of the American Dietetic Association on Food Insecurity and Hunger in the United States. *J Am Diet Assoc*. 2006;106:446-458.
4. Position of the American Dietetic Association: Food and water safety. *J Am Diet Assoc*. 2003;103:1203-1218.

*** Denotes indicator is used for nutrition assessment only. Other indicators are used for both nutrition assessment and nutrition monitoring and evaluation.

Breastfeeding (FH-6.1)

Definition
Degree to which breastfeeding plans and experience meet nutritional and other needs of the infant and mother

Nutrition Assessment and Monitoring and Evaluation
Indicators

Initiation of breastfeeding
- Breastfeeding attempts (number)

Duration of breastfeeding (specify, e.g., weeks, months, years)

Exclusive breastfeeding (yes/no)

Breastfeeding problems
- Evaluation of latch (correct/incorrect)
- Evaluation of mothers nipples (Not irritated/irritated)
- Evaluation of sucking (minutes rhythmic sucking per feeding)
- Presence of milk in baby's mouth when unlatched from breast (yes/no)
- Evaluation of mother's breasts (specify, e.g., full/firm prior to feeding, soft after feeding)
- Mother's evaluation of baby's satisfaction after feeding (specify, e.g., still hungry/satisfied)
- Other (specify)

Note: Infant/child growth can be found on the Body Composition/Growth/Weight History reference sheet.

Breastfeeding self-efficacy and intention to breastfeed can be found on the Beliefs and Attitudes reference sheet.

Examples of the measurement methods or data sources for this indicator: Patient/client report, practitioner observation of breastfeeding, self-monitoring records, infant weight trends

Typically used to determine and monitor and evaluate change in the following domains of nutrition interventions: Nutrition education, nutrition counseling, coordination of nutrition care

Typically used to determine and to monitor and evaluate change in the following nutrition diagnoses: Maternal breastfeeding difficulty, food- and nutrition-related knowledge deficit, harmful beliefs/attitudes about food- or nutrition-related topics, involuntary weight loss, inadequate fluid intake

Clinical judgment must be used to select indicators and determine the appropriate measurement techniques and reference standards for a given patient population and setting. Once identified, these indicators, measurement techniques, and reference standards should be identified in policies and procedures or other documents for use in patient/client records, quality or performance improvement, or in formal research projects.

*** Denotes indicator is used for nutrition assessment only. Other indicators are used for both nutrition assessment and nutrition monitoring and evaluation.

Assessment

Breastfeeding (FH-6.1)

Evaluation

Criteria for evaluation

Comparison to Goal or Reference Standard:

    1) Goal (tailored to patient/client's needs)

       OR

    2) Reference standard

Patient/Client Example(s)

Example(s) of one or two of the Nutrition Care Indicators (includes sample initial and reassessment documentation for one of the indicators)

Indicator(s) selected

Initiation of breastfeeding

Criteria for evaluation

Comparison to Goal or Reference Standard:

    1) Goal: Patient/client currently fears her breast milk supply is not adequate and worries about how she will manage when she returns to work in four weeks. Goal is for mother to breastfeed for six-months.

       OR

    2) Reference standard: No validated standard exists.

Sample nutrition assessment and monitoring and evaluation documentation

Initial encounter with patient/client	Postpartum patient/client states she is planning to use a combination of formula and breastfeeding and start solids at 3 months. Will educate and refer to lactation support group.
Reassessment after nutrition intervention	Patient/client reports she has exclusively breast fed for three months and plans to delay introduction of solids. Will reinforce and educate. Continue to monitor.

References

The following are some suggested references for indicators, measurement techniques, and reference standards for the outcome; other references may be appropriate.

1. Riordan, J. *Breastfeeding and Human Lactation.* 3rd ed. Sudbury, MA: Jones and Bartlett Publishers; 2005:219.
2. Leff EW, Gagne MP, Jefferis SC. Maternal perceptions of successful breastfeeding. *J Hum Lact.* 2004;10:99-104.
3. Avery M, Duckett L, Dodgson J, Savik K, Henly SJ. Factors associated with very early weaning among primiparas intending to breastfeed. *Maternal Child Health J.* 1998;2:167-179.
4. American Academy of Pediatrics. Policy statement: Breastfeeding and the use of human milk, section on breastfeeding. *Pediatrics.* 2005;115:496-506.
5. CAPPA Position Paper. The lactation educator's role in providing breastfeeding information and support. 2002. Available at: http://www.cappa.net. Accessed March13, 2007.
6. James DCS, Dobson B. Position of the American Dietetic Association: Promoting and Supporting Breastfeeding. *J Am Diet Assoc.* 2005;105(5): 810-818.

*** Denotes indicator is used for nutrition assessment only. Other indicators are used for both nutrition assessment and nutrition monitoring and evaluation.

Nutrition-Related Activities of Daily Living and Instrumental Activities of Daily Living (FH-6.2)

Definition
Level of cognitive and physical ability to perform nutrition-related activities of daily living and instrumental activities of daily living by older and/or disabled persons

Nutrition Assessment and Monitoring and Evaluation
Indicators

Physical ability to complete tasks for meal preparation (plan meals, shop for meals, finances, meal preparation) (yes/no)

Physical ability to self-feed (yes/no)

Ability to position self within 12-18 inches from mouth to plate (yes/no)

Does not receive assistance with intake (yes/no)

Ability to use adaptive eating devices that have been deemed necessary and that improve self-feeding skills (yes/no)

Cognitive ability to complete tasks for meal preparation (planning meals, shopping for meals, finances, meal preparation) (yes/no)

Remembers to eat, recalls eating (yes/no)

Mini Mental State Examination Score (score)

Nutrition-related activities of daily living (ADL) score (score)

Nutrition-related instrumental activities of daily living (IADL) score (score)

Note: Sufficient intake of food can be found on the Food Intake Reference Sheet.
   Sufficient intake of fluid can be found on the Fluid/Beverage Intake Reference Sheet.
   Food security and ability to maintain sanitation can be found on the Safe Food/Meal Availability Reference Sheet.
   Ability to maintain weight can be found on the Body Composition/Growth/Weight History Reference Sheet.

Examples of the measurement methods or data sources for these outcome indicators: Self-report, caregiver report, home visit, targeted questionnaires and monitoring devices, ADL and/or IADL measurement tool, congregate meal site attendance records

Typically used with the following domains of nutrition interventions: Coordination of nutrition care

*** *Denotes indicator is used for nutrition assessment only. Other indicators are used for both nutrition assessment and nutrition monitoring and evaluation.*

Assessment

Food/Nutrition-Related History Domain – Physical Activity and Function

Nutrition-Related Activities of Daily Living and Instrumental Activities of Daily Living (FH-6.2)

Typically used to determine and to monitor and evaluate change in the following nutrition diagnoses: Inability to manage self-care, impaired ability to prepare foods/meals

Clinical judgment must be used to select indicators and determine the appropriate measurement techniques and reference standards for a given patient population and setting. Once identified, these indicators, measurement techniques, and reference standards should be identified in policies and procedures or other documents for use in patient/client records, quality or performance improvement, or in formal research projects.

Evaluation

Criteria for evaluation
Comparison to Goal or Reference Standard:
   1) Goal (tailored to patient/client's needs)
      OR
   2) Reference standard

Patient/Client Example(s)

Example(s) of one or two of the Nutrition Care Indicators (includes sample initial and reassessment documentation for one of the indicators)

Indicator(s) selected
Nutrition-related instrumental activities of daily living (IADL) score

Criteria for evaluation
Comparison to Goal or Reference Standard:
   1) Goal: Patient/client with decreased food intake due to an inability to drive, no close relatives living in the vicinity, and difficulty in performing meal preparation tasks due to weakness.
      OR
   2) Reference standard: No validated standard exists.

*** *Denotes indicator is used for nutrition assessment only. Other indicators are used for both nutrition assessment and nutrition monitoring and evaluation.*

Nutrition-Related Activities of Daily Living and Instrumental Activities of Daily Living (FH-6.2)

Sample nutrition assessment and monitoring and evaluation documentation

Initial encounter with patient/client	Patient/client with inadequate food intake due to inability to drive, no close relative living in vicinity, subsequent weight loss and difficulties in performing ADLs and IADLs due to weakness. Client is to use new strategies and community resources to facilitate attendance at senior center congregate meals 5 times per week, use of community provided transportation offered to grocery store 1 x per week, and attendance in strength training at senior center.
Reassessment after nutrition intervention	Significant progress in nutrition-related activities of daily living. Patient/client able to attend senior center for meals and strength training 3 times this week. Goal is 5 times. Will continue to assess at next encounter. Client going to grocery store 1 x per week.

References

The following are some suggested references for indicators, measurement techniques, and reference standards for the outcome; other references may be appropriate.

1. ADL/IADL evaluation tools used for Administration on Aging (AoA) nutrition programs available from AoA. Performance Outcomes Management Project, Physical Functioning and Health Survey. Available at: https://www.gpra.net/PFmain.asp. Accessed March 18, 2007.

2. Kretser A, Voss T, Kerr W, Cavadini C, Friedmann J. Effects of two models of nutritional intervention on homebound older adults at nutritional risk. *J Am Diet Assoc.* 2003;103:329-336.

3. Sorbye LW, Schroll M, Finne Soveri H, Jonsson PV, Topinkova E, Ljunggren G, Bernabei R. Unintended weight loss in the elderly living at home: the Aged in Home Care Project (AdHOC). *J Nutr Health Aging.* 2008;12:10-6.

4. Folstein, M., Folstein, S.E., McHugh, P.R. (1975). "Mini-Mental State" a Practical Method for Grading the Cognitive State of Patients for the Clinician. *Journal of Psychiatric Research*, 12(3); 189-198.

5. U.S. Department of Health and Human Services, Administration on Aging. Older American Act Nutrition Program Fact Sheet, 2003. Available from: http://www.aoa.gov/press/fact/pdf/fs_nutrition.pdf Accessed 1-14-08, Assessed January 15, 2008.

6. Russell C, Dining Skills: Practical Interventions for Caregivers of Older Adults with Eating Problems. Consultant Dietitians in Health Care Facilities, A Dietetic Practice Group of the American Dietetic Association, Chicago, IL, 2001.

*** Denotes indicator is used for nutrition assessment only. Other indicators are used for both nutrition assessment and nutrition monitoring and evaluation.*

Assessment

Physical Activity (FH-6.3)

Definition
Level of physical activity and/or amount of exercise performed

Nutrition Assessment and Monitoring and Evaluation
Indicators

       Physical activity history*** (e.g., activities, preferences, attitudes)

       Consistency (yes/no)

       Frequency (number times/week)

       Duration (number minutes/session, number of total minutes/day)

       Intensity (e.g., talk test, Borg Rating of Perceived Exertion, % of predetermined max heart rate)

       Type of physical activity (e.g., cardiovascular, muscular strength/endurance, flexibility; lifestyle, programmed)

       Strength (grip strength)

       TV/screen time (minutes/day)

       Other sedentary activity time (e.g., commuting; sitting at desk, in meetings, at sporting or arts events) (minutes/day)

       Involuntary physical movement (present/absent)***

Examples of the measurement methods or data sources for these outcome indicators: History interview/questionnaire, physical activity log, step counter, accelerometer, attendance at strength training, balance training (for older adults), and/or aerobic classes, caretaker records, medical record

Typically used with the following domains of nutrition interventions: Nutrition education, nutrition counseling

Typically used to determine and to monitor and evaluate change in the following nutrition diagnoses: Physical inactivity, excessive exercise, underweight, overweight/obesity, involuntary weight loss or weight gain

Clinical judgment must be used to select indicators and determine the appropriate measurement techniques and reference standards for a given patient population and setting. Once identified, these indicators, measurement techniques, and reference standards should be identified in policies and procedures or other documents for use in patient/client records, quality or performance improvement, or in formal research projects.

*** Denotes indicator is used for nutrition assessment only. Other indicators are used for both nutrition assessment and nutrition monitoring and evaluation.

Physical Activity (FH-6.3)

Evaluation

Criteria for evaluation
Comparison to Goal or Reference Standard:
  1) Goal (tailored to patient/client's needs)
      OR
  2) Reference standard

Patient/Client Example(s)

Example(s) of one or two of the Nutrition Care Indicators (includes sample initial and reassessment documentation for one of the indicators)

Indicator(s) selected
Consistency and duration

Criteria for evaluation
Comparison to Goal or Reference Standard:
  1) Goal: Patient/client typically walks approximately 10 minutes, twice per week. Patient/client goal is to walk approximately 15 minutes, 5 days per week.
      OR
  2) Reference standard: Patient/client's typical 10-minute walk, twice a week is well below the recommended at least 30 minutes of moderate-intensity physical activity (in bouts 10 minutes or longer), 5 days per week or at least 20 minutes of vigorous intensity physical activity (in bouts 10 minutes or longer), 3 days per week (ACSM/AHA Physical Activity Guidelines for Public Health for adults and seniors)

Sample nutrition assessment and monitoring and evaluation documentation

Initial encounter with patient/client	Based upon exercise log, patient/client doing moderate-intensity physical activities 30 minutes/day, 2 days/week. Goal is to do at least 30 minutes/day (in bouts 10 minutes or longer), moderate-intensity activities, 5 or more days/wk. Will monitor physical activity level at next appointment.
Reassessment after nutrition intervention	Significant progress toward goal of exercising at 30 minutes/day, moderate-intensity activities, 5 or more days/wk. Patient/client reports doing moderate-intensity activities 30 minutes per day, 4 days/week.

*** *Denotes indicator is used for nutrition assessment only. Other indicators are used for both nutrition assessment and nutrition monitoring and evaluation.*

Assessment

Food/Nutrition-Related History Domain – Physical Activity and Function

Physical Activity (FH-6.3)

References

The following are some suggested references for indicators, measurement techniques, and reference standards for the outcome; other references may be appropriate.

1. Haskell WL, Lee IM, Pate RR, Powell KE, Blair SN, Franklin BA, Macera CA, Heath GW, Thompson PD, Bauman A. Physical activity and public health: Updated recommendation for adults from the American College of Sports Medicine and the American Heart Association. *Medicine and Science in Sports and Exercise*. 2007;39:8:1423-1434.

2. Nelson ME, Rejeski WJ, Blair SN, Duncan PW, Judge JO, King AC, Macera CA, Castaneda-Sceppa C. Physical activity and public health in older adults. Recommendation from the American College of Sports Medicine and the American Heart Association. *Medicine and Science in Sports and Exercise*. 2007;39:8:1435-1445.

3. American College of Sports Medicine Position Stands. Available at: http://www.acsm-msse.org. Accessed March 14, 2007.

4. Department of Health and Human Services, Centers for Disease Control and Prevention, Growing Stronger–Strength Training for Older Adults. Available at: http://www.cdc.gov/nccdphp/dnpa/physical/growing_stronger/index.htm. Accessed March 18, 2007.

5. American College of Sports Medicine, National Blueprint: Increasing physical activity among adults aged 50 and older. Available at: http://www.agingblueprint.org/overview.cfm. Accessed March 18, 2007.

6. Exercise Guidelines During Pregnancy. American Pregnancy Association. Available at: http://www.americanpregnancy.org/pregnancyhealth/exerciseguidelines.html. Accessed March 14, 2007.

7. Fabricatore AN. Behavior therapy and cognitive-behavioral therapy of obesity: Is there a difference? *J Am Diet Assoc*. 2007:107:92-99.

*** *Denotes indicator is used for nutrition assessment only. Other indicators are used for both nutrition assessment and nutrition monitoring and evaluation.*

Nutrition Quality of Life* (FH-7.1)

Definition
Extent to which the Nutrition Care Process impacts a patient/client's physical, mental and social well-being related to food and nutrition

Nutrition Assessment and Monitoring and Evaluation
Indicators
Nutrition quality of life responses

Note: A nutrition quality of life instrument has been developed and is being validated (Barr JT, et al 2003). Focused questioning around the six indicators using the 50 NQOL statements is recommended.

Examples of the measurement methods or data sources for these outcome indicators: Nutrition Quality of Life measurement tool, other quality of life tools

Typically used with the following domains of nutrition interventions: Food and/or nutrient delivery, supplements, nutrition education, nutrition counseling, coordination of nutrition care

Typically used to determine and to monitor and evaluate change in the following nutrition diagnoses: Poor nutrition quality of life, inadequate or excessive energy or macronutrient intake, underweight, involuntary weight loss, overweight/obesity, involuntary weight gain, disordered eating pattern, inability or lack of desire to manage self-care, swallowing difficulty, chewing difficulty, self-feeding difficulty, altered GI function, limited access to food

Clinical judgment must be used to select indicators and determine the appropriate measurement techniques and reference standards for a given patient population and setting. Once identified, these indicators, measurement techniques, and reference standards should be identified in policies and procedures or other documents for use in patient/client records, quality or performance improvement, or in formal research projects.

Evaluation

Criteria for evaluation
Comparison to Goal or Reference Standard:
1) Goal (tailored to patient/client's needs)
   OR
2) Reference standard

* This nutrition outcome is currently under development and included to encourage further research.

*** Denotes indicator is used for nutrition assessment only. Other indicators are used for both nutrition assessment and nutrition monitoring and evaluation.

Assessment

Food/Nutrition-Related History Domain – Nutrition-Related Patient/Client Centered Measures

Nutrition Quality of Life* (FH-7.1)

Patient/Client Example(s)

Example(s) of one or two of the Nutrition Care Indicators (includes sample initial and reassessment documentation for one of the indicators)

Indicator(s) selected

Nutrition quality of life score

Criteria for evaluation

Comparison to Goal or Reference Standard:

1) Goal: Patient/client with chronic renal disease currently reports poor nutrition quality of life, especially decreased walking ability (physical) and limited food choices on renal diet (food impact). The goal of medical nutrition therapy is to educate and coach patient and his family on options and strategies to significantly enhance his nutrition quality of life.

OR

2. Reference standard: No validated standard exists.

Sample nutrition assessment and monitoring and evaluation documentation

Initial encounter with patient/client	Patient/client with chronic renal disease reports poor nutrition quality of life, particularly in physical and food impact aspects. Patient/client to receive intensive medical nutrition therapy with a goal to improve client's overall nutrition quality of life over a 6-month period. Will monitor nutrition quality of life in 6 months.
Reassessment after nutrition intervention	Some progress toward goal. Patient/client's nutrition quality of life is increased, but further improvement is desired in the physical dimension. Will continue medical nutrition therapy and reassess in 3 months.

References

The following are some suggested references for indicators, measurement techniques, and reference standards for the outcome; other references may be appropriate.

1. Barr JT, Schumacher GE. The need for a nutrition-related quality-of-life measure. J Am Diet Assoc. 2003;103:177–180.
2. Barr JT, Schumacher GE. Using focus groups to determine what constitutes quality of life in clients receiving medical nutrition therapy: First steps in the development of a nutrition quality-of-life survey. J Am Diet Assoc. 2003;103:844-851.
3. Ware JE, Sherbourne CD. The MOS 36-item short-form health survey (SF-36), I: Conceptual framework and item selection. Med Care. 1992;30:473-483.
4. Moorehead M, Ardelt-Gattinger E, Lechner H, Oria H. The validation of the Moorehead-Ardelt Quality of Life Questionnaire II. Obes Surg. 2003;13:684-692.
5. Groll D, Vanner S, Depew W, DaCosta L, Simon J, Groll A, Roblin N, Paterson W. The IBS-36: a new quality of life measure for irritable bowel syndrome. Am J Gastroenterol. 2002;97:962-971.
6. Diabetes Control and Complications Trial Research Group. Reliability and validity of a diabetes quality of life measure for the Diabetes Control and Complications Trial (DCCT). Diabetes Care. 1988;11:725–732.
7. Niedert KC. Position of the American Dietetic Association: Liberalization of the Diet Prescription Improves Quality of Life for Older Adults in Long-Term Care. J Am Diet Assoc. 2005;105(12):1955-1965.

* This nutrition outcome is currently under development and included to encourage further research.

*** Denotes indicator is used for nutrition assessment only. Other indicators are used for both nutrition assessment and nutrition monitoring and evaluation.

Body Composition/Growth/Weight History (AD-1.1)

Definition
Comparative measures of the body, including fat, muscle, and bone components and growth

Nutrition Assessment and Monitoring and Evaluation
Indicators

Height/length
- Height/length (in/cm)
- Birth length (in/cm)***
- Pre-amputation height (in/cm)***
- Estimated height
  - Knee height (cm)
  - Arm span (in/cm)

Weight
- Weight (lbs, oz, kg, g)
- Measured
- Stated
- Usual body weight (UBW) (lbs/kg)***
- UBW percentage (%)
- Birth weight***
- Dosing weight (lbs, oz, kg, g)
- Dry weight (lbs, oz, kg, g)

Frame size
- Frame size (small/medium/large)

Weight change
- Weight change (specify lbs, kg, oz, g, %)
  Specify timeframe: _____
- Intent (intentional/unintentional)***
- Weight change, interdialytic (% dry weight)
- Weight change, gestational (lbs, oz, kg, g)
  Specify timeframe: _____

Body mass index
- Body mass index (BMI) (kg/m^2)
- BMI prime (actual BMI/upper limit BMI)

Growth pattern indices/percentile ranks
- Corrected age for prematurity
- BMI percentile/age (percentile rank)
- Head circumference (cm or in)
- Head circumference-for-age (percentile rank)
- Length/stature-for-age (percentile rank)
- Weight-for-length/stature (percentile rank)
- Weight-for-age (percentile rank)

Body compartment estimates
- Body fat percentage (%)
- Body surface area (m^2)
- Bone age (years)
- Bone mineral density (units)
- Mid-arm muscle circumference (percentile rank)
- Triceps skin fold (percentile rank)
- Waist circumference (in or cm)
- Waist hip ratio (ratio)

*** Denotes indicator is used for nutrition assessment only. Other indicators are used for both nutrition assessment and nutrition monitoring and evaluation.

Assessment

Anthropometric Measures Domain – Anthropometric Data

Body Composition/Growth/Weight History (AD-1.1)

Examples of the measurement methods or data sources for these outcome indicators: Referring health care provider or agency, direct measurement, patient/client report, medical record

Typically used with the following domains of nutrition interventions: Food and nutrient delivery, nutrition education, nutrition counseling, coordination of nutrition care

Typically used to determine and monitor and evaluate change in the following nutrition diagnoses: Excess or inadequate intake of energy, fat, protein, carbohydrate, alcohol, and/or mineral intake; underweight, overweight, physical inactivity, excessive exercise

Clinical judgment must be used to select indicators and determine the appropriate measurement techniques and reference standards for a given patient population and setting. Once identified, these indicators, measurement techniques, and reference standards should be identified in policies and procedures or other documents for use in patient/client records, quality or performance improvement, or in formal research projects.

Evaluation

Criteria for evaluation
Comparison to Goal or Reference Standard:
   1) Goal (tailored to patient/client's needs)
      OR
   2) Reference standard

Patient/Client Example(s)

Example(s) of one or two of the Nutrition Care Indicators (includes sample initial and reassessment documentation for one of the indicators)

Indicator(s) selected
Weight change/day
BMI percentile/age

Criteria for evaluation
Comparison to Goal or Reference Standard:
   1) Goal: The infant is only gaining, on average, 10 grams per day compared with a goal weight gain of 20–30 grams per day.
      OR
   2) Reference standard: Child's (> age 3 years) BMI percentile/age per growth curves has crossed 2 percentiles from 50% to 10% in last 6 months.

*** *Denotes indicator is used for nutrition assessment only. Other indicators are used for both nutrition assessment and nutrition monitoring and evaluation.*

Body Composition/Growth/Weight History (AD-1.1)

Sample nutrition assessment and monitoring and evaluation documentation

Initial nutrition assessment with patient/client	Child's BMI percentile/age per growth curves has crossed 2 percentiles from 50% to 10% in last 6 months. Will monitor BMI percentile/age at next encounter.
Reassessment after nutrition intervention	Child's BMI percentile/age per growth curves is unchanged from baseline measure.

References

The following are some suggested references for indicators, measurement techniques, and reference standards for the outcome; other references may be appropriate.

1. McDowell MA, Fryar CD, Hirsch R, Ogden CL. Anthropometric Reference Data for Children and Adults: U.S. Population, 1999-2002. *Advanced data from vital health statistics*; no 361. Hyattsville, MD: National Center for Health Statistics. 2005. Available at: http://www.cdc.gov/nchs/data/ad/ad361.pdf Accessed: February 29, 2008.

2. CDC. National Center for Health Statistics. National Health and Nutrition Examination Survey. 2000 CDC Growth Charts: United States. Available at: http://www.cdc.gov/growthcharts/ Accessed: February 29, 2008.

3. *ACSM's Guidelines for Exercise Testing and Prescription*. 6th ed. Indianapolis, IN: American College of Sports Medicine; 2000.

4. Charney P, Malone A, eds. *ADA Pocket Guide to Nutrition Assessment*. Chicago, IL: American Dietetic Association; 2004.

5. American Dietetic Association. Adult Weight Management Evidence-Based Nutrition Practice Guideline, 2006. Available at: http://www.adaevidencelibrary.com/topic.cfm?cat=2798. Accessed December 28, 2006.

6. Barlow SE and the Expert Committee. Expert committee recommendations regarding the prevention, assessment, and treatment of child and adolescent overweight and obesity: Summary report. *Pediatrics*. 2007;120:S164-S192.

7. Bone Health and Osteoporosis: A Report of the Surgeon General. Available at: http://www.surgeongeneral.gov/library/bonehealth/. Accessed December 10, 2006.

8. Callaway CW et al. Circumferences. In: Lohman TG et al. *Anthropometric Standardization Reference Manual*. Champaign, IL: Human Kinetics, 1988: 39-54.

9. Centers for Disease Control, Bone Health Campaign. Powerful Bones. Powerful Girls. Available at: http://www.cdc.gov/nccdphp/dnpa/bonehealth/. Accessed December 10, 2006.

10. Frankel HM. Body mass index graphic for children. Pediatrics. 2004;113:425-426.

11. Going S. Optimizing techniques for determining body composition. Available at: http://www.gssiweb.com/Article_Detail.aspx?articleid=720. Accessed on December 29, 2006.

12. Guidelines for the use of parenteral and enteral nutrition in adult and pediatric patients: Normal requirements—adults. J Parenter Enteral Nutr. 2002;26(Suppl):S22-S24.

13. Guidelines for the use of parenteral and enteral nutrition in adult and pediatric patients: Normal requirements—pediatrics. J Parenter Enteral Nutr. 2002;26(Suppl):S25-S32.

14. Heyward V, Wagner D, eds. *Applied Body Composition and Assessment*. 2nd ed. Champaign, IL: Human Kinetics; 2004.

15. The Johns H Johns Hopkins Hospital. *The Harriet Lane Handbook: A Manual for Pediatric House Officers*. 17th ed. St. Louis, MO: Mosby; 2005.

16. Kleinman RE, ed. *Pediatric Nutrition Handbook*. 5th ed. Chicago, IL: American Academy of Pediatrics; 2004.

17. Leonberg BL. *ADA Pocket Guide to Pediatric Nutrition Assessment*. Chicago, IL: American Dietetic Association; 2008.

18. Modlesky CM. Assessment of body size and composition. In: Dunford M *Sports Nutrition: A Practice Manual for Professionals*. 4th ed. Chicago, IL: American Dietetic Association; 2006.

17. Institute of Medicine. *Dietary Reference Intakes for Calcium, Phosphorus, Magnesium, Vitamin D, and Fluoride*. Washington, DC: National Academy Press; 1997.

18. NIDDK Weight control information network. Available at: http://win.niddk.nih.gov/publications/tools.htm. Accessed October 24, 2006.

19. NHLBI Guidelines on Overweight and Obesity, Online Textbook, 1998. Available at: http://www.nhlbi.nih.gov/guidelines/obesity/e_txtbk/index.htm. Accessed October 24, 2006.

20. NIH, National Center for Health Statistics (NCHS). Clinical Growth Charts, 2000. Available at: www.cdc.gov/nchs/about/major/nhanes/growthcharts/clinical_charts.htm. Accessed October 25, 2006.

*** Denotes indicator is used for nutrition assessment only. Other indicators are used for both nutrition assessment and nutrition monitoring and evaluation.

Assessment

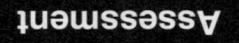

Anthropometric Measures Domain – Anthropometric Data

Body Composition/Growth/Weight History (AD-1.1)

References, cont'd

21. Nevin-Folino N. *Pediatric Manual of Clinical Dietetics*. 2nd ed. Chicago, IL: American Dietetic Association; 2003.

22. World Health Organization, Child Growth Standards. Available at: http://www.who.int/childgrowth/standards/chts_wfa_boys_p/en/index.html Accessed March 28, 2007.

23. Committee on Nutrition Status During Pregnancy and Lactation. Institute of Medicine. Nutrition During Pregnancy: Part I: Weight Gain, Part II: Nutrient Supplements. (1990). Available at: http://www.nap.edu/openbook.php?record_id=1451. Accessed on June 21, 2008.

24. Bouillanne O, Morineau G, Dupont C, Coulombel I, Vincent JP, Nicolis I, Benazeth S, Cynober L, Aussel C. Geriatric Nutritional Risk Index: a new index for evaluating at-risk elderly medical patients. *Am J Clin Nutr*. 2005;82:777-783.

25. Cogil B. *Anthropometric Indicators Measurement Guide*. Washington, DC: Food and Nutrition Technical Assistance Project, Academy of Educational Development; 2003

26. Samson-Fang LJ, Stevenson RD. Identification of malnutrition in children with cerebral palsy: poor performance of weight-for-height centiles. *Developmental Medicine & Child Neurology*. 2000;42:162-168.

27. Zemel BS, Riley EM, Stallings VA. Evaluation of methodology for nutritional assessment in children: Anthropometry, body composition, and energy expenditure. *Ann Rev of Nutr*. 1997;17:211-235.

24. Mitchell CO, Lipschitz DA. Arm length measurement as an alternative to height in the nutrition assessment of the elderly. *JPEN J Parenter Enteral Nutr*. 1982;6:226-229.

25. Cronk CE, Stallings VA, Spender Q, Ross JL, Widdoes HD. Measurement of short-term growth with a new knee height-measuring device. *Am J Hum Biol*. 1989. 31(2):206-14.

*** *Denotes indicator is used for nutrition assessment only. Other indicators are used for both nutrition assessment and nutrition monitoring and evaluation.*

Acid Base Balance (BD-1.1)

Definition
Balance between acids and bases in the body fluids. The pH (hydrogen ion concentration) of the arterial blood provides an index for the total body acid-base balance (1).

Nutrition Assessment
Indicators

> pH (number)***
>
> Arterial bicarbonate, HCO_3 (mmol/L)***
>
> Partial pressure of carbon dioxide in arterial blood, $PaCO_2$ (mmHg)***
>
> Partial pressure of oxygen in arterial blood, PaO_2 (mmHg)***
>
> Venous pH (number)
>
> Venous bicarbonate, CO_2 (mmol/L)
>
> *Note: Sodium and chloride can be found on the Electrolyte and Renal Profile reference sheet*

Examples of the measurement methods or data sources for these indicators: Biochemical measurement, laboratory report

Typically used with the following domains of nutrition interventions: Food and/or nutrient delivery, coordination of nutrition care

Typically used to determine and to monitor and evaluate change in the following nutrition diagnoses: Altered nutrition-related laboratory values

Clinical judgment must be used to select indicators and determine the appropriate measurement techniques and reference standards for a given patient population and setting. Once identified, these indicators, measurement techniques, and reference standards should be identified in policies and procedures or other documents for use in patient/client records, quality or performance improvement, or in formal research projects.

Evaluation

Criteria for evaluation
Comparison to Goal or Reference Standard:
> 1) Goal (tailored to patient/client's needs)
>   OR
> 2) Reference standard

*** *Denotes indicator is used for nutrition assessment only. Other indicators are used for both nutrition assessment and nutrition monitoring and evaluation.*

Assessment

Biochemical Data, Medical Tests and Procedures Domain – Biochemical and Medical Tests

Acid Base Balance (BD-1.1)

Patient/Client Example
Example(s) of one or two of the Nutrition Care Indicators (includes sample initial and reassessment documentation for one of the indicators)

Indicator(s) selected
pH, serum (number)

Criteria for evaluation
Comparison to Goal or Reference Standard:
1) Goal: Not generally used.
   OR
2) Reference standard: The patient/client pH is 7.48 which is above (above, below, or within expected range) the reference standard (7.35-7.45).

Sample nutrition assessment documentation

Initial nutrition assessment with patient/client	Patient/client's pH is 7.48, which is above expected range. Will monitor change in pH at next arterial blood gas.
Reassessment after nutrition intervention	Significant progress toward reference standard. Patient/client's pH is 7.40, within expected range.

References
The following are some suggested references for indicators, measurement techniques, and reference standards; other references may be appropriate.

1. National Library of Medicine - Medical Subject Headings. 2008 MeSH, MeSH Descriptor Data. Available at: http://www.nlm.nih.gov/cgi/mesh/2008/MB_cgi?mode=&index=130&field=all&HM=&II=&PA=&form=&input=. Accessed on March 4, 2008.

2. Pamela Charney, Ainsley Malone, eds. *ADA Pocket Guide to Nutrition Assessment*. Chicago, IL: American Dietetic Association; 2004.

3. The Johns H Johns Hopkins Hospital. *The Harriet Lane Handbook: A manual for Pediatric House Officers*, 17th ed. St. Louis MO: Mosby; 2005.

4. Dennis L. Kasper, Eugene Braunwald, Anthony S. Fauci, Stephen L. Hauser, Dan L. Longo, J. Larry Jameson, and Kurt J. Isselbacher, eds. *Harrison's Principle of Internal Medicine*, 16th ed. Columbus, OH: The McGraw-Hill Co.; 2005.

*** *Denotes indicator is used for nutrition assessment only. Other indicators are used for both nutrition assessment and nutrition monitoring and evaluation.*

Electrolyte and Renal Profile (BD-1.2)

Definition
Laboratory measures associated with electrolyte balance and kidney function

Nutrition Assessment and Monitoring and Evaluation
Indicators

BUN (mg/dL)

Creatinine (mg/dL)

BUN:creatinine ratio (ratio number)

Glomerular filtration rate (mL/min/1.73 m^2)

Sodium (mEq/L)

Chloride (mEq/L)

Potassium (mEq/L)

Magnesium (mEq/L)

Calcium, serum (mg/dL)

Calcium, ionized (mg/dL)

Phosphorus (mg/dL)

Serum osmolality (mOsm/kg)

Parathyroid hormone (pg/mL)

Note: Bicarbonate can be found on the Acid Base Balance reference sheet.

Serum albumin can be found on the Protein Profile Reference Sheet for adjustment of serum calcium.

Examples of the measurement methods or data sources for these indicators: Biochemical measurement, laboratory report

Typically used with the following domains of nutrition interventions: Food and/or nutrient delivery, coordination of nutrition care

Typically used to determine and to monitor and evaluate change in the following nutrition diagnoses: Excess or inadequate intake of protein or minerals

Clinical judgment must be used to select indicators and determine the appropriate measurement techniques and reference standards for a given patient population and setting. Once identified, these indicators, measurement techniques, and reference standards should be identified in policies and procedures or other documents for use in patient/client records, quality or performance improvement, or in formal research projects.

Evaluation

Criteria for evaluation
Comparison to Goal or Reference Standard:
1) Goal (tailored to patient/client's needs)
    OR
2) Reference standard

*** *Denotes indicator is used for nutrition assessment only. Other indicators are used for both nutrition assessment and nutrition monitoring and evaluation.*

Assessment

Biochemical Data, Medical Tests and Procedures Domain – Biochemical and Medical Tests

Electrolyte and Renal Profile (BD-1.2)

Patient/Client Example

Example(s) of one or two of the Nutrition Care Indicators (includes sample initial and reassessment documentation for one of the indicators)

Indicator(s) selected

Potassium (mEq/L)

Criteria for evaluation

Comparison to Goal or Reference Standard:

1) Goal: A goal of serum K+ 3.5-5.5 mEq/L in patient/client on medications that block the renin-angiotensin system.

   OR

2) Reference standard: The patient/client's potassium is 2.9 mEq/L which is below (above, below, within expected range) the expected range (3.5-5.0 mEq/L).

Sample nutrition assessment and monitoring and evaluation documentation

Initial nutrition assessment with patient/client	Patient/client's serum potassium is 2.9 mEq/L, which is below the expected range. Will monitor change in potassium at next encounter.
Reassessment after nutrition intervention	Regression from reference standard. Patient/client's potassium is 2.7 mEq/L, below the expected range.

References

The following are some suggested references for indicators, measurement techniques, and reference standards; other references may be appropriate.

1. Pamela Charney, Ainsley Malone, eds. *ADA Pocket Guide to Nutrition Assessment*. Chicago, IL: American Dietetic Association; 2004.

2. American Dietetic Association. *Chronic kidney disease (non-dialysis) medical nutrition therapy protocol*. Chicago (IL): American Dietetic Association; 2002 May.

3. ADA Nutrition Care Manual. 2004. Available at: www.nutritioncaremanual.org. Accessed December 11, 2006.

4. The Johns H Johns Hopkins Hospital. *The Harriet Lane Handbook A manual for Pediatric House Officers*, 17th ed. St. Louis MO: Mosby; 2005.

5. National Institutes of Health, Clinical Center Test Guide. Available at: http://cclnprod.cc.nih.gov/dlm/testguide.nsf/TestIndex?OpenForm&Count=5000. Accessed October 19, 2006.

6. National Kidney Foundation K/DOQI. Clinical practice guidelines for nutrition in chronic renal failure. *Am J Kid Dis*. 2000;35(6):S1-S104.

7. National Kidney Foundation K/DOQI Workgroup. National Kidney Foundation K/DOQI Guidelines on bone metabolism and disease in chronic kidney disease. *Am J Kid Dis*. 2003;42(4 Suppl 3):S1-S201.

8. National Kidney Foundation K/DOQI. Clinical Practice Guidelines on Hypertension and Antihypertensive Agents in Chronic Kidney Disease. *Am J Kid Dis*. 2004; 43 (5 Suppl 1) S1-S290).

9. Wiggins KL. *Guidelines for Nutrition Care of Renal Patients*. Chicago, Il.: American Dietetic Association Renal Practice Group; 2001.

*** Denotes indicator is used for nutrition assessment only. Other indicators are used for both nutrition assessment and nutrition monitoring and evaluation.

Essential Fatty Acid Profile (BD-1.3)

Definition
Laboratory measures of essential fatty acids

Nutrition Assessment and Monitoring and Evaluation
Indicators
> Triene:Tetraene ratio (ratio number)

Examples of the measurement methods or data sources for these indicators: Biochemical measurement, laboratory report/record

Typically used with the following domains of nutrition interventions: Food and/or nutrient delivery, coordination of nutrition care

Typically used to determine and to monitor and evaluate change in the following nutrition diagnoses: Inadequate intake of fat, parenteral nutrition; inappropriate intake of parenteral nutrition; altered nutrition-related laboratory values; impaired nutrient utilization

Clinical judgment must be used to select indicators and determine the appropriate measurement techniques and reference standards for a given patient population and setting. Once identified, these indicators, measurement techniques, and reference standards should be identified in policies and procedures or other documents for use in patient/client records, quality or performance improvement, or in formal research projects.

Evaluation

Criteria for evaluation
Comparison to Goal or Reference Standard:
  1) Goal (tailored to patient/client's needs)
     OR
  2) Reference standard

Patient/Client Example
Example(s) of one or two of the Nutrition Care Indicators (includes sample initial and reassessment documentation for one of the indicators)

Indicator(s) selected
Triene:Tetraene ratio (ratio number)

*** *Denotes indicator is used for nutrition assessment only. Other indicators are used for both nutrition assessment and nutrition monitoring and evaluation.*

Assessment

Biochemical Data, Medical Tests and Procedures Domain – Biochemical and Medical Tests

Essential Fatty Acid Profile (BD-1.3)

Criteria for evaluation

Comparison to Goal or Reference Standard:

1) Goal: Not generally used.

OR

2) Reference standard: The patient/client Triene:Tetraene ratio is 0.45 which is (above, below, or within expected range) above expected range (> 0.2-0.4 essential fatty acid deficiency).

Sample nutrition assessment and monitoring and evaluation documentation

Initial nutrition assessment with patient/client	Patient/client's Triene:Tetraene ratio is 0.45, above the expected range (essential fatty acid deficiency). Will monitor change in Triene:Tetraene ratio at next encounter.
Reassessment after nutrition intervention	Significant progress toward the expect range. Patient/client's Triene:Tetraene ratio is 0.1.

References

The following are some suggested references for indicators, measurement techniques, and reference standards; other references may be appropriate.

1. Pamela Charney, Ainsley Malone, eds. *ADA Pocket Guide to Nutrition Assessment*. Chicago, IL: American Dietetic Association; 2004.

2. Hise ME, Brown JC. Lipids. In: Gottschlich MM, ed. *The A.S.P.E.N. Nutrition Support Core Curriculum: A Case-Based Approach – the Adult Patient*. Silver Spring, MD :A.S.P.E.N.; 2007:48-70.

*** *Denotes indicator is used for nutrition assessment only. Other indicators are used for both nutrition assessment and nutrition monitoring and evaluation.*

Gastrointestinal Profile (BD-1.4)

Definition
Laboratory measures and medical tests associated with function of the gastrointestinal tract and related organs

Nutrition Assessment and Monitoring and Evaluation
Indicators

Alkaline phophatase (U/L)

Alanine aminotransferase, ALT (U/L)

Aspartate aminotransferase, AST (U/L)

Gamma glutamyl transferase, GGT (U/L)

Gastric residual volume (mL)

Bilirubin, total (mg/dL)

Ammonia, serum (μg/dL)

Toxicology report, including alcohol (by report)***

Prothrombin time, PT (seconds)

Partial thromboplastin time, PTT (seconds)

INR (ratio)

Fecal fat

Amylase (U/L)

Lipase(U/L)

Other digestive enzymes, specify***

D-xylose(blood mg/dL; urine % or grams)***

Hydrogen breath test(points)***

Intestinal biopsy (by report)***

Stool culture (by report)***

Gastric emptying time(minutes)***

Abdominal films (by report)***

Swallow study (by report)***

Examples of the measurement methods or data sources for these indicators: Biochemical measurement, laboratory report

Typically used with the following domains of nutrition interventions: Food and/or nutrient delivery, nutrition education, nutrition counseling

Typically used to determine and to monitor and evaluate change in the following nutrition diagnoses: Altered nutrition-related laboratory values, excess intake of protein or fat

Clinical judgment must be used to select indicators and determine the appropriate measurement techniques and reference standards for a given patient population and setting. Once identified, these indicators, measurement techniques, and reference standards should be identified in policies and procedures or other documents for use in patient/client records, quality or performance improvement, or in formal research projects.

*** Denotes indicator is used for nutrition assessment only. Other indicators are used for both nutrition assessment and nutrition monitoring and evaluation.*

Assessment

Gastrointestinal Profile (BD-1.4)

Evaluation

Criteria for evaluation

Comparison to Goal or Reference Standard:

> 1) Goal (tailored to patient/client's needs)
>   OR
> 2) Reference standard

Patient/Client Example

Example(s) of one or two of the Nutrition Care Indicators (includes sample initial and reassessment documentation for one of the indicators)

Indicator(s) selected

Ammonia, serum (μg/dL)

Criteria for evaluation

Comparison to Goal or Reference Standard:

> 1) Goal: The patient/client's serum ammonia is 105 μg/dL, which is above the goal (< 75 μg/dL) for this patient/client with end-stage liver disease.
>   OR
> 2) Reference standard: The patient/client serum ammonia is 85 μg/dL which is above (above, below, or percent of) the expected range (11-35 μg/dL).

Sample nutrition assessment and monitoring and evaluation documentation for this outcome

Initial nutrition assessment with patient/client	Patient/client's serum ammonia is 85 μg/dL, above the expected range. Will monitor change in serum ammonia at next encounter.
Reassessment after nutrition intervention	Significant progress toward expected range. Patient/client's serum ammonia 45 μg/dL.

References

The following are some suggested references for indicators, measurement techniques, and reference standards; other references may be appropriate.

1. National Institutes of Health, Clinical Center Test Guide. Available at: http://cclnprod.cc.nih.gov/dlm/testguide.nsf/TestIndex?OpenForm&Count=5000. Accessed October 19, 2006.

2. The Johns Hopkins Hospital. *The Harriet Lane Handbook: A manual for Pediatric House Officers*, 17th ed. St. Louis MO: Mosby; 2005.

*** *Denotes indicator is used for nutrition assessment only. Other indicators are used for both nutrition assessment and nutrition monitoring and evaluation.*

Glucose/Endocrine Profile (BD-1.5)

Definition
Laboratory measures associated with glycemic control and endocrine findings

Nutrition Assessment and Monitoring and Evaluation
Indicators

>Glucose, fasting (mg/dL)
>
>Glucose, casual (mg/dL)
>
>HgbA1c (%)
>
>Preprandial capillary plasma glucose (mg/dL)
>
>Peak postprandial capillary plasma glucose (mg/dL)
>
>Cortisol level (μg/dL)***
>
>IGF-binding protein (ng/mL)***
>
>Thyroid function tests***—TSH, Thyroid stimulating hormone (mIU/L); T4, Thyroxine test (mcg/dL); T3, Triiodothyronine (ng/dL)

Examples of the measurement methods or data sources for these indicators: Biochemical measurement, laboratory report

Typically used with the following domains of nutrition interventions: Food and/or nutrient delivery, nutrition education, nutrition counseling

Typically used to determine and to monitor and evaluate change in the following nutrition diagnoses: Excess or inadequate intake of carbohydrate, energy; inappropriate intake of types of carbohydrates; or inconsistent carbohydrate intake

Clinical judgment must be used to select indicators and determine the appropriate measurement techniques and reference standards for a given patient population and setting. Once identified, these indicators, measurement techniques, and reference standards should be identified in policies and procedures or other documents for use in patient/client records, quality or performance improvement, or in formal research projects.

*** *Denotes indicator is used for nutrition assessment only. Other indicators are used for both nutrition assessment and nutrition monitoring and evaluation.*

Assessment

Biochemical Data, Medical Tests and Procedures Domain – Biochemical and Medical Tests

Glucose/Endocrine Profile (BD-1.5)

Evaluation

Criteria for evaluation
Comparison to Goal or Reference Standard:
    1) Goal (tailored to patient/client's needs)
        OR
    2) Reference standard

Patient/Client Example
Example(s) of one or two of the Nutrition Care Indicators (includes sample initial and reassessment documentation for one of the indicators)

Indicator(s) selected
HgbA1c (%)

Criteria for evaluation
Comparison to Goal or Reference Standard:
    1) Goal: The patient/client's HgbA1c is 7.8%, which is above the expected limit, but is an acceptable goal in a pediatric patient.
        OR
    2) Reference standard: The patient/client's HgbA1c is 11% which is above (above, below, expected limit or range) the expected limit (< 6%).

Sample nutrition assessment and monitoring and evaluation documentation

Initial nutrition assessment with patient/client	Patient/client's HgbA1c is 9%, which is above the expected limit. Will monitor change in HgbA1c at next encounter.
Reassessment after nutrition intervention	Regression from the expected limit. Patient/client's HgbA1c is 10%.

References
The following are some suggested references for indicators, measurement techniques, and reference standards; other references may be appropriate.

1. American Diabetes Association. Diagnosis and classification of diabetes mellitus. Diabetes Care; 29:2006:S43-S48. Available at: http://care.diabetesjournals.org/cgi/content/full/29/suppl_1/s43. Accessed on October 20, 2006.
2. American Diabetes Association. Standards of medical care in diabetes. Diabetes Care; 29:2006:S4-S42. Available at: http://care.diabetesjournals.org/cgi/content/full/29/suppl_1/s4. Accessed on October 20, 2006.
3. American Dietetic Association. Critical illness evidence-based nutrition guideline, 2006. Available at: http://www.adaevidencelibrary.com/topic.cfm?cat=2809. Accessed November 1, 2006.
4. International Diabetes Center. Type 2 diabetes practice guidelines, 2003. Available at: http://www.guideline.gov/summary/summary.aspx?doc_id=4159&nbr=3187. Accessed November 1, 2006.
5. Joslin Diabetes Center. Clinical Guidelines for Adults. Available at: http://www.joslin.org/managing_your_diabetes_joslin_clinical_guidelines.asp. Accessed January 10, 2007.

*** *Denotes indicator is used for nutrition assessment only. Other indicators are used for both nutrition assessment and nutrition monitoring and evaluation.*

Inflammatory Profile (BD-1.6)

Definition
Laboratory measures of inflammatory proteins

Nutrition Assessment
Indicators
C-reactive protein, highly sensitive or hs-CRP (mg/L) [cardiovascular disease]***

Examples of the measurement methods or data sources for these indicators: Direct measurement, medical record

Typically used with the following domains of nutrition interventions: Food and/or nutrient delivery

Typically used to determine the following nutrition diagnoses: Increased nutrient need; inappropriate intake of food fats; excessive exercise

Clinical judgment must be used to select indicators and determine the appropriate measurement techniques and reference standards for a given patient population and setting. Once identified, these indicators, measurement techniques, and reference standards should be identified in policies and procedures or other documents for use in patient/client records, quality or performance improvement, or in formal research projects.

Evaluation

Criteria for evaluation
Comparison to Goal or Reference Standard:
1) Goal (tailored to patient/client's needs)
   OR
2) Reference standard

Patient/Client Example
Example(s) of one or two of the Nutrition Care Indicators (includes sample initial and reassessment documentation for one of the indicators)

Indicator(s) selected
C-reactive protein (mg/L)

*** *Denotes indicator is used for nutrition assessment only. Other indicators are used for both nutrition assessment and nutrition monitoring and evaluation.*

Assessment

Biochemical Data, Medical Tests and Procedures Domain – Biochemical and Medical Tests

Inflammatory Profile (BD-1.6)

Criteria for evaluation

Comparison to Goal or Reference Standard:

1) Goal: Not generally used.

   OR

2) Reference standard: A patient/client has a C-reactive protein level of 4.0 mg/L, which is above (above, below, within expected range) the expected range of 1.0-3.0 mg/L.

Sample nutrition assessment documentation

Nutrition assessment with patient/client	Patient/client's C-reactive protein level is 4.0 mg/L, which is above (above, below, within expected range) the expected range of 1.0-3.0 mg/L.

References:

The following are some suggested references for indicators, measurement techniques, and reference standards; other references may be appropriate.

1. American Heart Association. Inflammation, Heart Disease and Stroke: The Role of C-Reactive Protein. Available at: http://www.americanheart.org/presenter.jhtml?identifier=4648 Accessed on November 26, 2007.

2. NHLBI Workshop Report. C-Reactive Protein: Basic and Clinical Research Needs. Available at: http://www.nhlbi.nih.gov/meetings/workshops/crp/report.htm. Accessed on November 26, 2007.

3. Position of the American Dietetic Association and Dietitians of Canada: Dietary Fatty Acids. *J Amer Diet Assoc*. 2007;107:1599-1611.

*** Denotes indicator is used for nutrition assessment only. Other indicators are used for both nutrition assessment and nutrition monitoring and evaluation.

Lipid Profile (BD-1.7)

Definition
Laboratory measures associated with lipid disorders

Nutrition Assessment and Monitoring and Evaluation
Indicators

Cholesterol, serum (mg/dL)

Cholesterol, HDL (mg/dL)

Cholesterol, LDL (mg/dL)

Cholesterol, non-HDL (mg/dL)

Total cholesterol:HDL cholesterol

LDL:HDL

Triglycerides, serum (mg/dL)

Examples of the measurement methods or data sources for these indicators: Biochemical measurement, laboratory report, patient/client report

Typically used with the following domains of nutrition interventions: Nutrition education, nutrition counseling

Typically used to determine and to monitor and evaluate change in the following nutrition diagnoses: Excess or inadequate intake of fat, energy

Clinical judgment must be used to select indicators and determine the appropriate measurement techniques and reference standards for a given patient population and setting. Once identified, these indicators, measurement techniques, and reference standards should be identified in policies and procedures or other documents for use in patient/client records, quality or performance improvement, or in formal research projects.

Evaluation

Criteria for evaluation
Comparison to Goal or Reference Standard:
1) Goal (tailored to patient/client's needs)
   OR
2) Reference standard

*** *Denotes indicator is used for nutrition assessment only. Other indicators are used for both nutrition assessment and nutrition monitoring and evaluation.*

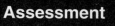

Assessment

Biochemical Data, Medical Tests and Procedures Domain – Biochemical and Medical Tests

Lipid Profile (BD-1.7)

Patient/Client Example
Example(s) of one or two of the Nutrition Care Indicators (includes sample initial and reassessment documentation for one of the indicators)

Indicator(s) selected
LDL cholesterol (mg/dL)

Criteria for evaluation
Comparison to Goal or Reference Standard:
1) Goal: The patient/client's LDL cholesterol is 200 mg/dL compared to a goal of < 100 mg/dL. (Note: While reference standards are generally used for laboratory measures, a goal might be used in a special situation such as this example. The patient/client has a familial hypercholesterolemia where a normal reference standard may not be realistic.)
   OR
2) Reference standard: The patient/client's LDL cholesterol is 159 mg/dL, which is above the expected limit of the NHLBI recommendation of < 100 mg/dL.

Sample nutrition assessment and monitoring and evaluation documentation

Initial nutrition assessment with patient/client	The patient/client LDL cholesterol is 159 mg/dL compared to the NHLBI recommended level of < 100 mg/dL. Will monitor LDL cholesterol at next encounter.
Reassessment after nutrition intervention	Some progress toward goal/reference standard as patient/client's LDL cholesterol is 145 mg/dL.

References
The following are some suggested references for indicators, measurement techniques, and reference standards; other references may be appropriate.

1. Grundy S, Cleeman JI, Bairey Merz CN, Brewer HB, Clark LT, Hunninghake DB, Pasternak RC, Smith SC, Stone NJ, for the Coordinating Committee of the National Cholesterol Education Program, Endorsed by the National Heart, Lung, and Blood Institute, American College of Cardiology Foundation, and American Heart Association. Implications of recent clinical trials for the National Cholesterol Education Program Adult Treatment Panel III guidelines. *Circulation.* 2004; 110: 227-239.

2. Ingelsson E, Schaefer EJ, Contois JH, McNamara JR, Sullivan L, Keyes MJ, Pencina MJ, Schoonmaker C, Wilson PW, D'Agostino RB, Vasan RS. Clinical utility of different lipid measures for prediction of coronary heart disease in men and women. *JAMA.* 2007 Aug 15;298(7):776-85.

3. Nam BH, Kannel WB, D'Agostino RB. Search for an optimal atherogenic lipid risk profile: from the Framingham Study. *Am J Cardiol.* 2006 Feb 1;97(3):372-5.

4. National Institutes of Health, National Heart, Lung, and Blood Institute (NHLBI). Third Report of the Expert Panel on Detection, Evaluation, and Treatment of High Cholesterol in Adults, May 2001. Available at: http://www.nhlbi.nih.gov/guidelines/cholesterol/index.htm. Accessed on October 18, 2006.

5. National Kidney Foundation, K/DOQI Guidelines, 2000. Maintenance Dialysis, Evaluation of Protein-Energy Nutrition Status. Available at: http://www.kidney.org/professionals/kdoqi/guidelines/nut_a06.html. Accessed on October 28, 2006.

*** *Denotes indicator is used for nutrition assessment only. Other indicators are used for both nutrition assessment and nutrition monitoring and evaluation.*

Lipid Profile (BD-1.7)

References, cont'd

6. Onder G, Landi F, Volpato S, Fellin R, Carbonin P, Gambassi G, Bernabei R. Serum cholesterol levels and in-hospital mortality in the elderly. *Am J Med.* 2003;115:265-71.

7. Position of the American Dietetic Association and Dietitians of Canada: Nutrition intervention in the care of persons with human immunodeficiency virus infection. *J Am Diet Assoc.* 2004;104:1425-1441.

8. Ridker PM, Rifai N, Cook NR, Bradwin G, Buring JE. Non-HDL cholesterol, apolipoproteins A-I and B100, standard lipid measures, lipid ratios, and CRP as risk factors for cardiovascular disease in women. *JAMA.* 2005 Jul 20;294(3):326-33.

9. Wang TD, Chen WJ, Chien KL, Seh-Yi Su SS, Hsu HC, Chen MF, Liau CS, Lee YT. Efficacy of cholesterol levels and ratios in predicting future coronary heart disease in a Chinese population. *Am J Cardiol.* 2001 Oct 1;88(7):737-43.

*** *Denotes indicator is used for nutrition assessment only. Other indicators are used for both nutrition assessment and nutrition monitoring and evaluation.*

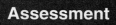
Assessment

Metabolic Rate Profile (BD-1.8)

Definition
Measures associated with or having implications for assessing metabolic rate

Nutrition Assessment and Monitoring and Evaluation
Indicators

Resting metabolic rate, measured (calories/day)***

Respiratory quotient (RQ = CO_2 produced/O_2 consumed)

Note: Use of RQ is considered valid if respiratory factors (hyper-or hypoventilation), equipment failure, measurement protocol violations, or operator errors have not occurred.

Examples of the measurement methods or data sources for these indicators: Direct measurement (indirect calorimetry), medical record

Typically used with the following domains of nutrition interventions: Food and/or nutrient delivery

Typically used to determine the following nutrition diagnoses: Excessive or inadequate intake of parenteral/enteral nutrition; inappropriate infusion of enteral/parenteral nutrition; excessive energy intake; excessive mineral intake; disordered eating pattern; excessive exercise, increased energy expenditure, increased nutrient needs (energy), inadequate protein-energy intake.

Clinical judgment must be used to select indicators and determine the appropriate measurement techniques and reference standards for a given patient population and setting. Once identified, these indicators, measurement techniques, and reference standards should be identified in policies and procedures or other documents for use in patient/client records, quality or performance improvement, or in formal research projects.

Evaluation
Criteria for evaluation
Comparison to Goal or Reference Standard:
1) Goal (tailored to patient/client's needs)
   OR
2) Reference standard

*** *Denotes indicator is used for nutrition assessment only. Other indicators are used for both nutrition assessment and nutrition monitoring and evaluation.*

Metabolic Rate Profile (BD-1.8)

Patient/Client Example

Example(s) of one or two of the Nutrition Care Indicators (includes sample initial and reassessment documentation for one of the indicators)

Indicator(s) selected

Respiratory quotient

Criteria for evaluation

Comparison to Goal or Reference Standard:

1) Goal: Not generally used.

   OR

2) Reference standard: A patient/client on parenteral nutrition support with an RQ of 1.04 which is above (above, below, within expected range) the expected range (0.7-1.0) with no apparent errors in the measurement.

Sample nutrition assessment and/or monitoring and evaluation documentation

Initial nutrition assessment with patient/client	Patient/client's RQ is 1.04, with energy intake from parenteral nutrition 400 kcal higher than measured metabolic rate. No apparent respiratory factors (hyper-or hypoventilation), equipment failure, measurement protocol violations, or operator errors. Will adjust content of parenteral nutrition and re-measure RQ.
Reassessment after nutrition intervention	RQ has dropped to 0.92 with no apparent measurement error. Metabolic rate and calorie intake are matched. Parenteral nutrition has been appropriately adjusted to equal patient's energy requirement.

References

The following are some suggested references for indicators, measurement techniques, and reference standards; other references may be appropriate.

1. American Dietetic Association. Critical Illness Adult Weight Management Evidence-Based Nutrition Practice Guideline. Available at: http://www.adaevidencelibrary.com/topic.cfm?cat=2799. Accessed December 19, 2006.

2. Compher C, Frankenfield D, Keim N, Roth-Yousey L. Best practice methods to apply to measurement of resting metabolic rate in adults: A systematic review. *J Amer Diet Assoc*. 2006;106:881-903.

3. Guidelines for the use of parenteral and enteral nutrition in adult and pediatric patients: Specific guidelines for disease - adults. *J Parenter Enteral Nutr*. 2002;26(Suppl):S61-S96.

4. Guidelines for the use of parenteral and enteral nutrition in adult and pediatric patients: Specific guidelines for disease - pediatrics. *J Parenter Enteral Nutr*. 2002;26(Suppl):S111-S138.

5. McClave SA, Lowen CC, Kleber MJ, McConnell JW, Jung LY, Goldsmith LJ. Clinical use of the respiratory quotient obtained from indirect calorimetry. *J Parenter Enteral Nutr*. 2003;27:21-26.

*** Denotes indicator is used for nutrition assessment only. Other indicators are used for both nutrition assessment and nutrition monitoring and evaluation.

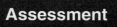

Assessment

Mineral Profile (BD-1.9)

Definition
Laboratory measures associated with body mineral status

Nutrition Assessment and Monitoring and Evaluation
Indicators

Copper, serum or plasma (µg/dL)

Iodine, urinary excretion (µg/24hr)

Zinc, serum or plasma (µg/dL)

Other:

Manganese, urinary excretion (µg/L), blood µg/L, plasma µg/L

Selenium, serum (µmol/L), urinary excretion µg/L or µg/day

Note: Other measures of body mineral status, such as urinary manganese excretion, are provided to offer complete information in the reference sheet. These are rarely used in practice, but may be warranted in limited circumstances.

Calcium, magnesium, phosphorus, and potassium can be found on the Electrolyte and Renal Profile reference sheet.

Serum iron, serum ferritin, and transferrin saturation can be found on the Nutritional Anemia Profile reference sheet.

Thyroid stimulating hormone (↑ TSH as an indicator of excess iodine supplementation) can be found on the Glucose/Endocrine Profile reference sheet.

Examples of the measurement methods or data sources for these indicators: Biochemical measurement, laboratory record

Typically used with the following domains of nutrition interventions: Food and/or nutrient delivery, nutrition education, nutrition counseling

Typically used to determine and to monitor and evaluate change in the following nutrition diagnoses: Excess or inadequate intake of minerals, parenteral nutrition

Clinical judgment must be used to select indicators and determine the appropriate measurement techniques and reference standards for a given patient population and setting. Once identified, these indicators, measurement techniques, and reference standards should be identified in policies and procedures or other documents for use in patient/client records, quality or performance improvement, or in formal research projects.

*** Denotes indicator is used for nutrition assessment only. Other indicators are used for both nutrition assessment and nutrition monitoring and evaluation.*

Mineral Profile (BD-1.9)

Evaluation

Criteria for evaluation

Comparison to Goal or Reference Standard:

    1) Goal (tailored to patient/client's needs)

        OR

    2) Reference standard

Patient/Client Example

Example(s) of one or two of the Nutrition Care Indicators (includes sample initial and reassessment documentation for one of the indicators)

Indicator(s) selected

Zinc, plasma (µg/dL)

Criteria for evaluation

Comparison to Goal or Reference Standard:

    1) Goal: There is no goal generally associated with mineral status.

        OR

    2) Reference standard: The patient/client's plasma zinc is 40 µg/dL which is below (above, below, within expected range) the expected range (66-110 µg/dL) for adults.

Sample nutrition assessment and monitoring and evaluation documentation

Initial nutrition assessment with patient/client	Patient/client's plasma zinc is 40 µg/dL, which is below the expected range for adults. Will monitor change in plasma zinc at next encounter.
Reassessment after nutrition intervention	Goal/reference standard achieved as patient/client's plasma zinc is 90 µg/dL.

References

The following are some suggested references for indicators, measurement techniques, and reference standards; other references may be appropriate.

    1. National Academy of Sciences, Institute of Medicine. *Dietary Reference Intakes for Calcium, Phosphorus, Magnesium, Vitamin D, and Fluoride.* Washington, DC: National Academy Press; 1997.

    2. National Academy of Sciences, Institute of Medicine. *Dietary Reference Intakes for Vitamin A, Vitamin K, Arsenic, Boron, Chromium, Copper, Iodine, Iron, Manganese, Molybdenum, Nickel, Silicon, Vanadium, Zinc.* Washington, DC: National Academy Press; 2001.

    3. National Academy of Sciences, Institute of Medicine. *Dietary Reference Intakes for Vitamin C, Vitamin E, Selenium, and Carotenoids.* Washington, DC: National Academy Press; 2000.

    4. National Academy of Sciences, Institute of Medicine. *Dietary Reference Intakes for Water, Potassium, Sodium, Chloride, and Sulfate.* Washington DC: National Academy Press; 2004.

*** Denotes indicator is used for nutrition assessment only. Other indicators are used for both nutrition assessment and nutrition monitoring and evaluation.

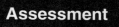
Assessment

Biochemical Data, Medical Tests and Procedures Domain – Biochemical and Medical Tests

Nutritional Anemia Profile (BD-1.10)

Definition
Laboratory measures associated with nutritional anemias

Nutrition Assessment and Monitoring and Evaluation
Indicators

Hemoglobin (g/dL)

Hematocrit (%)

Mean corpuscular volume, MCV (fL)

RBC folate (ng/mL)

Red cell distribution width, RDW (%)

Serum B12 (pg/mL)

Serum methylmalonic acid, MMA (nmol/L)

Serum folate (ng/mL)

Serum homocysteine (µmol/L)

Serum ferritin (ng/mL)

Serum iron (µg/dL)

Total iron-binding capacity (µg/dL)

Transferrin saturation (%)

Examples of the measurement methods or data sources for these indicators: Biochemical measurement, patient/client laboratory record; national/state/local nutrition monitoring and surveillance data

Typically used with the following domains of nutrition interventions: Food and/or nutrient delivery, nutrition education, nutrition counseling, coordination of nutrition care

Typically used to determine and to monitor and evaluate change in the following nutrition diagnoses: Excess or inadequate intake of vitamins or minerals (e.g., iron, B12, folate); altered nutrition-related laboratory values; impaired nutrient utilization

Clinical judgment must be used to select indicators and determine the appropriate measurement techniques and reference standards for a given patient population and setting. Once identified, these indicators, measurement techniques, and reference standards should be identified in policies and procedures or other documents for use in patient/client records, quality or performance improvement, or in formal research projects.

Evaluation

Criteria for evaluation
Comparison to Goal or Reference Standard:
1) Goal (tailored to patient/client's needs)
   OR
2) Reference standard

*** *Denotes indicator is used for nutrition assessment only. Other indicators are used for both nutrition assessment and nutrition monitoring and evaluation.*

Nutritional Anemia Profile (BD-1.10)

Patient/Client Example

Example(s) of one or two of the Nutrition Care Indicators (includes sample initial and reassessment documentation for one of the indicators)

Indicator(s) selected

Hemoglobin (gm/dL)

Serum ferritin (ng/mL)

Criteria for evaluation

Comparison to Goal or Reference Standard:

1) Goal: The patient/client's hemoglobin and hematocrit are below the expected limits for adult males, but are within the goal range for a patient/client receiving hemodialysis.

    OR

2) Reference standard: The patient/client's serum ferritin is 8 ng/mL which is below (above, below, or within expected range) the expected range for adult females.

Sample nutrition assessment and monitoring and evaluation documentation

Initial nutrition assessment with patient/client	Patient/client's serum ferritin is 8 ng/mL, which is below the expected range for adult females. Will monitor change in serum ferritin at next encounter.
Reassessment after nutrition intervention	Patient/client's serum ferritin is 10.9 ng/mL, within the expected range.

References

The following are some suggested references for indicators, measurement techniques, and reference standards; other references may be appropriate.

1. American Dietetic Association. Pamela Charney, Ainsley Malone, eds. *ADA Pocket Guide to Nutrition Assessment*. Chicago, IL: American Dietetic Association; 2004.

2. Centers for Disease Control and Prevention. Recommendations to prevent and control iron deficiency anemia in the United States. *Morb Mortal Wkly Rep*. 2002;51:897-899.

3. The Johns H Johns Hopkins Hospital. *The Harriet Lane Handbook: A manual for Pediatric House Officers*. 17th ed. St. Louis MO: Mosby; 2005.

4. National Kidney Foundation, Dialysis Outcomes Quality Initiative. Available at http://kidney.niddk.nih.gov/kudiseases/pubs/anemia/index.htm#diagnosis. Accessed October 23, 2006.

5. National Library of Medicine and NIH, Medline Plus Medical Encyclopedia. Available at http://www.nlm.nih.gov/medlineplus/encyclopedia.html. Accessed October 25, 2006.

6. US Department of Health and Human Services. *Healthy People 2010* (Conference Edition, in Two Volumes). Washington, DC: January 2000.

*** Denotes indicator is used for nutrition assessment only. Other indicators are used for both nutrition assessment and nutrition monitoring and evaluation.

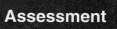

Assessment

Biochemical Data, Medical Tests and Procedures Domain – Biochemical and Medical Tests

Protein Profile (BD-1.11)

Definition
Laboratory measures associated with hepatic and circulating proteins

Nutrition Assessment and Monitoring and Evaluation
Indicators

Albumin (g/dL)

Prealbumin (mg/dL)

Transferrin (mg/dL)

Phenylalanine, plasma (mg/dL)

Tyrosine, plasma (100 µmol/L)

Amino acid, other (by report)***

Note: Heptatic proteins may be useful when monitoring nutritional status over time in conjunction with other markers/information about nutritional status (e.g., body weight, weight change, nutrient intake).

Examples of the measurement methods or data sources for these indicators: Biochemical measurement, laboratory report

Typically used with the following domains of nutrition interventions: Food and/or nutrient delivery, nutrition education, nutrition counseling, coordination of nutrition care

Typically used to determine and to monitor and evaluate change in the following nutrition diagnoses: Increased nutrient needs, evident protein-energy malnutrition, inadequate intake of enteral/parenteral nutrition

Clinical judgment must be used to select indicators and determine the appropriate measurement techniques and reference standards for a given patient population and setting. Once identified, these indicators, measurement techniques, and reference standards should be identified in policies and procedures or other documents for use in patient/client records, quality or performance improvement, or in formal research projects.

Evaluation

Criteria for evaluation
Comparison to Goal or Reference Standard:
1) Goal (tailored to patient/client's needs)
   OR
2) Reference standard

*** *Denotes indicator is used for nutrition assessment only. Other indicators are used for both nutrition assessment and nutrition monitoring and evaluation.*

Protein Profile (BD-1.11)

Patient/Client Example
Example(s) of one or two of the Nutrition Care Indicators (includes sample initial and reassessment documentation for one of the indicators)

Indicator(s) selected
Prealbumin (mg/dL)

Criteria for evaluation
Comparison to Goal or Reference Standard:

    1) Goal: Not generally used.

       OR

    2) Reference standard: The patient/client's prealbumin is 7 mg/dL (above, below, or within expected range), which is below the expected range (16-40 mg/dL) for adults.

Sample nutrition assessment and monitoring and evaluation documentation

Initial nutrition assessment with patient/client	Patient/client's prealbumin is 7.0 mg/dL below the expected range (16-40 mg/dL) for adults. Will monitor change in prealbumin at next encounter.
Reassessment after nutrition intervention	Significant progress toward expected range as patient/client's serum prealbumin is 13.0 mg/dL.

References
The following are some suggested references for indicators, measurement techniques, and reference standards; other references may be appropriate.

1. American Dietetic Association. Pamela Charney, Ainsley Malone, eds. *ADA Pocket Guide to Nutrition Assessment*. Chicago, IL: American Dietetic Association; 2004.
2. ADA Nutrition Care Manual. 2004. Available at: www.nutritioncaremanual.org. Accessed December 10, 2006.
3. Fuhrman MP, Charney P, Mueller CM. Hepatic proteins and nutrition assessment. *J Am Diet Assoc*. 2004;104:1258-1264.
4. The Johns Hopkins Hospital. *The Harriet Lane Handbook: A Manual for Pediatric House Officers*. 17th ed. St. Louis MO: Mosby; 2005.
5. National Kidney Foundation, Clinical Practice Guidelines for Nutrition in Chronic Renal Failure, 2000. Available at http://www.kidney.org/professionals/kdoqi/guidelines/doqi_nut.html. Accessed October 19, 2006.

*** Denotes indicator is used for nutrition assessment only. Other indicators are used for both nutrition assessment and nutrition monitoring and evaluation.

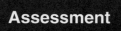

Assessment

Biochemical Data, Medical Tests and Procedures Domain – Biochemical and Medical Tests

Urine Profile (BD-1.12)

Definition
Physical and/or chemical properties of urine

Nutrition Assessment and Monitoring and Evaluation
Indicators
Urine color (by visualization)

Urine osmolality (mOsm/kg H_2O)

Urine specific gravity (number)

Urine tests (e.g., calcium mg/day and/or presence/absence of ketones, sugar, protein)

Urine volume (mL/24 hours; however, in certain populations (e.g., infants) this indicator may be reported in number of wet diapers/day)

Examples of the measurement methods or data sources for these indicators: Observation, biochemical measurement, laboratory report, patient/client report

Typically used with the following domains of nutrition interventions: Food and/or nutrient delivery, coordination of nutrition care

Typically used to determine and to monitor and evaluate change in the following nutrition diagnoses: Inadequate or excessive fluid intake; inadequate or excessive enteral/parenteral nutrition

Clinical judgment must be used to select indicators and determine the appropriate measurement techniques and reference standards for a given patient population and setting. Once identified, these indicators, measurement techniques, and reference standards should be identified in policies and procedures or other documents for use in patient/client records, quality or performance improvement, or in formal research projects.

Evaluation

Criteria for evaluation
Comparison to Goal or Reference Standard:
1) Goal (tailored to patient/client's needs)
   OR
2) Reference standard

*** *Denotes indicator is used for nutrition assessment only. Other indicators are used for both nutrition assessment and nutrition monitoring and evaluation.*

Urine Profile (BD-1.12)

Patient/Client Example

Example(s) of one or two of the Nutrition Care Indicators (includes sample initial and reassessment documentation for one of the indicators)

Indicator(s) selected

Urine specific gravity

Criteria for evaluation

Comparison to Goal or Reference Standard:

    1) Goal: Not generally used for this indicator.

      OR

    2) Reference standard: The patient/client's urine specific gravity is 1.050, which is above (above, below, within expected range) the expected range (1.003-1.030).

Sample nutrition assessment and monitoring and evaluation documentation

Initial nutrition assessment with patient/client	Patient/client's urine specific gravity is 1.050, which is above the expected range. Will monitor change in urine specific gravity at next encounter.
Reassessment after nutrition intervention	Significant progress toward goal, patient/client's urine specific gravity is 1.035, which is within the expected range.

References

The following are some suggested references for indicators, measurement techniques, and reference standards; other references may be appropriate.

    1. American Dietetic Association. Pamela Charney, Ainsley Malone, eds. *ADA Pocket Guide to Nutrition Assessment*. Chicago, IL: American Dietetic Association; 2004.

    2. Armstrong, LE. Hydration assessment techniques. *Nutr Rev*. 2005;63(6 pt 2):S40-54.

    3. National Institutes of Health, Clinical Center Test Guide. Available at: http://cclnprod.cc.nih.gov/dlm/testguide.nsf/TestIndex?OpenForm&Count=5000. Accessed October 27, 2006.

*** Denotes indicator is used for nutrition assessment only. Other indicators are used for both nutrition assessment and nutrition monitoring and evaluation.

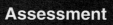

Assessment

Biochemical Data, Medical Tests and Procedures Domain – Biochemical and Medical Tests

Vitamin Profile (BD-1.13)

Definition
Laboratory measures associated with body vitamin status

Nutrition Assessment and Monitoring and Evaluation
Indicators

Vitamin A, serum or plasma retinol (µg/dL)

Vitamin C, plasma or serum (mg/dL)

Vitamin D, 25-hydroxy (ng/mL)

Vitamin E, plasma alpha-tocopherol (mg/dL)

Thiamin, activity coefficient for erythrocyte transketolase activity (µg/mL/hr)

Riboflavin, activity coefficient for erythrocyte glutathione reductase activity (IU/g hemoglobin)

Niacin, urinary N'methyl-nicotinamide concentration (µmol/day)

Vitamin B6, plasma or serum pyridoxal 5'phosphate concentration (ng/mL)

Other:

> Pantothenic acid, urinary pantothenate excretion (mg/day)
>
> Biotin, urinary 3-hydroxyisovaleric acid excretion (mmol/mmol creatinine) or lymphocyte propionyl-CoA carboxylase in pregnancy [pmol/(min × mg)]
>
> Choline, serum alanine amino transferase (units/L)

Note: Other measures of body vitamin status, such as urinary panothenate excretion, are provided to offer complete information in the reference sheet. These are rarely used in practice, but may be warranted in limited circumstances.

Measures for folate and Vitamin B12 can be found on the Nutritional Anemia Profile reference sheet.

Measures related to Vitamin K (PT, PTT, INR) can be found on the GI Profile reference sheet.

Examples of the measurement methods or data sources for these indicators: Biochemical measurement, patient/client record

Typically used with the following domains of nutrition interventions: Food and/or nutrient delivery, coordination of nutrition care

*** Denotes indicator is used for nutrition assessment only. Other indicators are used for both nutrition assessment and nutrition monitoring and evaluation.*

Vitamin Profile (BD-1.13)

Typically used to determine and to monitor and evaluate change in the following nutrition diagnoses: Excess or inadequate intake of vitamins

Clinical judgment must be used to select indicators and determine the appropriate measurement techniques and reference standards for a given patient population and setting. Once identified, these indicators, measurement techniques, and reference standards should be identified in policies and procedures or other documents for use in patient/client records, quality or performance improvement, or in formal research projects.

Evaluation

Criteria for evaluation
Comparison to Goal or Reference Standard:
  1) Goal (tailored to patient/client's needs)
     OR
  2) Reference standard

Patient/Client Example

Example(s) of one or two of the Nutrition Care Indicators (includes sample initial and reassessment documentation for one of the indicators)

Indicator(s) selected:
Vitamin A, serum retinol (µg/dL)

Criteria for evaluation
Comparison to Goal or Reference Standard:
  1) Goal: Not generally used for this indicator.
     OR
  2) Reference standard: The patient/client's serum retinol is 95 µg/dL which is above (above, below, within expected range) the expected range (10-60 µg/dL).

Sample nutrition assessment and monitoring and evaluation documentation

Initial nutrition assessment with patient/client	Patient/client's serum retinol is 95 µg/dL, which is above the expected range. Will monitor change in serum retinol at next encounter, along with vitamin A and beta-carotene intake.
Reassessment after nutrition intervention	Significant progress toward expected range. Patient/client's retinol is 70 µg/dL.

*** Denotes indicator is used for nutrition assessment only. Other indicators are used for both nutrition assessment and nutrition monitoring and evaluation.

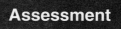

Assessment

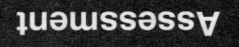

Biochemical Data, Medical Tests and Procedures Domain – Biochemical and Medical Tests

Vitamin Profile (BD-1.13)

References

The following are some suggested references for indicators, measurement techniques, and reference standards; other references may be appropriate.

1. ADA Nutrition Care Manual. 2004. Available at: www.nutritioncaremanual.org. Accessed December 11, 2006.

2. Grooper SS, Smith JL, Groff JL. *Advanced nutrition and human metabolism*. Thomson Wadsorth, 2005.

3. Guidelines for the use of parenteral and enteral nutrition in adult and pediatric patients: Normal requirements - adults. *J Parenter Enteral Nutr*. 2002;26(Suppl):S22-S24.

4. Guidelines for the use of parenteral and enteral nutrition in adult and pediatric patients: Normal requirements - pediatrics. *J Parenter Enteral Nutr*. 2002;26(Suppl):S25-S32.

5. McMahon RJ. Biotin in metabolism and molecular biology. *Ann Rev Nutr*. 2002;22:221-239.

6. Monsen ER. Dietary Reference Intakes for the antioxidant nutrients: Vitamin C, vitamin E, selenium, and carotenoids. *J Am Diet Assoc*. 2000; 100:637-640.

7. National Academy of Sciences, Institute of Medicine. *Dietary Reference Intakes for Calcium, Phosphorus, Magnesium, Vitamin D, and Fluoride. Washington*, DC: National Academy Press; 1997.

8. National Academy of Sciences, Institute of Medicine. *Dietary Reference Intakes: Thiamin, riboflavin, niacin, vitamin B6, folate, vitamin B12, pantothenic acid, biotin, and choline*. National Academy Press. Washington, DC, 1998.

9. National Academy of Sciences, Institute of Medicine. *Dietary Reference Intakes for Vitamin A, Vitamin K, Arsenic, Boron, Chromium, Copper, Iodine, Iron, Manganese, Molybdenum, Nickel, Silicon, Vanadium, and Zinc*. National Academy Press, Washington, DC, 2001.

10. National Academy of Sciences, Institute of Medicine. *Dietary Reference Intakes: Vitamin C, Vitamin E, Selenium, and Carotenoids*. National Academy Press, Washington, DC, 2000.

11. Stratton SL, Bogusiewicz A, Mock MM, Mock NI, Wells AM, Mock DM. Lymphoctye propionyl-CoA carboxylase and its activation by biotin are sensitive indicators of marginal biotin deficiency in humans. *Am J Clin Nutr*. 2006;84:384-388.

12. The Johns Hopkins Hospital. *The Harriet Lane Handbook: A manual for Pediatric House Officers*, 17th ed. St. Louis MO: Mosby; 2005.

13. Trumbo P, Yates A, Schlicker S, Poos M. Dietary Reference Intakes: Vitamin A, Vitamin K, Arsenic, Boron, Chromium, Copper, Iodine, Iron, Manganese, Molybdenum, Nickel, Silicon, Vanadium, and Zinc. *J Am Diet Assoc*. 2001;101:294-301.

14. Yates A, Schlicker SA, Suitor CW. Dietary Reference Intakes: The new basis for recommendations for calcium and related nutrients, B vitamins, and choline. *J Am Diet Assoc*. 1998;98:699-706.

15. Zempleni J, Mock DM. Biotin biochemistry and human requirements. *J Nutr Biochem*. 1999;10:128-138.

*** *Denotes indicator is used for nutrition assessment only. Other indicators are used for both nutrition assessment and nutrition monitoring and evaluation.*

Nutrition-Focused Physical Findings (PD-1.1)

Definition
Nutrition-related physical characteristics associated with pathophysiological states derived from a nutrition-focused physical exam, interview, or the medical record

Nutrition Assessment and Monitoring and Evaluation
Indicators (Note: Presence or absence unless otherwise specified)

- Overall appearance***
  - Body positioning, e.g., muscle contractures***
  - Body habitus, specify***
  - Cushingoid appearance***
  - Amputations, specify***
  - Ability to communicate***
  - Affect, specify***
  - Tanner stage, specify***
- Body language (note: varies by culture), specify***
- Cardiovascular-pulmonary system
  - edema, pulmonary; crackles or rales
  - shortness of breath***
- Extremities, muscles and bones
  - bones, specify, obvious prominence, fragility, widening at ends
  - change in how clothes fit, specify
  - edema, peripheral, specify

- fat, subcutaneous, specify loss or excess
- fatigue
- feeling cold all of the time
- hands/feet, specify, cyanosis, tingling and numbness
- joint, arthralgia, effusions***
- joint mobility, wrist/digit/arm/knee/hip movement***
- muscle mass, specify
- muscle soreness or weakness
- nails, nail beds, specify, blue, clubbing, pale, other
- Russell's sign
- Digestive system (mouth to rectum):
  - belching, excessive
  - cheilosis
  - dry mucus membranes, xerostomia
  - feeling of food "stuck" in throat
  - gingivitis***
  - heart burn
  - hoarse or wet voice***

- ketone smell on breath, halitosis
- lesions, oral or esophageal
- lips, specify (dry or cracked, poor closure, drooling)***
- malformations, oral, e.g., cleft palate or other***
- mastication, altered, specify***
- mucosal edema***
- parotid glands, swollen***
- polydipsia
- pouching***
- stomatitis
- swallow function, compromised or painful***
- suck, swallow, breath coordination (infants)***
- taste alterations, specify
- teeth, specify (edentulous, partially or completely)***
- tongue, specify, bright red, magenta, dry cracked, glossitis, impaired movement, frenulum abnormality***

*** *Denotes indicator is used for nutrition assessment only. Other indicators are used for both nutrition assessment and nutrition monitoring and evaluation.*

Edition: 2009

Assessment

Nutrition-Focused Physical Findings (PD-1.1)

- Digestive system (mouth to rectum), cont'd:
  - abdominal distension, bloating, cramping, pain
  - appetite, specify***
  - ascites
  - bowel function, including flatus, specify, e.g., type, frequency, volume
  - bowel sounds, specify, normal, hyperactive, hypoactive***
  - epigastric pain
  - nausea
  - satiety, specify
  - vomiting
- Eyes and head
  Eyes:
  - bitot's spots
  - night blindness
  - sclera, jaundiced***
  - sunken eyes
  - vision, specify***
  - xerophthalmia

- Head:
  - fontanelle, bulging or sunken***
  - hair, specify, brittle, lifeless, coiled, loss
  - headache
  - lanugo hair formation
  - nasal mucosa, dry
  - olfactory sense, altered, specify***
  - temporal wasting
- Nerves and cognition
  - confusion, loss of concentration
  - cranial nerve evaluation, specify***
  - dizziness***
  - motor, gait disturbance
  - neurological changes, other, specify***
  - vibratory and position sense, specify
- Skin
  - acanthanosis nigricans
  - calcinosis
  - changes consistent with nutrient deficiency/excess, specify

- dermatitis
- dry, scaly
- ecchymosis
- erythema, scaling and peeling
- fistula output, specify volume
- follicular hyperkeratosis
- integrity, turgor, specify
- jaundice***
- perifolicular hemorrhages
- petechiae
- pressure ulcers, specify location and stage
- pruritis***
- seborrheic dermatitis
- wound healing, specify
- xanthomas
- Vital signs
  - blood pressure (mmHg)
  - heart rate (beats/min)***
  - respiratory rate (breaths/min)
  - temperature (degrees)***

Examples of the measurement methods or data sources for these indicators: Direct observation, patient/client report, medical record

Typically used with the following domains of nutrition interventions: Food and nutrient delivery, nutrition education, nutrition counseling, coordination of care

*** Denotes indicator is used for nutrition assessment only. Other indicators are used for both nutrition assessment and nutrition monitoring and evaluation.

Nutrition-Focused Physical Findings (PD-1.1)

Typically used to determine and to monitor and evaluate change in the following nutrition diagnoses: Excess or inadequate intake of sodium, vitamins/minerals, fluid, parenteral/enteral nutrition; overweight/obesity, underweight, unintentional weight loss

Clinical judgment must be used to select indicators and determine the appropriate measurement techniques and reference standards for a given patient population and setting. Once identified, these indicators, measurement techniques, and reference standards should be identified in policies and procedures or other documents for use in patient/client records, quality or performance improvement, or in formal research projects.

Evaluation

Criteria for evaluation

Comparison to Goal or Reference Standard:

    1) Goal (tailored to patient/client's needs)

       OR

    2) Reference standard

Patient/Client Example

Example(s) of one or two of the Nutrition Care Indicators (includes sample initial and reassessment documentation for one of the indicators)

Indicator(s) selected

Blood pressure (mmHg)

Criteria for evaluation

Comparison to Goal or Reference Standard:

    1) Goal: The patient/client has reduced blood pressure to goal of 135/85 mmHg with weight loss.

       OR

    2) Reference standard: The patient/client's blood pressure is 150/90 mmHg, which is above (above, below) the expected limit (<120/80 mmHg) consistent with Stage I Hypertension.

Sample nutrition assessment and monitoring and evaluation documentation

Initial nutrition assessment with patient/client	Patient/client's blood pressure is 150/90 mmHg, which is above the expected limit consistent with Stage I hypertension. Will monitor change in blood pressure at next encounter.
Reassessment after nutrition intervention	Significant progress toward expected limit. Patient/client's blood pressure is 135/82 mmHg.

*** *Denotes indicator is used for nutrition assessment only. Other indicators are used for both nutrition assessment and nutrition monitoring and evaluation.*

Assessment

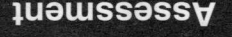
Nutrition-Focused Physical Findings (PD-1.1)

References

The following are some suggested references for indicators, measurement techniques, and reference standards; other references may be appropriate.

1. American Dietetic Association. Critical illness evidence-based nutrition guideline, 2006. Available at: http://www.adaevidencelibrary.com/topic.cfm?cat=2809. Accessed November 5, 2006.

2. Pamela Charney, Ainsley Malone, eds. *ADA Pocket Guide to Nutrition Assessment*. Chicago, IL: American Dietetic Association; 2004.

3. Centers for Medicare and Medicaid Services. Minimum Data Set (MDS)-Version 2.0 for Nursing Home Resident Assessment and Care Screening Basic Assessment Tracking Form. Available at: http://www.cms.hhs.gov/MDS20SWSpecs/Downloads/MDS%20Tracking%20Form.pdf. Accessed November 14, 2006.

4. Mackle TJ, Touger-Decker R, Maillet JO, Holland BK. Registered dietitians' use of physical assessment parameters in professional practice. *J Am Diet Assoc*. 2003;103:1632-1638.

5. National Institutes of Health, National Heart, Lung, and Blood Institute. The Seventh Report of the Joint National Committee on Prevention, Detection, Evaluation, and Treatment of High Blood Pressure. Available at: http://www.nhlbi.nih.gov/guidelines/hypertension/express.pdf. Accessed October 24, 2006.

6. Position of the American Dietetic Association: Oral health and nutrition. *J Amer Diet Assoc*. 2003;103:615-625.

7. Radler DR and Touger-Decker R. Nutrition Screening in Oral Health. *Topics in Clinical Nutrition* 2005;20(3):181-188.

8. U.S. Preventive Services Task Force (USPSTF). Screening for high blood pressure: recommendations and rationale. Rockville (MD): Agency for Healthcare Research and Quality (AHRQ), 2003. Available at: http://www.guideline.gov/summary/summary.aspx?doc_id=3853&nbr=003068&string=AHRQ+AND+guideline. Accessed on November 14, 2006.

*** *Denotes indicator is used for nutrition assessment only. Other indicators are used for both nutrition assessment and nutrition monitoring and evaluation.*

Personal Data (CH-1.1)

Definition

General patient/client information such as age, gender, race/ethnicity, occupation, tobacco use, and physical disability

Nutrition Assessment:

Indicators

Age***
- Age in days (neonates)***
- Age in months (up to 36 months)***
- Age in years***
- Other (e.g., age adjusted)***

Gender***
- Female***
- Male***

Race/ethnicity***
- White***
- Black/African American***
- Hispanic ethnicity***
- Asian***
- Other (specify)***

Language***
- English***
- Spanish***
- Other (specify)***

Literacy factors***
- Language barrier***
- Low literacy***

Education***
- Years of education (Year of education)***

Role in family***
- specify***

Tobacco use***
- Yes***
  - Average number cigarettes smoked per day (number/day)***
  - Total number of other tobacco products used/day (number/day)***
  - Number years tobacco products used on a regular basis (years)***
- No***

Physical disability***
- Eyesight impaired***
- Hearing impaired***
- Other (specify)***

Mobility***
- House bound***
- Bed or chair bound***
- Tremors (Parkinson's)***
- Other (specify)***

Examples of the measurement methods or data sources for these outcome indicators: Patient/client report, medical record, referring health care provider or agency, surveys, administrative data sets

Typically used with following domains of nutrition interventions: Food and/or Nutrient Delivery, nutrition education, nutrition counseling, coordination of nutrition care

*** *Denotes indicator is used for nutrition assessment only. Other indicators are used for both nutrition assessment and nutrition monitoring and evaluation.*

Assessment

Client History Domain – Personal History

Personal Data (CH-1.1)

Typically used to determine the following nutrition diagnoses: N/A

Clinical judgment must be used to select indicators and determine the appropriate measurement techniques and reference standards for a given patient population and setting. Once identified, these indicators, measurement techniques, and reference standards should be identified in policies and procedures or other documents for use in patient/client records, quality or performance improvement, or in formal research projects.

Evaluation

Criteria for evaluation
Comparison to Goal or Reference Standard:
1) Goal (tailored to patient/client's needs)
   OR
2) Reference standard

Patient/Client Example(s)
Example(s) of one or two of the Nutrition Care Indicators (includes sample initial assessment documentation for one of the indicators)

Indicator(s) selected
Age, race/ethnicity, gender and education level

Criteria for evaluation
Comparison to Goal or Reference Standard:
1) Goal: Not typically used
   OR
2) Reference standard: No standard exists

Sample nutrition assessment documentation

Initial nutrition assessment with patient/client	Patient/client is a 40-year-old African American male with new onset type 2 diabetes, education level 7th grade

References
The following are some suggested references for indicators, measurement techniques, and reference standards for the outcome; other references may be appropriate.

1. Charney P, Malone A eds. *ADA Pocket Guide to Nutrition Assessment*. Chicago, IL, The Amercian Dietetic Association; 2004.
2. Loenberg BL. *ADA Pocket Guide to Pediatric Nutriton Assessment*. Chicago, IL, The Amercian Dietetic Association; 2004.

*** Denotes indicator is used for nutrition assessment only. Other indicators are used for both nutrition assessment and nutrition monitoring and evaluation.

Patient/Client or Family Nutrition-Oriented Medical/Health History (CH-2.1)

Definition
Patient/client or family member disease states, conditions, and illnesses that may impact nutritional status

Nutrition Assessment
Indicators

Patient/client chief nutrition complaint (specify)***

Cardiovascular***
- Cardiovascular disease***
- Congestive heart failure***
- Hyperlipidemia***
- Hypertension***
- Stroke***
- Other***

Endocrine/metabolism***
- Cystic fibrosis***
- Diabetes mellitus***
- Diabetes, gestational***
- Inborn errors***
- Malnutrition/failure to thrive***
- Metabolic syndrome***
- Obesity***
- Overweight***
    Specify duration:***
- Other (specify)***

Excretory***
- Dehydration***
- Renal failure, acute***
- Renal failure, chronic***
- Other (specify)***

Gastrointestinal***
- Crohn's disease***
- Diverticulitis/osis***
- Dyspepsia***
- Inflammatory bowel disease***
- Lactase deficiency***
- Liver disease***
- Pancreatic disease (specify)***
- Other (specify)***

Gynecological***
- Amenorrhea***
- Lactating***
- Mastitis***
- Perimenopausal/postmenopausal***
- Pregnant***
    - Gestational age (weeks)***
    - Single fetuses***
    - Multiple fetus (specify)***
- Other (specify)***

Hematology/oncology***
- Anemia (specify)***
- Cancer (specify)***
- Other (specify)***

Immune***
- AIDS/HIV***

Food allergies***
- Sepsis/severe infection***
- Other (specify)***

Integumentary***
- Burns***
- Other (specify)***

Musculo-skeletal***
- Multiple trauma/fractures***
- Osteoporosis***
- Other (specify)***

Neurological***
- Developmental delay***
- Other (specify) ***

Psychological***
- Alcoholism***
- Cognitive impairment***
- Dementia/Alzheimer's***
- Depression***
- Eating disorder (specify)***
- Psychosis***
- Other (specify)***

Respiratory***
- Chronic obstructive pulmonary disease***
- Other (specify)***

*** Denotes indicator is used for nutrition assessment only. Other indicators are used for both nutrition assessment and nutrition monitoring and evaluation.

Edition: 2009

169

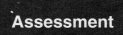

Patient/Client or Family Nutrition-Oriented Medical/Health History (CH-2.1)

Examples of the measurement methods or data sources for these outcome indicators: Medical record, referring health care provider or agency

Typically used with following domains of nutrition interventions: Nutrition education, nutrition counseling

Typically used to determine the following nutrition diagnoses: All

Clinical judgment must be used to select indicators and determine the appropriate measurement techniques and reference standards for a given patient population and setting. Once identified, these indicators, measurement techniques, and reference standards should be identified in policies and procedures or other documents for use in patient/client records, quality or performance improvement, or in formal research projects.

Evaluation

Criteria for evaluation
Comparison to Goal or Reference Standard:
  1) Goal (tailored to patient/client's needs)
     OR
  2) Reference standard

Patient Example(s)
Example(s) of one or two of the Nutrition Care Indicators (includes sample initial assessment documentation for one of the indicators)

Indicator(s) selected
Cardiovascular disease (CVD)

Criteria for evaluation
Comparison to Goal or Reference Standard:
  1) Goal: Not typically used
     OR
  2) Reference standard: No reference standard exists.

Sample nutrition assessment documentation

Initial nutrition assessment with patient/client	Patient/client with history of CVD. Recommend the Therapeutic Lifestyle Changes (TLC) diet in accordance with National Cholesterol Education Program Adult Treatment Panel III guidelines

*** *Denotes indicator is used for nutrition assessment only. Other indicators are used for both nutrition assessment and nutrition monitoring and evaluation.*

Patient/Client or Family Nutrition-Oriented Medical/Health History (CH-2.1)

References
The following are some suggested references for indicators, measurement techniques, and reference standards for the outcome; other references may be appropriate.

1. Charney P, Malone A eds. *ADA Pocket Guide to Nutrition Assessment*. Chicago, IL, The Amercian Dietetic Association; 2004.

2. American Heart Association Nutrition Committee: Lichtenstein, A, Appel, L, Brands M, Carnethon M, Daniels S, Franch HA, Franklin B, Kris-Etherton P, Harris WS, Howard B, Karanja N, Lefevre M, Rudel L, Sacks F, Van Horn L, Winston M, Wylie-Rosett J. Diet and lifestyle recommendations revision 2006: a scientific statement from the American Heart Association Nutrition Committee. *Circulation*. 2006;114:82-96.

3. Bantle JP, Wylie-Rosett J, Albright AL, Apovian CM, Clark NG, Franz MJ, Hoogwerf BJ, Lichtenstein AH, Mayer-Davis E, Mooradian AD, Wheeler ML. Nutrition recommendations and interventions for diabetes-2006: a position statement of the American Diabetes Association. *Diabetes Care*. 2006;29:2140-2157.

4. US Departments of Agriculture and Health and Human Services. Dietary Guidelines for Americans 2005. Available at: www.healthierus.gov/dietaryguidelines/.

5. US Department of Health and Human Services. National Institutes of Health. National Heart, Lung and Blood Institute. *Third Report of the Expert Panel on Detection, Evaluation, and Treatment of High Blood Cholesterol in Adults (Adult Treatment Panel III)*. Bethesda, MD: National Institutes of Health; 2001

6. ADA Nutrition Care Manual. 2006. Available at: www.nutritioncaremanual.org. Accessed December 11, 2006.

7. Murray KO, Holli BB, Calabrese RJ. *Communication & Education Skills for Dietetics Professionals*, 4th Ed. Philadelphia: Lippincott Williams & Wilkins, 2003.

*** *Denotes indicator is used for nutrition assessment only. Other indicators are used for both nutrition assessment and nutrition monitoring and evaluation.*

Assessment

Client History Domain – Patient/Client/Family Medical/Health History

Treatments/Therapy/Complementary/Alternative Medicine (CH-2.2)

Definition
Documented medical or surgical treatments, complementary and alternative medicine that may impact nutritional status of the patient

Nutrition Assessment
Indicators

Medical treatment/therapy***
- Chemotherapy***
- Dialysis***
- Mechanical ventilation***
- Ostomy (specify)***
- Radiation therapy***
- Other (specify, e.g., speech, OT, PT)***

Surgical treatment***
- Coronary artery bypass (CABG)***
- Gastric bypass (specify type)***

- Intestinal resection***
- Joint/orthopedic surgery/replacement***
- Limb amputation***
- Organ transplant (specify)***
- Total gastrectomy***
- Other (specify)***

Complementary/alternative medicine, specify (e.g., homeopathy, ayurveda, yoga)***

Examples of the measurement methods or data sources for these indicators: Patient/client interview, medical record, referring health care provider or agency

Typically used with following domains of nutrition interventions: Food and/or Nutrient Delivery, nutrition education, nutrition counseling, coordination of nutrition care

Typically used to determine the following nutrition diagnoses: Impaired nutrient utilization, increased nutrient needs, altered gastrointestinal function, biting/chewing (masticatory) difficulty, involuntary weight loss.

Clinical judgment must be used to select indicators and determine the appropriate measurement techniques and reference standards for a given patient population and setting. Once identified, these indicators, measurement techniques, and reference standards should be identified in policies and procedures or other documents for use in patient/client records, quality or performance improvement, or in formal research projects.

*** Denotes indicator is used for nutrition assessment only. Other indicators are used for both nutrition assessment and nutrition monitoring and evaluation.

Treatments/Therapy/Complementary/Alternative Medicine (CH-2.2)

Evaluation

Criteria for evaluation
Comparison to Goal or Reference Standard:
1) Goal (tailored to patient/client's needs)
   OR
2) Reference standard

Patient/Client Example(s)
Example(s) of one or two of the Nutrition Care Indicators (includes sample initial assessment documentation for one of the indicators)

Indicator(s) selected
Radiation therapy

Criteria for evaluation
Comparison to Goal or Reference Standard:
1) Goal: Patient/client receiving radiation therapy for lung cancer, experiencing decreased appetite and pain with eating. Goal is to optimize nutrition during radiation therapy.
   OR
2) Reference standard: No standards exist.

Sample nutrition assessment documentation

Initial nutrition assessment with patient/client	Patient/client receiving radiation therapy for lung cancer, experiencing decreased appetite due to fatigue and pain with eating.

References
The following are some suggested references for indicators, measurement techniques, and reference standards for the outcome; other references may be appropriate.
1. Charney P, Malone A eds. *ADA Pocket Guide to Nutrition Assessment.* Chicago, IL, The Amercian Dietetic Association; 2004.
2. ADA Nutrition Care Manual. 2006. Available at: www.nutritioncaremanual.org. Accessed December 11, 2006.
3. ADA Oncology Nutrition Practice Group, Elliott L, Molseed LL, McCallum PD, Grant B. *The clinical guide to oncology nutrition,* 2nd ed. Chicago, IL: American Dietetic Association; 2006.
4. ADA Evidence Analysis Library. Accessed on: 10/28/2006 from http://www.ada.portalxm.com/eal/category.cfm?cid=5&cat=0
5. U.S. National Library of Medicine, National Institutes of Health, Medline Plus. Accessed on: 12/18/2007 from http://www.nlm.nih.gov/medlineplus/canceralternativetherapies.html
6. National Institutes of Health and the National Center for Complementary and Alternative Medicine. Accessed on: 11/ 29/2007 from http://nccam.nih.gov/health/.

*** Denotes indicator is used for nutrition assessment only. Other indicators are used for both nutrition assessment and nutrition monitoring and evaluation.

Edition: 2009   173

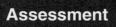

Assessment

Social History (CH-3.1)

Definition

Patient/client information such as socioeconomic factors, housing situation, medical support, occupation, religion, history of recent crisis and involvement in social groups

Nutrition Assessment

Indicators

Socioeconomic factors***
- Economic constraints (major/minor)***
- Access to medical care (full/limited/none)***
- Diverts food money to other needs***
- Other (specify)***

Living/housing situation***
- Lives alone***
- Lives with family member/caregiver***
- Homeless***

Domestic issues***
- Specify***

Social and medical support***
- Family members***
- Caregivers***
- Community group/senior center/church***
- Support group attendance (e.g., weight control, substance abuse, etc)***
- Other (specify)***

Geographic location of home***
- Urban***
- Rural***
- Limited exposure to sunlight (vitamin D)***
- Other (specify)***

Occupation***
- Stay-at-home mother***
- Student***
- Retired***
- Specify***

Religion***
- Catholic***
- Jewish***
- Protestant***
    Specify***
- Islam***
- Specify***

History of recent crisis***
- Job loss***
- Family member death***
- Trauma, surgery***
- Other (specify)***

Daily stress level (high, moderate, low)***

*** Denotes indicator is used for nutrition assessment only. Other indicators are used for both nutrition assessment and nutrition monitoring and evaluation.

Social History (CH-3.1)

Examples of the measurement methods or data sources for these outcome indicators: Patient/client report, medical record, referring health care provider or agency

Typically used with following domains of nutrition interventions: Food and/or Nutrient Delivery, nutrition education, nutrition counseling, coordination of nutrition care

Typically used to determine the following nutrition diagnoses: All

Clinical judgment must be used to select indicators and determine the appropriate measurement techniques and reference standards for a given patient population and setting. Once identified, these indicators, measurement techniques, and reference standards should be identified in policies and procedures or other documents for use in patient/client records, quality or performance improvement, or in formal research projects.

Evaluation

Criteria for evaluation
Comparison to Goal or Reference Standard:
    1) Goal (tailored to patient/client's needs)
       OR
    2) Reference standard

Patient/Client Example(s)

Example(s) of one or two of the Nutrition Care Indicators (includes sample initial assessment documentation for one of the indicators)

Indicator(s) selected
Age, race/ethnicity and gender

Criteria for evaluation
Comparison to Goal or Reference Standard:
    1) Goal: Not typically used
       OR
    2) Reference standard: No reference standard exists.

*** *Denotes indicator is used for nutrition assessment only. Other indicators are used for both nutrition assessment and nutrition monitoring and evaluation.*

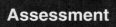

Assessment

Client History Domain – Social History

Social History (CH-3.1)

Sample nutrition assessment documentation

Initial nutrition assessment with patient/client	Patient/client is house bound, lives in a rural area and receives one meal/day from Meals on Wheels.

References

The following are some suggested references for indicators, measurement techniques, and reference standards for the outcome; other references may be appropriate.

1. Charney P, Malone A eds. *ADA Pocket Guide to Nutrition Assessment*. Chicago, IL, The Amercian Dietetic Association; 2004.
2. Loenberg BL. *ADA Pocket Guide to Pediatric Nutriton Assessment*. Chicago, IL, The Amercian Dietetic Association; 2004.
3. Murray KO, Holli BB, Calabrese RJ. *Communication & Education Skills for Dietetics Professionals*, 4t Ed. Philadelphia: Lippincott Williams & Wilkins, 2003.

*** *Denotes indicator is used for nutrition assessment only. Other indicators are used for both nutrition assessment and nutrition monitoring and evaluation.*

Estimated Energy Needs (CS-1.1)

Definition
Estimated quantity of total energy needed for nutritional adequacy.

Purpose
Identify appropriate reference standard of energy intake needs for individual patients/clients. Utilized as a basis of comparison to assess adequacy or excessiveness of patient/client's estimated total energy intake as compared to estimated needs and for development of the nutrition prescription.

Indicators

Total estimated energy needs assumed to be consistent with the Dietary Reference Intakes unless otherwise specified: (specify, e.g., calories/day, calories/kg/day)

	EAR	**RDA**	**AI**	**UL**	**Other**
Energy*					Formula

EAR — Estimated Average Requirement
RDA — Recommended Dietary Allowance
AI — Adequate Intake
UL — Tolerable Upper Intake Level
See DRI Interpretation Table on page 35.

Method for estimating energy needs:

- Estimated (specify, e.g., patient/client goal or nutrition prescription, equation/method and adjustments for activity, stress, pregnancy, breastfeeding, and/or fever)
- Measured (specify assessment method)

References
The following are some suggested references; other references may be appropriate.

1. American Dietetic Association. Pamela Charney, Ainsley Malone, eds. *ADA Pocket Guide to Nutrition Assessment.* Chicago, IL: American Dietetic Association; 2004.

2. American Dietetic Association. Beth Leonberg, ed. *ADA Pocket Guide to Pediatric Nutrition Assessment.* Chicago, IL: American Dietetic Association; 2008.

3. American Dietetic Association Evidenced-based Library. Available at: http://www.adaevidencelibrary.com/.

4. American Dietetic Association. Nutrition Care Manual. 2004. Available at: www.nutritioncaremanual.org.

5. American Society for Parenteral and Enteral Nutrition Board of Directors and The Clinical Guidelines Task Force. Guidelines for the use of parenteral and enteral nutrition in adult and pediatric patients. *J Parenter Enteral Nutr.* 2002;26(Suppl):S1-S138.

6. Compher C. Frankenfield D, Keim N, Roth-Yousey L. Best practice methods to apply to measurement of resting metabolic rate in adults: A systematic review. *J Am Diet Assoc.* 2006;106:881-903.

7. Frankenfield D, Roth-Yousey L, Compher C. Comparison of predictive equations for resting metabolic rate in healthy nonobese adults: A systematic review. *J Am Diet Assoc.* 2005;105:775-789.

8. Institute of Medicine, Food and Nutrition Board. *Dietary Reference Intakes for Energy, Carbohydrate, Fiber, Fat, Fatty Acids, Cholesterol, Protein and Amino Acids.* Food and Nutrition Board. National Academy of Sciences. Washington, DC: National Academy Press; 2002. Available at: www.iom.edu/Object.File/Master/21/372/DRI%20Tables%20after%20electrolytes%20plus%20micro-macroEAR_2.pdf.

9. Nevin Folino N., ed. *Pediatric Manual of Clinical Dietetics.* American Dietetic Association. Chicago, IL: 2003

10. Otten JJ, Hellwig JP, et al., eds. *Dietary Reference Intakes. The Essential Guide to Nutrient Requirements.* Washington, D.C.: The National Academy of Sciences; 2006.

11. USDA Nutrient Data Laboratory, National Nutrient Database for Standard Reference. Available at: http://www.nal.usda.gov/fnic/foodcomp/search/. Accessed on December 1, 2007.

Edition: 2009

Estimated Fat Needs (CS-2.1)

Definition

Estimated quantity of total and/or type fat intake needed for nutritional adequacy.

Purpose

Identify appropriate reference standard of fat intake needs for individual patients/clients. Utilized as a basis of comparison to assess adequacy or excessiveness of patient/client's estimated total fat intake as compared to needs and for development of the nutrition prescription.

Indicators

Total fat needs, assumed to be consistent with the Dietary Reference Intakes unless otherwise specified: (specify, e.g., grams/day, grams/kg/day, percent of calories)

Types of fat needed (specify, e.g., grams/day, grams/kg/day, percent of calories)

Macronutrients*	EAR	RDA	AI	UL	Other
Fat			X Infants only		Acceptable Macronutrient Distribution Range (AMDR) (children and adults)
n-6 polyunsaturated fatty acids (linoleic acid)			X (All ages)		Acceptable Macronutrient Distribution Range (AMDR) (children and adults)
n-3 polyunsaturated fatty acids (α-linolenic acid)			X (All ages)		
Dietary cholesterol Trans fatty acids Saturated fatty acids					As low as possible while consuming a nutritionally adequate diet

EAR — Estimated Average Requirement
RDA — Recommended Dietary Allowance
AI — Adequate Intake
UL — Tolerable Upper Intake Level
See DRI Interpretation Table on page 35.

Method for estimating fat needs (specify, e.g., patient/client goal or nutrition prescription, disease/condition-based reference standard, Dietary Reference Intake)

References

The following are some suggested references; other references may be appropriate.

1. American Dietetic Association. Pamela Charney, Ainsley Malone, eds. *ADA Pocket Guide to Nutrition Assessment*. Chicago, IL: American Dietetic Association; 2004.

2. American Dietetic Association. Beth Leonberg, ed. *ADA Pocket Guide to Pediatric Nutrition Assessment*. Chicago, IL: American Dietetic Association; 2008.

3. American Dietetic Association Evidence Analysis Library. http://www.adaevidencelibrary.com/.

4. American Dietetic Association Nutrition Care Manual. 2004. Available at: www.nutritioncaremanual.org.

5. American Heart Association Nutrition Committee: Lichtenstein, A, Appel, L, Brands M, Carnethon M, Daniels S, Franch HA, Franklin B, Kris-Etherton P, Harris WS, Howard B, Karanja N, Lefevre M, Rudel L, Sacks F, Van Horn L, Winston M, Wylie-Rosett J. Diet and lifestyle recommendations revision 2006: a scientific statement from the American Heart Association Nutrition Committee. *Circulation*. 2006, 114(1) 82-96.

Estimated Fat Needs (CS-2.1)

References, cont'd

6. American Society for Parenteral and Enteral Nutrition Board of Directors and The Clinical Guidelines Task Force. Guidelines for the use of parenteral and enteral nutrition in adult and pediatric patients. *J Parenter Enteral Nutr*. 2002;26(Suppl):S1-S138.

7. Bantle JP, Wylie-Rosett J, Albright AL, Apovian CM, Clark NG, Franz MJ, Hoogwerf BJ, Lichtenstein AH, Mayer-Davis E, Mooradian AD, Wheeler ML. Nutrition recommendations and interventions for diabetes-2006: a position statement of the American Diabetes Association. Diabetes Care, 2006, 29(9):2140-2157.

8. Committee on Nutrient Relationships in Seafood – National Academies. *Seafood choices: Balancing Benefits and Risks*. National Academies Press. 2006.

9. Institute of Medicine, Food and Nutrition Board. *Dietary Reference Intakes for Energy, Carbohydrate, Fiber, Fat, Fatty Acids, Cholesterol, Protein and Amino Acids*. Food and Nutrition Board. National Academy of Sciences. Washington, DC: National Academy Press; 2002. Available at: www.iom.edu/Object.File/Master/21/372/DRI%20Tables%20after%20electrolytes%20plus%20micro-macroEAR_2.pdf.

10. Nevin Folino N., ed. *Pediatric Manual of Clinical Dietetics*. American Dietetic Association. Chicago, IL: 2003

11. US Departments of Agriculture and Health and Human Services. Dietary Guidelines for Americans 2005. Available at: www.healthierus. gov/dietaryguidelines/.

12. US Department of Health and Human Services. National Institutes of Health. National Heart, Lung and Blood Institute. *Third Report of the Expert Panel on Detection, Evaluation, and Treatment of High Blood Cholesterol in Adults (Adult Treatment Panel III)*, 2001.

13. USDA Nutrient Data Laboratory, National Nutrient Database for Standard Reference. Available at: http://www.nal.usda.gov/fnic/foodcomp/search/. Accessed December 1, 2007.

Edition: 2009

Estimated Protein Needs (CS-2.2)

Definition

Estimated quantity and/or type of protein needed for nutritional adequacy.

Purpose

Identify appropriate reference standard of protein intake needs for individual patients/clients. Utilized as a basis of comparison to assess adequacy or excessiveness of patient/client's estimated total protein intake as compared to estimated needs and for development of the nutrition prescription.

Indicators

Total estimated protein needs, assumed to be consistent with the Dietary Reference Intakes unless otherwise specified: (specify, e.g., grams/day, grams/kg/day, percent of calories)

Macronutrient*	EAR	RDA	AI	UL	Other
Protein	X All except infants 0-6 months	X All except infants 0-6 months	X Infants 0-6 months		Acceptable Macronutrient Distribution Range (children and adults)

EAR — Estimated Average Requirement
RDA — Recommended Dietary Allowance
AI — Adequate Intake
UL — Tolerable Upper Intake Level
*See DRI Interpretation Table on page 35.

Types of protein/amino acids needed (specify, e.g., grams/day, grams/kg/day, percent of total protein, percent of calories)

Method for estimating protein needs (specify, e.g., patient/client goal or nutrition prescription, disease/condition-based reference standard, Dietary Reference Intake)

References

The following are some suggested references; other references may be appropriate.

1. American Dietetic Association. Pamela Charney, Ainsley Malone, eds. *ADA Pocket Guide to Nutrition Assessment*. Chicago, IL: American Dietetic Association; 2004.

2. American Dietetic Association. Beth Leonberg, ed. *ADA Pocket Guide to Pediatric Nutrition Assessment*. Chicago, IL: American Dietetic Association; 2008.

3. ADA Nutrition Care Manual. 2004. Available at: www.nutritioncaremanual.org.

4. American Society for Parenteral and Enteral Nutrition Board of Directors and The Clinical Guidelines Task Force. Guidelines for the use of parenteral and enteral nutrition in adult and pediatric patients. *J Parenter Enteral Nutr*. 2002;26(Suppl):S1-S138.

5. Institute of Medicine, Food and Nutrition Board. Dietary Reference Intakes for Energy, Carbohydrate, Fiber, Fat, Fatty Acids, Cholesterol, Protein and Amino Acids. Food and Nutrition Board. National Academy of Sciences. Washington, DC: National Academy Press; 2002. Available at: www.iom.edu/Object.File/Master/21/372/DRI%20Tables%20after%20electrolytes%20plus%20micro-macroEAR_2.pdf

6. Nevin Folino N., ed. *Pediatric Manual of Clinical Dietetics*. American Dietetic Association. Chicago, IL: 2003

7. USDA Nutrient Data Laboratory, National Nutrient Database for Standard Reference. Available at: http://www.nal.usda.gov/fnic/foodcomp/search/. Accessed on December 1, 2007.

Estimated Carbohydrate Needs (CS-2.3)

Definition
Estimated quantity of total and/or type of carbohydrates needed for nutritional adequacy.

Purpose
Identify appropriate reference standard of carbohydrate intake needs for individual patients/clients. Utilized for assessing the adequacy or excessiveness of patient/client's estimated total carbohydrate intake as compared to estimated needs and for development of the nutrition prescription.

Indicators

Total estimated carbohydrate needs assumed to be consistent with the Dietary Reference Intakes unless otherwise specified: (specify, e.g., grams/day, grams or mg/kg/min, percent of calories)

Types of carbohydrate needed (specify, e.g., grams/day, grams or mg/kg/min, percent of carbohydrate, percent of calories)

Macronutrients*	EAR	RDA	AI	UL	Other
Carbohydrates		X	X infants		Acceptable Macronutrient Distribution Range (children and adults)
					Added sugars – limit to no more than 25% of total energy (All ages)

EAR — Estimated Average Requirement
RDA — Recommended Dietary Allowance
AI — Adequate Intake
UL — Tolerable Upper Intake Level
*See DRI Interpretation Table on page 35.

Method for estimating carbohydrate needs (specify, e.g., patient/client goal or nutrition prescription, disease/condition-based reference standard, Dietary Reference Intake)

References
The following are some suggested references; other references may be appropriate.

1. American Diabetes Association. Standards of Medical Care in Diabetes–2006. *Diabetes Care.* 2006;29:S4-S42.

2. American Dietetic Association. Pamela Charney, Ainsley Malone, eds. *ADA Pocket Guide to Nutrition Assessment.* Chicago, IL: American Dietetic Association; 2004.

3. American Dietetic Association. Beth Leonberg, ed. *ADA Pocket Guide to Pediatric Nutrition Assessment.* Chicago, IL: American Dietetic Association; 2008.

4. American Dietetic Association Nutrition Care Manual. 2004. Available at: www.nutritioncaremanual.org.

5. American Dietetic Association Evidenced-based Library. Available at: http://www.adaevidencelibrary.com/.

6. American Society for Parenteral and Enteral Nutrition Board of Directors and The Clinical Guidelines Task Force. Guidelines for the use of parenteral and enteral nutrition in adult and pediatric patients. *J Parenter Enteral Nutr.* 2002;26(Suppl):S1-S138.

7. Institute of Medicine, Food and Nutrition Board. *Dietary Reference Intakes for Energy, Carbohydrate, Fiber, Fat, Fatty Acids, Cholesterol, Protein and Amino Acids.* Food and Nutrition Board. National Academy of Sciences. Washington, DC: National Academy Press; 2002. Available at: www.iom.edu/Object.File/Master/21/372/DRI%20Tables%20after%20electrolytes%20plus%20micro-macroEAR_2.pdf

8. Nevin Folino N., ed. *Pediatric Manual of Clinical Dietetics.* American Dietetic Association. Chicago, IL: 2003

9. US Departments of Agriculture and Health and Human Services. Dietary Guidelines for Americans 2005. Available at: www.healthierus.gov/dietaryguidelines/

10. USDA Nutrient Data Laboratory, National Nutrient Database for Standard Reference. Available at: http://www.nal.usda.gov/fnic/foodcomp/search/. Accessed on December 1, 2007.

Edition: 2009

Estimated Fiber Needs (CS-2.4)

Definition

Estimated quantity of total and/or type of fiber needed for nutritional adequacy.

Purpose

Identify appropriate reference standard of fiber intake needs for individual patients/clients. Utilized as a basis of comparison to assess adequacy or excessiveness of patient/client's estimated total fiber intake as compared to estimated needs and for development of the nutrition prescription.

Indicators

Total estimated fiber needs, assumed to be consistent with the Dietary Reference Intakes unless otherwise specified: (specify, e.g., grams/day, grams/1000 kcal/day)

Macronutrients*	EAR	RDA	AI	UL	Other
Fiber			X Children and adults		

EAR — Estimated Average Requirement
RDA — Recommended Dietary Allowance
AI — Adequate Intake
UL — Tolerable Upper Intake Level
See DRI Interpretation Table on page 35.

Types of fiber needed (specify, e.g., grams/day, percent of total fiber)

Method for estimating fiber needs (specify, e.g., patient/client goal or nutrition prescription, disease/condition-based reference standard, Dietary Reference Intake)

References

The following are some suggested references; other references may be appropriate.

1. American Dietetic Association. Pamela Charney, Ainsley Malone, eds. *ADA Pocket Guide to Nutrition Assessment.* Chicago, IL: American Dietetic Association; 2004.

2. American Dietetic Association. Beth Leonberg, ed. *ADA Pocket Guide to Pediatric Nutrition Assessment.* Chicago, IL: American Dietetic Association; 2008.

3. American Dietetic Association Nutrition Care Manual. 2004. Available at: www.nutritioncaremanual.org.

4. Institute of Medicine, Food and Nutrition Board. *Dietary Reference Intakes for Energy, Carbohydrate, Fiber, Fat, Fatty Acids, Cholesterol, Protein and Amino Acids.* Food and Nutrition Board. National Academy of Sciences. Washington, DC: National Academy Press; 2002. Available at: www.iom.edu/Object.File/Master/21/372/DRI%20Tables%20after%20electrolytes%20plus%20micro-macroEAR_2.pdf

5. Nevin Folino N., ed. *Pediatric Manual of Clinical Dietetics.* American Dietetic Association. Chicago, IL: 2003

6. US Department of Health and Human Services. National Institutes of Health. National Heart, Lung and Blood Institute. *Third Report of the Expert Panel on Detection, Evaluation, and Treatment of High Blood Cholesterol in Adults (Adult Treatment Panel III),* 2001

7. USDA Nutrient Data Laboratory, National Nutrient Database for Standard Reference. Available at: http://www.nal.usda.gov/fnic/foodcomp/search/. Accessed on December 1, 2007.

Comparative Standards

Estimated Fluid Needs (CS-3.1)

Definition
Estimated quantity of fluid needed for nutritional adequacy.

Purpose
Identify appropriate reference standard of fluid intake needs for individual patients/clients. Utilized as a basis of comparison to assess adequacy or excessiveness of patient/client's estimated total fluid intake as compared to estimated need and for development of the nutrition prescription.

Indicators

Total estimated fluid needs, assumed to be consistent with the Dietary Reference Intakes unless otherwise specified: (specify, e.g., mL or L/day, mL/kg/day, mL/calories expended, ml/m2/day, mL output)

Macronutrient*	EAR	RDA	AI	UL	Other
Total Water			X		

EAR — Estimated Average Requirement
RDA — Recommended Dietary Allowance
AI — Adequate Intake
UL — Tolerable Upper Intake Level
See DRI Interpretation Table on page 35.

Method for estimating fluid needs (specify, e.g., patient/client goal or nutrition prescription, disease/condition-based reference standard, Dietary Reference Intake and adjustments, if needed, e.g., patient/client goal or nutrition prescription, increased due to fever, sweating, hyperventilation, hyperthyroid, extraordinary gastric/renal losses, or decreased due to, for example, renal or liver disease)

References
The following are some suggested references; other references may be appropriate.

1. American Dietetic Association. Pamela Charney, Ainsley Malone, eds. *ADA Pocket Guide to Nutrition Assessment*. Chicago, IL: American Dietetic Association; 2004.

2. American Dietetic Association. Beth Leonberg, ed. *ADA Pocket Guide to Pediatric Nutrition Assessment*. Chicago, IL: American Dietetic Association; 2008.

3. American Dietetic Association Nutrition Care Manual. 2004. Available at: www.nutritioncaremanual.org. Accessed November 29, 2006.

4. American Dietetic Association. Evidence Analysis Library. Available at: http://www.ada.portalxm.com/eal/topic.cfm?cat=2820.

5. American Society for Parenteral and Enteral Nutrition Board of Directors and The Clinical Guidelines Task Force. Guidelines for the use of parenteral and enteral nutrition in adult and pediatric patients. *J Parenter Enteral Nutr.* 2002;26(Suppl):S1-S138.

6. Institute of Medicine, Food and Nutrition Board. *Dietary Reference Intakes for Energy, Carbohydrate, Fiber, Fat, Fatty Acids, Cholesterol, Protein and Amino Acids.* Food and Nutrition Board. National Academy of Sciences. Washington, DC: National Academy Press; 2002. Available at: www.iom.edu/Object.File/Master/21/372/DRI%20Tables%20after%20electrolytes%20plus%20micro-macroEAR_2.pdf.

7. Institute of Medicine. National Academy of Sciences. *Dietary Reference Intakes for Water, Potassium, Sodium, Chloride, and Sulfate.* Washington DC: National Academy Press; 2004.

8. Nevin Folino N., ed. Pediatric Manual of Clinical Dietetics. American Dietetic Association. Chicago, IL: 2003

9. Nutrient Data Laboratory, USDA National Nutrient Database for Standard Reference, Release 20, Nutrient Lists. Available at: http://www.ars.usda.gov/Main/docs.htm?docid=15869. Accessed on December 1, 2007.

Edition: 2009

Estimated Vitamin Needs (CS-4.1)

Definition
Estimated quantity of one or more vitamins needed for nutritional adequacy and avoidance of toxicity.

Purpose
Identify appropriate reference standard of vitamin intake needs for individual patients/clients. Utilized as a basis of comparison to assess adequacy or excessiveness of patient/client's estimated total vitamin intake as compared to estimated needs and for development of the nutrition prescription.

Indicators

Total estimated vitamin needs, assumed to be consistent with the Dietary Reference Intakes unless otherwise specified:

Micronutrients - Vitamins*	EAR	RDA	AI	UL
Vitamin A (µg/day)	X	X	X Infants	X
Vitamin C (mg/day)	X	X	X Infants	X Children and adults
Vitamin D (µg/day)			X	X
Vitamin E (mg/day)	X	X	X Infants	X Children and adults
Vitamin K (µg/day)			X	
Thiamin (mg/day)	X	X	X Infants	
Riboflavin (mg/day)	X	X	X Infants	
Niacin (mg/day)	X	X	X Infants	X Children and adults
Vitamin B6 (mg/day)	X	X	X Infants	X Children and adults
Folate (µg/day)	X	X	X Infants	X Children and adults
Vitamin B12 (µg/day)	X	X	X Infants	
Pantothenic acid (mg/day)			X	
Biotin (µg/day)			X	
Choline (mg/d)			X	X Children and adults

EAR — Estimated Average Requirement
RDA — Recommended Dietary Allowance
AI — Adequate Intake
UL — Tolerable Upper Intake Level
*See DRI Interpretation Table on page 35.

Method for estimating vitamin needs (specify, e.g., patient/client goal or nutrition prescription, disease/condition-based reference standard, any adjustments for special conditions or situations, Dietary Reference Intake)

Estimated Vitamin Needs (CS-4.1)

References

The following are some suggested references; other references may be appropriate.

1. American Dietetic Association. Pamela Charney, Ainsley Malone, eds. *ADA Pocket Guide to Nutrition Assessment*. Chicago, IL: American Dietetic Association; 2004.

2. American Dietetic Association. Beth Leonberg, ed. *ADA Pocket Guide to Pediatric Nutrition Assessment*. Chicago, IL: American Dietetic Association; 2008.

3. American Dietetic Association Evidenced-based Library. Available at: http://www.adaevidencelibrary.com/.

4. American Dietetic Association Nutrition Care Manual. 2004. Available at: www.nutritioncaremanual.org

5. American Society for Parenteral and Enteral Nutrition Board of Directors and The Clinical Guidelines Task Force. Guidelines for the use of parenteral and enteral nutrition in adult and pediatric patients. *J Parenter Enteral Nutr*. 2002;26(Suppl):S1-S138.

6. Barr SI, Murphy SP, Poos MI. Interpreting and using the dietary reference intakes in dietary assessment of individuals and groups. *J Am Diet Assoc*. 2002; 102:780-788.

7. Gartner LM, Greer FR, American Academy of Pediatrics Committee on Nutrition. Prevention of rickets and vitamin D deficiency: new guidelines for vitamin D Intake. *Pediatrics*. 2003:111:908-10.

8. Institute of Medicine, Food and Nutrition Board. *Dietary Reference Intakes for Energy, Carbohydrate, Fiber, Fat, Fatty Acids, Cholesterol, Protein and Amino Acids*. Food and Nutrition Board. National Academy of Sciences. Washington, DC: National Academy Press; 2002. Available at: www.iom.edu/Object.File/Master/21/372/DRI%20Tables%20after%20electrolytes%20plus%20micro-macroEAR_2.pdf.

9. Institute of Medicine, National Academy of Sciences. *Dietary reference intakes: Applications in Dietary Assessment*. Washington, DC: National Academies Press; 2000.

10. Institute of Medicine. National Academy of Sciences. *Dietary Reference Intakes for Calcium, Phosphorus, Magnesium, Vitamin D, and Fluoride*. Washington, DC: National Academy Press; 1997.

11. Institute of Medicine. National Academy of Sciences. *Dietary Reference Intakes: Thiamin, riboflavin, niacin, vitamin B6, folate, vitamin B12, pantothenic acid, biotin, and choline*. National Academy Press. Washington, DC, 1998.

12. Institute of Medicine. National Academy of Sciences. *Dietary Reference Intakes for Vitamin A, Vitamin K, Arsenic, Boron, Chromium, Copper, Iodine, Iron, Manganese, Molybdenum, Nickel, Silicon, Vanadium, and Zinc*. National Academy Press, Washington, DC, 2001.

13. Institute of Medicine. National Academy of Sciences. *Dietary Reference Intakes: Vitamin C, Vitamin E, Selenium, and Carotenoids*. National Academy Press, Washington, DC, 2000.

14. Murphy SP, Poos MI. *Dietary Reference Intakes: Summary of applications in dietary assessment*. Public Health Nutr. 2002;5:843-849.

15. Nevin Folino N., ed. *Pediatric Manual of Clinical Dietetics*. American Dietetic Association. Chicago, IL: 2003

16. USDA Nutrient Data Laboratory, National Nutrient Database for Standard Reference. Available at: http://www.nal.usda.gov/fnic/foodcomp/search/. Accessed on December 1, 2007.

Comparative
Standards

Estimated Mineral/Element Needs (CS-4.2)

Definition

Estimated quantity of one or more minerals needed for nutritional adequacy and avoidance of toxicity.

Purpose

Identify appropriate reference standard of mineral intake needs for individual patients/clients. Utilized as a basis of comparison to assess adequacy or excessiveness of patient/client's estimated mineral intake as compared to estimated needs and for development of the nutrition prescription.

Indicators

Total estimated mineral needs, assumed to be consistent with the Dietary Reference Intakes unless otherwise specified:

Micronutrients - Minerals/elements*	EAR	RDA	AI	UL	Other
Calcium (mg/day)			X	X Children and adults	
Chloride (g/day)			X	X Children and adults	
Chromium (µg/day)			X		
Copper (µg/day)	X	X	X Infants	X Children and adults	
Fluoride (mg/day)			X	X	
Iodine (µg/day)	X	X	X Infants	X Children and adults	
Iron (mg/day)	X	X	X Infants 0-6 mos.	X	
Magnesium (mg/day)	X	X	X Infants	X Children and adults	
Manganese (mg/d)			X	X Children and adults	
Phosphorus (mg/day)	X	X	X Infants	X Children and adults	
Potassium (g/day)			X		

Estimated Mineral/Element Needs (CS-4.2)

Indicators, cont'd

Micronutrients - Minerals/elements,* cont'd	EAR	RDA	AI	UL	Other
Selenium (µg/day)	X	X	X Infants	X	
Sodium (g/day)			X	X Children and adults	
Zinc (mg/day)	X	X	X Infants 0-6 mos.	X	

EAR — Estimated Average Requirement
RDA — Recommended Dietary Allowance
AI — Adequate Intake
UL — Tolerable Upper Intake Level
See DRI Interpretation Table on page 35.

Method for estimating mineral needs (specify, e.g., patient/client goal or nutrition prescription, disease/condition-based reference standard, any adjustments for special conditions or situations, Dietary Reference Intake)

References

The following are some suggested references; other references may be appropriate.

1. American Dietetic Association. Pamela Charney, Ainsley Malone, eds. *ADA Pocket Guide to Nutrition Assessment.* Chicago, IL: American Dietetic Association; 2004.

2. American Dietetic Association. Beth Leonberg, ed. *ADA Pocket Guide to Pediatric Nutrition Assessment.* Chicago, IL: American Dietetic Association; 2008.

3. American Dietetic Association Adult Weight Management Evidence-Based Guideline, 2006. Available at: http://www.adaevidencelibrary.com/topic.cfm?cat=2798. Accessed on December 1, 2007.

4. American Dietetic Association Nutrition Care Manual. 2004. Available at: www.nutritioncaremanual.org.

5. American Society for Parenteral and Enteral Nutrition Board of Directors and The Clinical Guidelines Task Force. Guidelines for the use of parenteral and enteral nutrition in adult and pediatric patients. *J Parenter Enteral Nutr.* 2002;26(Suppl):S1-S138.

6. Appel LJ, Moore TJ, Obarzanek E, Vollmer WM, Svetkey LP, Sacks FM, Bray GA, Vogt TM, Cutler JA, Windhauser MM, Lin P, Karanja N, Simons-Morton D, McCullough M, Swain J, Steele P, Evans MA, Miller ER, Harsha DW. A clinical trial of the effects of dietary patterns on blood pressure. *NEJM.* 1997;336:1117-1124.

7. Dietary Guidelines for Americans, 2005. Available at: http://www.health.gov/dietaryguidelines/dga2005/document/html/executivesummary.htm. Accessed October 27, 2006.

8. Institute of Medicine, Food and Nutrition Board. *Dietary Reference Intakes for Energy, Carbohydrate, Fiber, Fat, Fatty Acids, Cholesterol, Protein and Amino Acids.* Food and Nutrition Board. National Academy of Sciences. Washington, DC: National Academy Press; 2002. Available at: www.iom.edu/Object.File/Master/21/372/DRI%20Tables%20after%20electrolytes%20plus%20micro-macroEAR_2.pdf.

9. Institute of Medicine. National Academy of Sciences. *Dietary Reference Intakes for Calcium, Phosphorus, Magnesium, Vitamin D, and Fluoride.* Washington, DC: National Academy Press; 1997.

10. Institute of Medicine. National Academy of Sciences. *Dietary Reference Intakes for Vitamin A, Vitamin K, Arsenic, Boron, Chromium, Copper, Iodine, Iron, Manganese, Molybdenum, Nickel, Silicon, Vanadium, Zinc.* Washington, DC: National Academy Press; 2001.

11. Institute of Medicine. National Academy of Sciences. Dietary *Reference Intakes for Vitamin C, Vitamin E, Selenium, and Carotenoids.* Washington, DC: National Academy Press; 2000.

12. Institute of Medicine. National Academy of Sciences. *Dietary Reference Intakes for Water, Potassium, Sodium, Chloride, and Sulfate.* Washington DC: National Academy Press; 2004.

13. Nevin Folino N., ed. *Pediatric Manual of Clinical Dietetics.* American Dietetic Association. Chicago, IL: 2003

14. USDA Nutrient Data Laboratory, National Nutrient Database for Standard Reference. Available at: http://www.nal.usda.gov/fnic/foodcomp/search/. Accessed on December 1, 2007.

Edition: 2009

Recommended Body Weight/Body Mass Index/Growth (5.1)

Definition

Estimated reference ideal body weight (known as desirable body weight), body mass index and/or growth parameter used to evaluate nutritional status

Purpose

Identify appropriate reference standard for body weight for individual patients/clients. Utilized as a basis of comparison to assess patient/client's body weight as compared to recommendations and for development of the nutrition prescription

Indicators (Measures)

Ideal/reference body weight

- Method for determining ideal body weight (IBW)/desirable body weight (specify, e.g., Hamwi equation, growth chart)
- IBW adjustment (e.g., spinal cord injury, amputees)
- % IBW

Recommended Body Mass Index (BMI)* (kg/m^2)

- Normal range BMI (specify if using adjustment for South East Asian body types)

Desired growth pattern (based on individual health, growth pattern and genetic potential)

- 0-36 months
  - Weight-for-age (percentile rank)
  - Length-for-age (percentile rank)
  - Weight-for-length (percentile rank)
  - Head circumference-for-age (percentile rank)
- 2-5 years
  - Weight-for-stature (percentile rank)
- 2-20 years
  - Weight-for-age (percentile rank)
  - Stature-for-age (percentile rank)
  - BMI-for-age (percentile rank)
- Specialized and disease-specific growth charts (specify, e.g., type chart and percentile rank)

Note: Estimated stature and corrected age for prematurity are found on the body composition/growth/weight history reference sheet.

*BMI is a measure of the weight of an individual scaled according to height. It is a common method for assessing body fat in the clinical setting and is compared to a population standard (e.g., U.S. National Institutes of Health guidelines or World Health Organization guidelines). BMI was designed for use within a physically inactive population.

Recommended Body Weight/Body Mass Index/Growth (5.1)

References

The following are some suggested references; other references may be appropriate.

1. National Heart Lung and Blood Institute. Obesity Guidelines. Body mass index table Available at: http://www.nhlbi.nih.gov/guidelines/obesity/bmi_tbl.htm Accessed on February 29, 2008.

2. World Health Organization. Growth reference 5-19 years. Available at: http://www.who.int/growthref/who2007_height_for_age/en/index.html Assessed February 29, 2008.

3. Hamwi GJ. Changing dietary concepts. In: Donowski TS, ed. *Diabetes Mellitus: Diagnosis and Treatment.* New York, NY: American Diabetes Association; 1964:73-78.

4. Charney P, Malone A, eds. *ADA Pocket Guide to Nutrition Assessment.* Chicago, IL: American Dietetic Association; 2004.

5. Leonberg BL. *ADA Pocket Guide to Pediatric Nutrition Assessment.* Chicago, IL: American Dietetic Association; 2008.

6. Nevin-Folino NF, ed. *Pediatric Manual of Clinical Dietetics.* 2nd ed. Chicago, Ill: American Dietetic Association; 2003:763-810.

7. Campell J, Conkin C, Montgomery C, Phillips S, Wade K. eds. *Texas Children's Hospital Pediatric Nutrition Reference Guide. 2005.* 7th ed. Houston, Texas: Texas Children's Hospital; 2005.

8. McDowell MA, Fryar CD, Hirsch R, Ogden CL. Anthropometric Reference Data for Children and Adults: U.S. Population, 1999-2002. Advanced data from vital health statistics; no 361. Hyattsville, MD: National Center for Health Statistics. 2005. Available at: http://www.cdc.gov/nchs/data/ad/ad361.pdf Accessed: February 29, 2008.

9. Centers for Disease Control and Prevention. 2000 CDC Growth Charts: United States. Available at: http://www.cdc.gov/growthcharts/ Accessed: February 29, 2008.

10. Centers for Disease Control and Prevention. Epi Info. Available at: http://www.cdc.gov/epiinfo. Accessed March 12, 2008.

11. Abbott Laboratories, Inc., Ross Product Division. IHDP Growth Percentiles. Columbus, Ohio: Abbott Laboratories, Inc., Ross Product Division; 1999.

12. Cronk C, Crocker AC, Pueschel SM, Shea AM, Zachai E, Pickens G. Growth charts for children with Down syndrome: 1 month to 18 years of age. *Pediatrics.* 1988;81: 102-110.

13. Lyon AF, Preece MA, Grant DB. Growth curves for girls with Turner Syndrome. *Arch Dis Child.* 1985;60:932-935.

14. Krick J, Murphy-Miller P, Zeger S, Wright E. Pattern of growth in children with cerebral palsy. *J Am Diet Assoc.* 1996;96:680-685.

15. Butler MG, Meaney EJ. Standards for selected anthropometric measurements in Prader-Willi syndrome. *Pediatrics.* 1991;88:853.

16. Horton WA, Rotter JI, Rimoin DL, Scott CI, Hall JG. Standard growth curves for achondroplasia. *J Pediatr.* 1978;93:435-438

17. Witt DR, Keena BA, Hall JG, Allanson JE. Growth curves for height in Noonan syndrome. *Clin Genet.* 1986;30:150-153

18. Morris CA, Demsey SA, Leonard CO, Dilts C, Blackburn BL. Natural history of Williams syndrome: physical characteristics. *J Pediatr.* 1988;113:318-326.

19. Kline AD, Barr M, Jackson LG. Growth manifestations in the Brachmann-de Lange syndrome. *Am J Med Genet.* 1993;47:1042-1049.

20. Stevens CA, Hennekam RC, Blackburn BL. Growth in the Rubinstein-Taybi syndrome. *Am J Med Genet.* 1990;6:51-55.

21. Peifer SC, Blust P, Leyson JF. Nutritional assessment of the spinal cord injured patient. *J Am Diet Assoc.* 1981;78:501-505.

24. *Nutritional Care for High Risk Newborns* Eds. Groh-Wargo S, Thompson M, Cox JH. Precept Press. Chicago, IL. 2000.

25. Mitchell CO, Lipschitz DA. Arm length measurement as an alternative to height in the nutrition assessment of the elderly. JPEN *J Parenter Enteral Nutr.* 1982;6:226-229.

26. Samson-Fang LJ, Stevenson RD. Identification of malnutrition in children with cerebral palsy: poor performance of weight-for-height centiles. *Developmental Medicine & Child Neurology.* 2000;42:162-168.

27. Cronk CE, Stallings VA, Spender Q, Ross JL, Widdoes HD. Measurement of short-term growth with a new knee height-measuring device. *Am. J. Hum. Biol.* 1989. 31(2):206-14.

28. Zemel BS, Riley EM, Stallings VA. Evaluation of methodology for nutritional assessment in children: Anthropometry, body composition, and energy expenditure. *Annual Review of Nutrition.* 1997;17:211-235.

Edition: 2009

NCP Step 2. Nutrition Diagnosis

What is the purpose of a Nutrition Diagnosis? The purpose is to identify and describe a specific nutrition problem that can be resolved or improved through treatment/nutrition intervention by a dietetics practitioner. A nutrition diagnosis (e.g., inconsistent carbohydrate intake) is different from a medical diagnosis (e.g., diabetes).

How does a dietetics practitioner determine a Nutrition Diagnosis? Dietetics practitioners use the data collected in the nutrition assessment to identify and label the patient/client's* nutrition diagnosis using standard nutrition diagnostic terminology. Each nutrition diagnosis has a reference sheet that includes its definition, possible etiology/causes and common signs or symptoms identified in the nutrition assessment step.

How are the Nutrition Diagnoses organized? In three categories:

Intake	Clinical	Behavioral-Environmental
Too much or too little of a food or nutrient compared to actual or estimated needs	*Nutrition problems that relate to medical or physical conditions*	*Knowledge, attitudes, beliefs, physical environment, access to food, or food safety*

How is the Nutrition Diagnosis documented? Dietetics practitioners write a PES statement to describe the problem, its root cause, and the assessment data that provide evidence for the nutrition diagnosis. The format for the PES statement is "Nutrition problem label related to ____ as evidenced by ____."

(P) Problem or Nutrition Diagnosis Label	**(E) Etiology**	**(S) Signs/Symptoms**
Describes alterations in the patient/client's nutritional status.	Cause/Contributing Risk Factors Linked to the nutrition diagnosis label by the words "related to."	Data used to determine that the patient/client has the nutrition diagnosis specified. Linked to the etiology by the words "as evidenced by."

What are the guidelines for selecting the nutrition diagnosis and writing a clear PES statement? The most important and urgent problem to be addressed is selected. When specifying the nutrition diagnosis and writing the PES statement; dietetics practitioners ask themselves a series of questions that help clarify the nutrition diagnosis. (See the critical thinking box).

Critical thinking during this step...

Evaluate your PES statement by using the following

P – Can the nutrition professional resolve or improve the nutrition diagnosis for this individual, group or population? When all things are equal and there is a choice between stating the PES statement using two nutrition diagnoses from different domains, consider the Intake nutrition diagnosis as the one more specific to the role of the RD.

E – Evaluate what you have used as your etiology to determine if it is the "root cause" or the most specific root cause that the RD can address with a nutrition intervention. If as an RD you can not resolve the problem by addressing the etiology, can the RD intervention at least lessen the signs and symptoms?

S – Will measuring the signs and symptoms indicate if the problem is resolved or improved? Are the signs and symptoms specific enough that you can monitor (measure/evaluate changes) and document resolution or improvement of the nutrition diagnosis?

PES Overall – Does the nutrition assessment data support a particular nutrition diagnosis with a typical etiology and signs and symptoms?

Are dietetics practitioners limited to the Nutrition Diagnosis terms? Nutrition diagnosis terms and definitions were developed with extensive input and should fit most situations; however, food and dietetics practitioners can submit proposals for additions or revisions using the Procedure for Nutrition Controlled Vocabulary/Terminology Maintenance/Review available from ADA.

Detailed information about this step can be found in the American Dietetic Association's International Dietetics and Nutrition Terminology (IDNT) Reference Manual: Standardized Language for the Nutrition Care Process, Second Edition.

Patient/client refers to individuals, groups, family members, and/or caregivers.

Diagnosis

Edition: 2009

Nutrition Care Process Step 2.
Nutrition Diagnosis

Introduction

The ADA has identified and defined nutrition diagnoses/problems to be used in the profession of dietetics. Nutrition diagnosis is identifying and labeling a nutritional problem that a dietetics practitioner is responsible for treating independently. The standardized language of nutrition diagnoses/problems is an integral component in the Nutrition Care Process. In fact, several other professions, including medicine, nursing, physical therapy, and occupational therapy, utilize care processes with defined terms for making nutrition diagnoses specific to their professional scope of practice.

ADA's Standardized Language Task Force developed a conceptual framework for the standardized nutrition language and identified the nutrition diagnoses/problems. The framework outlines the domains within which the nutrition diagnoses/problems fall and the flow of the Nutrition Care Process in relation to the continuum of health, disease, and disability.

The methodology for developing sets of terms such as these included systematically collecting data from multiple sources simultaneously. Data were collected from a select group of ADA-recognized leaders and award winners prior to starting the project. A 12-member task force developed the terms with input from groups of community, ambulatory, acute care, and long-term care practitioners and obtained feedback from experts concerning the research supporting the terms and definitions.

The methodology for continued development and refinement of these terms has been identified. As with the ongoing updating of the American Medical Association Current Procedural Terminology (CPT) codes, these will also be published on an annual basis. The terms are being studied in a number of research projects to assess their validity. Based upon the results of two content validation studies, the Committee recommended changes to the nutrition diagnoses (1 and E.B. Enrione personal communication, December 2006) and these were published in the First Edition. Further changes are anticipated as results of additional studies become available. The nutrition diagnostic terms are being incorporated into several research studies that explore use in ambulatory or inpatient settings or by specific types of practice, e.g., nutrition support and oncology.

As each of the research studies is completed, findings will be incorporated into future versions of these terms. Future iterations and changes to the nutrition diagnoses/problems and the reference sheets are expected as this standard language evolves. In addition, practitioners can submit suggested changes. The process for practitioners to submit suggested revisions to the nutrition diagnoses is included near the end of this reference manual.

ADA is working toward including the concepts from the Nutrition Care Process and these specific terms in standards for electronic health records and incorporation into standardized informatics languages and language systems, such as the Systematized Nomenclature of Medicine International (SNOMED), Logical Observation Identifiers Names and Codes (LOINC), and Unified Medical Language System (UMLS). ADA has already begun the dialogue with these groups to let them know the direction that the Association is headed and to keep them appraised of progress. Thus far, the feedback from the database and informatics groups has been quite positive, and they have expressed a need for documenting the unique nature of nutrition services.

What Is New in This Edition Related to Nutrition Diagnosis?

There are notable changes to the nutrition diagnosis section in this edition. One change concerns reorganization of the Signs/Symptoms individual nutrition diagnosis reference sheets. Other changes include revisions and clarifications to individual nutrition diagnosis reference sheets.

Reorganization of the Sign/Symptoms Reference Sheet Table

The changes related to reorganization of the Signs/Symptoms in individual nutrition diagnosis reference sheets affect the grouping of the terms, but do not influence the content of the nutrition diagnosis. There are four components of a nutrition diagnosis reference sheet—definition, etiology, signs/symptoms, and references—which are described in detail later in this chapter. Briefly, dietetics practitioners gather pertinent signs/symptoms during nutrition assessment to assist in identifying and labeling a nutrition diagnosis. With the reorganization and classification of the nutrition assessment terms and indicators, there are changes in placement of the signs/symptoms within the nutrition diagnosis sheets:

- In some cases, signs/symptoms gathered during the nutrition assessment are moved from one assessment domain or category, such as Client History, to another domain, such as Food/Nutrition-Related History. Again, these changes do not affect the content of the nutrition diagnosis, just the organization of the sign/symptoms.

Revisions and Clarifications

Changes in the nutrition diagnoses include revisions and clarifications to individual nutrition diagnosis reference sheets. First, specific changes to nutrition diagnosis labels, etiologies, and signs/symptoms were completed based upon practitioner questions and feedback and Committee review. Second, in response to questions about how to label and document inadequate intake, a note was added to the definition of the eleven nutrition diagnoses associated with inadequate intake. Since the note reminds practitioners to include additional supporting evidence (e.g., biochemical data, anthropometric data), nutrition-focused physical findings were added to two of the nutrition diagnoses. A chart for guiding interpretation of the DRIs was also added to the publication. Third, to assist practitioners with identifying the etiology (E) of a problem for use in the PES statement, the Committee developed a Nutrition Diagnosis Etiology Matrix.

Diagnosis Label, Etiologies, and Signs/Symptoms

Throughout the year, dietetics practitioners suggest additions or changes to the standardized language associated with the Nutrition Care Process (see the Procedure for Nutrition Controlled Vocabulary/Terminology Maintenance/Review available on ADA's website, www.eatright.org, in the Nutrition Care Process section). Below are highlights of the changes. A document detailing all of the specific changes to the nutrition diagnoses, the year in which the review or change occurred, and the rationale, is available in the Nutrition Care Process and Model Resource section of ADA's website at www.eatright.org in the Nutrition Care Process section. Editorial changes not affecting the content are not included in this document.

Evident Protein-Energy Malnutrition (NI-5.2):

- Revision of the Nutrition Diagnosis Label. The words "Evident Protein-Energy" were removed from the label, and this nutrition diagnosis is retitled Malnutrition (NI-5.2).

- Removal of the two signs/symptoms (biochemical measures) related to serum albumin. The following footnote is added to the nutrition diagnosis: "In the past, hepatic transport protein measures (e.g., albumin and prealbumin) were used as indicators of malnutrition. The sensitivity of these as nutrition indicators has been questioned. An ADA evidence-analysis project is evaluating the body of science."

- Modifications to the sign/symptoms (anthropometric measurements) of weight change in adults and growth rate in pediatrics were added for clarity.

Inadequate Fat Intake (NI-5.6.1):

- Addition of an etiology: Alteration in gastrointestinal tract structure and/or function; supporting signs/symptoms already listed in the nutrition diagnosis.

Inappropriate Intake of Food Fats (specify) (NI-5.6.3):

- Modification of the nutrition diagnosis label removing the word "food." The nutrition diagnosis includes inappropriate fat from any source, for example, food, EN/PN, formula, and intravenously.

Swallowing Difficulty (NC-1.1):

- Modification of an etiology to include altered suck, swallow, breathe patterns within the list of Motor causes for this nutrition diagnosis.

Altered Nutrition-Related Laboratory Values (specify) (NC-2.2):

- Addition of an etiology, Prematurity, as a potential cause/contributing factor for this nutrition diagnosis.

Underweight (NC-3.1):

- Addition of an etiology—Small for gestational age, intrauterine growth retardation/restriction and/or lack of progress/appropriate weight gain per day.

Food- and Nutrition-related Knowledge Deficit (NB-1.1):

- Addition of an etiology, Lack of understanding of infant/child cues to indicate hunger.

Excessive Exercise (NB-2.2):

- Excessive Exercise (NB-2.2) is now Excessive Physical Activity (NB-2.2) reflecting involuntary and voluntary physical activity/movement, and exercise.

- Modification of the definition to: Involuntary or voluntary physical activity or movement that interferes with energy needs, growth, or exceeds that which is necessary to achieve optimal health.

Inadequate Intake

Some dietetics practitioners have raised questions about the use of the nutrition diagnosis label "inadequate", when describing the intake of patients/clients. There is concern that this may pose an increased risk of litigation or legal exposure. Additional information regarding this issue can be found at www.eatright.org in the Nutrition Care Process section.

Critical to the understanding of this subject is the recognition of three issues:

1) It is very difficult to determine accurately a patient/client's intake even when enteral and/or parenteral nutrition is provided as the sole source of nutrition; these measures are estimates of intake.

2) When using the Dietary Reference Intakes (DRIs) to determine if nutrient intake is sufficient, it is not recommended to rely on nutrient intake data alone.

3) Inadequate nutrient intake does not necessarily equate to nutrient deficiency.

- As such, the Standardized Language Committee created a clarification statement that should be given professional consideration prior to identifying and labeling a patient/client with "Inadequate Intake," (e.g. inadequate vitamin intake, inadequate protein intake). The note is part of the definition for the eleven nutrition diagnoses with "Inadequate" in the label. An additional nutrition diagnosis with "inadequate" in the label, Inadequate Bioactive Substances NI-4.1, contains a special notation described below.

  *Note: Whenever possible, nutrient intake data should be considered in combination with clinical, biochemical, anthropometric information, medical diagnosis, clinical status, and/or other factors as well as diet to provide a valid assessment of nutritional status based on a totality of the evidence. (*Dietary Reference Intakes. Applications in Dietary Assessment. Institute of Medicine. Washington, D.C.: National Academy Press; 2000.)

- If a synonym, or alternate word with the same meaning, for the term "inadequate" is helpful or needed, an approved alternate is the word "suboptimal." Thus, a dietetics professional could use either the nutrition diagnosis label "Suboptimal Protein Intake" or "Inadequate Protein Intake."

- Bioactive substances are not addressed within the DRIs. Further, the Nutrition Assessment and Monitoring and Evaluation reference sheet notes that the criteria for evaluation of intake must be the nutrition prescription or goal because no validated reference standard exists. The nutrition prescription or goal would be based upon an individual goal or research, for example, the ADA Disorders of Lipid Metabolism Evidence-Based Guideline. Therefore, the note added to the definition of Inadequate Bioactive Substance Intake is:

  Note: Bioactive Substances are not included as part of the Dietary Reference Intakes, and therefore there are no established minimum requirements or Tolerable Upper Intake Levels. However, RDs can assess whether estimated intakes are adequate or excessive using the patient/client goal or nutrition prescription for comparison

Because nutrient intake data should be considered in combination with clinical, biochemical, and anthropometric information, medical diagnosis, and/or clinical status, two nutrition diagnoses, Inadequate Protein Intake NI-5.7.1 and Inadequate Fiber Intake NI-5.8.5, were revised. The Committee added signs/symptoms of nutrition-focused physical findings in addition to intake and client history data.

A document detailing all of the specific changes to the nutrition diagnoses, the year in which the review or change occurred, and the rationale, is available in the Nutrition Care Process and Model Resource section of ADA's website at www.eatright.org in the Nutrition Care Process section. Editorial changes not affecting the content are not included in this document.

Nutrition Diagnosis Etiology Matrix

As part of the review and development of the nutrition assessment standardized language, the etiologies associated with each nutrition diagnosis were examined. There are two significant changes regarding the nutrition diagnosis etiologies.

- **Nutrition Diagnosis and Etiology Matrix development.** A matrix of the etiologies and the nutrition diagnosis with which they are associated is available on ADA's website.

- **Refinement of the Etiologies for clarity.** In the First Edition, for example, Excessive Mineral Intake NI-5.10.2 includes the etiology "Lack of knowledge about management of diagnosed genetic disorders altering mineral homeostasis." This etiology is rephrased to be consistent with the other nutrition diagnoses. It now reads "Food and nutrition-related knowledge deficit concerning management of diagnosed genetic disorders altering mineral homeostasis." These edits represent changes for clarity and content was not changed unless indicated.

This matrix, due to space considerations, is available on ADA's website, www.eatright.org, in the Nutrition Care Process section.

Nutrition Care Process and Nutrition Diagnosis

Nutrition diagnosis is a critical step between nutrition assessment and nutrition intervention. The nutrition diagnosis is the identification and labeling of the specific nutrition problem that dietetics practitioners are responsible for treating independently.

Naming the nutrition diagnosis and identifying the etiology, and signs and symptoms provides a way to document the link between nutrition assessment and nutrition intervention and set realistic and measurable expected outcomes for each patient/client. Identifying the nutrition diagnosis also assists practitioners in establishing priorities when planning an individual patient/client's nutrition intervention.

> **Special Note:** The terms **patient/client** are used in association with the NCP; however, the process is also intended for use with groups. In addition, family members or caregivers are an essential asset to the patient/client and dietetics practitioner in the NCP. Therefore, **groups, families, and caregivers** of patients/clients are implied each time a reference is made to patient/client.

In simple terms, a nutrition practitioner identifies and labels a specific nutrition diagnosis (problem) that, in general, he or she is responsible for treating independently (e.g., excessive carbohydrate intake). With nutrition intervention, the nutrition diagnosis ideally resolves. In contrast, a medical diagnosis describes a disease or pathology of organs or body systems (e.g., diabetes). In some instances, such as the nutrition diagnosis Swallowing Difficulty NC-1.1, nutrition practitioners are labeling or diagnosing the functional problem that has a nutritional consequence. Nutrition practitioners do not identify medical diagnoses; they diagnose phenomena in the nutrition domain.

Categories of Nutrition Diagnostic Terminology

The 60 nutrition diagnoses/problems have been given labels that are clustered into three domains: intake, clinical, and behavioral-environmental. Each domain represents unique characteristics that contribute to nutritional health. Within each domain are classes and, in some cases, subclasses of nutrition diagnoses.

A definition of each follows:

> The **Intake** domain lists actual problems related to intake of energy, nutrients, fluids, or bioactive substances through oral diet, or nutrition support (enteral or parenteral nutrition).

Class: Energy Balance (1)—Actual or estimated intake of energy (kcal).

Class: Oral or Nutrition Support Intake (2)—Actual or estimated food and beverage intake from oral diet or nutrition support compared with patient/client's goal.

Class: Fluid Intake (3)—Actual or estimated fluid intake compared with patient/client's goal.

Class: Bioactive Substances Intake (4)—Actual or estimated intake of bioactive substances, including single or multiple functional food components, ingredients, dietary supplements, and alcohol.

Class: Nutrient Intake (5)—Actual or estimated intake of specific nutrient groups or single nutrients as compared with desired levels.

> Subclass: Fat and Cholesterol (5.6)
>
> Subclass: Protein (5.7)
>
> Subclass: Carbohydrate and Fiber (5.8)
>
> Subclass: Vitamin (5.9)
>
> Subclass: Mineral (5.10)

The **Clinical** domain is nutritional findings/problems identified as related to medical or physical conditions.

Class: Functional (1)—Change in physical or mechanical functioning that interferes with or prevents desired nutritional consequences.

Class: Biochemical (2)—Change in the capacity to metabolize nutrients as a result of medications, surgery, or as indicated by altered lab values.

Class: Weight (3)—Chronic weight or changed weight status when compared with usual or desired body weight.

The **Behavioral-Environmental** domain includes nutritional findings/problems identified that relate to knowledge, attitudes/beliefs, physical environment, access to food, and food safety.

Class: Knowledge and Beliefs (1)—Actual knowledge and beliefs as reported, observed, or documented.

Class: Physical Activity and Function (2)—Actual physical activity, self-care, and quality of life problems as reported, observed, or documented.

Class: Food Safety and Access (3)—Actual problems with food access or food safety.

Examples of nutrition diagnoses and their definitions include:

INTAKE DOMAIN • Energy Balance

Inadequate* energy intake NI-1.4

Energy intake that is less than energy expenditure, established reference standards, or recommendations based on physiological needs.

> *Note: May not be an appropriate nutrition diagnosis when the goal is weight loss, during end-of-life care, upon initiation of EN/PN, or acute stressed state (e.g., surgery, organ failure).*
>
> *Whenever possible, nutrient intake data should be considered in combination with clinical, biochemical, anthropometric information, medical diagnosis, clinical status, and/or other factors as well as diet to provide a valid assessment of nutritional status based on a totality of the evidence.* (Dietary Reference Intakes. Applications in Dietary Assessment. *Institute of Medicine. Washington, D.C.: National Academy Press; 2000.*)

Edition: 2009

Diagnosis

CLINICAL DOMAIN • Functional

Swallowing difficulty NC-1.1   Impaired movement of food and liquid from the mouth to the stomach.

BEHAVIORAL-ENVIRONMENTAL DOMAIN • Knowledge and Beliefs

Not ready for diet/lifestyle change NB-1.3   Lack of perceived value of nutrition-related behavior change compared to costs (consequences or effort required to make changes); conflict with personal value system; antecedent to behavior change.

The Nutrition Diagnosis Statement (or PES)

The nutrition diagnosis is summarized into a structured sentence named the nutrition diagnosis statement. This statement, also called a PES statement is composed of three distinct components: the problem (P), the etiology (E), and the signs and symptoms (S). The practitioner obtains the etiology and the signs and symptoms during the nutrition assessment phase of the Nutrition Care Process. The nutrition diagnosis is derived from the synthesis of nutrition assessment data, and the wording is obtained from the nutrition diagnoses reference sheets.

The generic format for the nutrition diagnosis statement is:

Problem (P) *related to* etiology (E) *as evidenced by* signs and symptoms (S).

Where:

The **Problem or Nutrition Diagnosis Label** describes alterations in the patient/client's nutritional status that dietetics practitioners are responsible for treating independently. A nutrition diagnosis allows the dietetics practitioner to identify realistic and measurable outcomes, formulate nutrition interventions, and monitor and evaluate change.	The **Etiology** (Cause/Contributing Risk Factors) are those factors contributing to the existence, or maintenance of pathophysiological, psychosocial, situational, developmental, cultural, and/or environmental problems. It is linked to the nutrition diagnosis label by the words "related to." Identifying the etiology will lead to the selection of a nutrition intervention aimed at resolving the underlying cause of the nutrition problem whenever possible.	The **Signs/Symptoms** (Defining Characteristics) consist of objective (signs) and/or subjective (symptoms) data used to determine whether the patient/client has the nutrition diagnosis specified. It is linked to the etiology by the words "as evidenced by." The clear identification of quantifiable data in the signs and symptoms will serve as the basis for monitoring and evaluating nutrition outcomes.
Select from terms on pages 213-337.	Usually free text, but can also use some terms from pages 213-337.	Usually free text, but can also use some terms from pages 213-337 as long as they are quantified.

A well-written nutrition diagnostic (PES) statement is:

- Simple, clear, and concise
- Specific to the patient/client or group
- Related to a single patient/client nutrition-related problem
- Accurately related to an etiology
- Based on reliable and accurate nutrition assessment data

Specific questions that dietetics practitioners should use in evaluating the PES they have developed are:

P – Can the nutrition professional resolve or improve the nutrition diagnosis for this individual, group or population? When all things are equal and there is a choice between stating the PES statement using two nutrition diagnoses from different domains, consider the Intake nutrition diagnosis as the one more specific to the role of the RD.

E – Evaluate what you have used as your etiology to determine if it is the "root cause" or the most specific root cause that the RD can address with a nutrition intervention. If as an RD you can not resolve the problem by addressing the etiology, can the RD intervention at least lessen the signs and symptoms?

S – Will measuring the signs and symptoms indicate if the problem is resolved or improved? Are the signs and symptoms specific enough that you can monitor (measure/evaluate changes) and document resolution or improvement of the nutrition diagnosis?

PES Overall – Does the nutrition assessment data support a particular nutrition diagnosis with a typical etiology and signs and symptoms?

Examples of nutrition diagnosis statements (PES) are:

Diagnosis or Problem		Etiology		Signs and/or Symptoms
Excessive fat intake	*Related to*	frequent consumption of fast-food meals	*As evidenced by*	serum cholesterol level of 230 mg/dL and 10 meals per week of hamburgers/sandwich and fries
Excessive energy intake	*Related to*	unchanged dietary intake and restricted mobility while fracture healing	*As evidenced by*	5 lb weight gain during last 3 weeks due to consumption of 500 kcal/day more than estimated needs
Inadequate* oral food/beverage intake	*Related to*	lack of GI access	*As evidenced by*	nothing by mouth (NPO) diet order x 7 days and absence of consistent bowel sounds
Disordered eating pattern	*Related to*	harmful belief about food and nutrition	*As evidenced by*	reported use of laxatives after meals and statements that calories are not absorbed when laxatives are used
Swallowing difficulty	*Related to*	post stroke complications	*As evidenced by*	results of swallowing tests and reports of choking during mealtime

* If a synonym, or alternate word with the same meaning, for the term "inadequate" is helpful or needed, an approved alternate is the word "suboptimal." Thus, a dietetics professional could use either the nutrition diagnosis label "Suboptimal oral food/beverage intake" or "Inadequate oral food/beverage intake."

Nutrition Diagnosis Reference sheet

A reference sheet is available for each nutrition diagnosis. Reference sheets contain four distinct components: nutrition diagnosis label, definition of nutrition diagnosis label, examples of common etiologies, and signs/symptoms. Following is a description of the four components of the reference sheet.

The **Problem or Nutrition Diagnosis Label** describes alterations in the patient/client's nutritional status that dietetics practitioners are responsible for treating independently. Nutrition diagnosis differs from medical diagnosis in that a nutrition diagnosis changes as the patient/client response changes. The medical diagnosis does not change as long as the disease or condition exists. A nutrition diagnosis allows the dietetics practitioner to identify realistic and measurable outcomes, formulate nutrition interventions, and monitor and evaluate change.

Edition: 2009

The **Definition** of Nutrition Diagnosis Label briefly describes the Nutrition Diagnosis Label to differentiate a discrete problem area.

The **Etiology** (Cause/Contributing Risk Factors) are those factors contributing to the existence, or maintenance of pathophysiological, psychosocial, situational, developmental, cultural, and/or environmental problems. It is linked to the Nutrition Diagnosis Label by the words *related to*.

The **Signs/Symptoms** (Defining Characteristics) consist of subjective and/or objective data used to determine whether the patient/client has the nutrition diagnosis specified. It is linked to the etiology by the words *as evidenced by*.

The signs and symptoms are gathered in Step 1 of the Nutrition Care Process: nutrition assessment. There are five categories of nutrition assessment data used to cluster the information on the nutrition diagnosis reference sheet— food/nutrition-related history; biochemical data, medical tests, and procedures; anthropometric measurements; nutrition-focused physical findings; and client history. Within each nutrition assessment category, potential indicators associated with the specific nutrition diagnosis are listed on the reference sheet.

Example
Swallowing Difficulty NC-1.1

Nutrition Assessment Category	Potential Indicator of this Nutrition Diagnosis
Nutrition-Focused Physical Finding	• Evidence of dehydration, e.g., dry mucous membranes, poor skin turgor

These reference sheets, following this chapter, will assist practitioners with identifying, consistently and correctly, the nutrition diagnoses.

Special Note: Laboratory parameters within the nutrition diagnosis reference sheets are provided only for guidance and practitioners:

- Should be aware that laboratory values may be different depending on the laboratory performing the test.

- Must recognize that there may not be scientific consensus on the best measure to use for testing and evaluating a particular lab or reference standard parameter.

- Need to evaluate laboratory findings for their significance or lack of significance depending on the patient/client population, disease severity, and/or treatment goals.

- Are responsible for keeping abreast of national, institutional, and regulatory guidelines that impact practice and applying them as appropriate to individual patient/clients.

Summary

Nutrition diagnosis is the critical link in the Nutrition Care Process between nutrition assessment and nutrition intervention. Nutrition interventions can then be clearly targeted to address either the etiology (E) or signs and symptoms (S) of the specific nutrition diagnosis/problem identified. Using a standardized terminology for identifying the nutrition diagnosis/problem will make one aspect of the critical thinking of dietetics practitioners visible to other professionals as well as provide a clear method of communicating among dietetics practitioners. Implementation of a standard language throughout the profession, with tools to assist practitioners, is making this language a success. Ongoing study and evaluation is critical as the standardized language is utilized by the profession.

References

1. Charney, P. J. (2006). *Reliability of nutrition diagnostic codes and their defining characteristics.* (Doctoral dissertation, University of Medicine and Dentistry of New Jersey, 2006.).

Diagnosis

INTAKE — NI

Defined as "actual problems related to intake of energy, nutrients, fluids, bioactive substances through oral diet or nutrition support"

Energy Balance (1)

Defined as "actual or estimated changes in energy (kcal) balance"

- ☐ Unused — NI-1.1
- ☐ Increased energy expenditure — NI-1.2
- ☐ Unused — NI-1.3
- ☐ Inadequate energy intake — NI-1.4
- ☐ Excessive energy intake — NI-1.5

Oral or Nutrition Support Intake (2)

Defined as "actual or estimated food and beverage intake from oral diet or nutrition support compared with patient goal"

- ☐ Inadequate oral food/ beverage intake — NI-2.1
- ☐ Excessive oral food/beverage intake — NI-2.2
- ☐ Inadequate intake from enteral/parenteral nutrition — NI-2.3
- ☐ Excessive intake from enteral/parenteral nutrition — NI-2.4
- ☐ Inappropriate infusion of enteral/parenteral nutrition (use with caution) — NI-2.5

Fluid Intake (3)

Defined as "actual or estimated fluid intake compared with patient goal"

- ☐ Inadequate fluid intake — NI-3.1
- ☐ Excessive fluid intake — NI-3.2

Bioactive Substances (4)

Defined as "actual or observed intake of bioactive substances, including single or multiple functional food components, ingredients, dietary supplements, alcohol"

- ☐ Inadequate bioactive substance intake — NI-4.1
- ☐ Excessive bioactive substance intake — NI-4.2
- ☐ Excessive alcohol intake — NI-4.3

Nutrient (5)

Defined as "actual or estimated intake of specific nutrient groups or single nutrients as compared with desired levels"

- ☐ Increased nutrient needs (specify) _____ — NI-5.1
- ☐ Malnutrition — NI-5.2
- ☐ Inadequate protein-energy intake — NI-5.3
- ☐ Decreased nutrient needs (specify) _____ — NI-5.4
- ☐ Imbalance of nutrients — NI-5.5

Fat and Cholesterol (5.6)

- ☐ Inadequate fat intake — NI-5.6.1
- ☐ Excessive fat intake — NI-5.6.2
- ☐ Inappropriate intake of fats (specify) _____ — NI-5.6.3

Protein (5.7)

- ☐ Inadequate protein intake — NI-5.7.1
- ☐ Excessive protein intake — NI-5.7.2
- ☐ Inappropriate intake of amino acids (specify) _____ — NI-5.7.3

Carbohydrate and Fiber (5.8)

- ☐ Inadequate carbohydrate intake — NI-5.8.1
- ☐ Excessive carbohydrate intake — NI-5.8.2
- ☐ Inappropriate intake of types of carbohydrate (specify) _____ — NI-5.8.3
- ☐ Inconsistent carbohydrate intake — NI-5.8.4
- ☐ Inadequate fiber intake — NI-5.8.5
- ☐ Excessive fiber intake — NI-5.8.6

Vitamin (5.9)

- ☐ Inadequate vitamin intake (specify) _____ — NI-5.9.1
  - ☐ A (1)
  - ☐ C (2)
  - ☐ D (3)
  - ☐ E (4)
  - ☐ K (5)
  - ☐ Thiamin (6)
  - ☐ Riboflavin (7)
  - ☐ Niacin (8)
  - ☐ Folate (9)
  - ☐ B6 (10)
  - ☐ B12 (11)
  - ☐ Other (specify) _____ (12)
- ☐ Excessive vitamin intake (specify) _____ — NI-5.9.2
  - ☐ A (1)
  - ☐ C (2)
  - ☐ D (3)
  - ☐ E (4)
  - ☐ K (5)
  - ☐ Thiamin (6)
  - ☐ Riboflavin (7)
  - ☐ Niacin (8)
  - ☐ Folate (9)
  - ☐ B6 (10)
  - ☐ B12 (11)
  - ☐ Other (specify) _____ (12)

Mineral (5.10)

- ☐ Inadequate mineral intake (specify) _____ — NI-5.10.1
  - ☐ Calcium (1)
  - ☐ Chloride (2)
  - ☐ Iron (3)
  - ☐ Magnesium (4)
  - ☐ Potassium (5)
  - ☐ Phosphorus (6)
  - ☐ Sodium (7)
  - ☐ Zinc (8)
  - ☐ Other (specify) _____ (9)
- ☐ Excessive mineral intake (specify) _____ — NI-5.10.2
  - ☐ Calcium (1)
  - ☐ Chloride (2)
  - ☐ Iron (3)
  - ☐ Magnesium (4)
  - ☐ Potassium (5)
  - ☐ Phosphorus (6)
  - ☐ Sodium (7)
  - ☐ Zinc (8)
  - ☐ Other (specify) _____ (9)

CLINICAL — NC

Defined as "nutritional findings/problems identified that relate to medical or physical conditions"

Functional (1)

Defined as "change in physical or mechanical functioning that interferes with or prevents desired nutritional consequences"

- ☐ Swallowing difficulty — NC-1.1
- ☐ Biting/Chewing (masticatory) difficulty — NC-1.2
- ☐ Breastfeeding difficulty — NC-1.3
- ☐ Altered GI function — NC-1.4

Biochemical (2)

Defined as "change in capacity to metabolize nutrients as a result of medications, surgery, or as indicated by altered lab values"

- ☐ Impaired nutrient utilization — NC-2.1
- ☐ Altered nutrition-related laboratory values (specify) _____ — NC-2.2
- ☐ Food-medication interaction — NC-2.3

Weight (3)

Defined as "chronic weight or changed weight status when compared with usual or desired body weight"

- ☐ Underweight — NC-3.1
- ☐ Involuntary weight loss — NC-3.2
- ☐ Overweight/obesity — NC-3.3
- ☐ Involuntary weight gain — NC-3.4

BEHAVIORAL-ENVIRONMENTAL — NB

Defined as "nutritional findings/problems identified that relate to knowledge, attitudes/beliefs, physical environment, access to food, or food safety"

Knowledge and Beliefs (1)

Defined as "actual knowledge and beliefs as related, observed or documented"

- ☐ Food- and nutrition-related knowledge deficit — NB-1.1
- ☐ Harmful beliefs/attitudes about food- or nutrition-related topics (use with caution) — NB-1.2
- ☐ Not ready for diet/lifestyle change — NB-1.3
- ☐ Self-monitoring deficit — NB-1.4
- ☐ Disordered eating pattern — NB-1.5
- ☐ Limited adherence to nutrition-related recommendations — NB-1.6
- ☐ Undesirable food choices — NB-1.7

Physical Activity and Function (2)

Defined as "actual physical activity, self-care, and quality-of-life problems as reported, observed, or documented"

- ☐ Physical inactivity — NB-2.1
- ☐ Excessive physical activity — NB-2.2
- ☐ Inability or lack of desire to manage self-care — NB-2.3
- ☐ Impaired ability to prepare foods/meals — NB-2.4
- ☐ Poor nutrition quality of life — NB-2.5
- ☐ Self-feeding difficulty — NB-2.6

Food Safety and Access (3)

Defined as "actual problems with food access or food safety"

- ☐ Intake of unsafe food — NB-3.1
- ☐ Limited access to food — NB-3.2

Diagnosis

Date Identified	Date Resolved

#1 Problem _____

    Etiology _____

    Signs/Symptoms _____

#2 Problem _____

    Etiology _____

    Signs/Symptoms _____

#3 Problem _____

    Etiology _____

    Signs/Symptoms _____

Edition: 2009

Nutrition Diagnosis Terms and Definitions

Nutrition Diagnostic Term	Term Number	Definition	Reference Sheet Page Numbers
DOMAIN: INTAKE	NI	Actual problems related to intake of energy, nutrients, fluids, bioactive substances through oral diet or nutrition support (enteral or parenteral nutrition).	
Class: Energy Balance (1)		Actual or estimated changes in energy (kcal) balance.	
Unused	NI-1.1		
Increased energy expenditure	NI-1.2	Resting metabolic rate (RMR) more than predicted requirements due to body composition, medications, body system, environmental, or genetic changes. *Note: RMR is the sum of metabolic processes of active cell mass related to the maintenance of normal body functions and regulatory balance during rest.*	213
Unused	NI-1.3		
Inadequate energy intake	NI-1.4	Energy intake that is less than energy expenditure, established reference standards, or recommendations based on physiological needs. *Note: May not be an appropriate nutrition diagnosis when the goal is weight loss, during end-of-life care, upon initiation of EN/PN, or acute stressed state (e.g., surgery, organ failure). Whenever possible, nutrient intake data should be considered in combination with clinical, biochemical, anthropometric information, medical diagnosis, clinical status, and/or other factors as well as diet to provide a valid assessment of nutritional status based on a totality of the evidence.* (Dietary Reference Intakes. Applications in Dietary Assessment. *Institute of Medicine. Washington, D.C.: National Academy Press; 2000.)*	214-215
Excessive energy intake	NI-1.5	Energy intake that exceeds energy expenditure, established reference standards, or recommendations based on physiological needs. *Note: May not be an appropriate nutrition diagnosis when weight gain is desired.*	216-217

Diagnosis

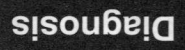
Nutrition Diagnosis Terms and Definitions

Nutrition Diagnostic Term	Term Number	Definition	Reference Sheet Page Numbers
Class: Oral or Nutrition Support Intake (2)		Actual or estimated food and beverage intake from oral diet or nutrition support compared with patient goal.	
Inadequate oral food/beverage intake	NI-2.1	Oral food/beverage intake that is less than established reference standards or recommendations based on physiological needs. *Note: May not be an appropriate nutrition diagnosis when the goal is weight loss, during end-of-life care, upon initiation of feeding, or during combined oral/EN/PN therapy. Whenever possible, nutrient intake data should be considered in combination with clinical, biochemical, anthropometric information, medical diagnosis, clinical status, and/or other factors as well as diet to provide a valid assessment of nutritional status based on a totality of the evidence.* (Dietary Reference Intakes. Applications in Dietary Assessment. *Institute of Medicine. Washington, D.C.: National Academy Press; 2000.)*	218-219
Excessive oral food/beverage intake	NI-2.2	Oral food/beverage intake that exceeds estimated energy needs, established reference standards, or recommendations based on physiological needs. *Note: May not be an appropriate nutrition diagnosis when weight gain is desired.*	220-221
Inadequate intake from enteral/parenteral nutrition	NI-2.3	Enteral or parenteral infusion that provides fewer calories or nutrients compared to established reference standards or recommendations based on physiological needs. *Note: May not be an appropriate nutrition diagnosis when recommendation is for weight loss, during end-of-life care, upon initiation of feeding, or during acute stressed states (e.g., surgery, organ failure). Whenever possible, nutrient intake data should be considered in combination with clinical, biochemical, anthropometric information, medical diagnosis, clinical status, and/or other factors as well as diet to provide a valid assessment of nutritional status based on a totality of the evidence.* (Dietary Reference Intakes. Applications in Dietary Assessment. *Institute of Medicine. Washington, D.C.: National Academy Press; 2000.)*	222-224
Excessive intake from enteral/parenteral nutrition	NI-2.4	Enteral or parenteral infusion that provides more calories or nutrients compared to established reference standards or recommendations based on physiological needs.	225-226

Nutrition Diagnosis Terms and Definitions

Nutrition Diagnostic Term	Term Number	Definition	Reference Sheet Page Numbers
Inappropriate infusion of enteral/ parenteral nutrition USE WITH CAUTION only after discussion with other members if the health care team	NI-2.5	Enteral or parenteral infusion that provides either fewer or more calories and/or nutrients or is of the wrong composition or type, parental nutrition that is not warranted because the patient is able to tolerate an enteral intake, or is unsafe because of the potential for sepsis or other complications	227-228
Class: Fluid Intake (3)		Actual or estimated fluid intake compared with patient goal.	
Inadequate fluid intake	NI-3.1	Lower intake of fluid-containing foods or substances compared to established reference standards or recommendations based on physiological needs. *Note: Whenever possible, nutrient intake data should be considered in combination with clinical, biochemical, anthropometric information, medical diagnosis, clinical status, and/or other factors as well as diet to provide a valid assessment of nutritional status based on a totality of the evidence. (Dietary Reference Intakes. Applications in Dietary Assessment. Institute of Medicine. Washington, D.C.: National Academy Press; 2000.)*	229-230
Excessive fluid intake	NI-3.2	Higher intake of fluid compared to established reference standards or recommendations based on physiological needs.	231-232
Class: Bioactive Substances (4)		Actual or observed intake of bioactive substances, including single or multiple functional food components, ingredients, dietary supplements, alcohol.	
Inadequate bioactive substance intake	NI-4.1	Lower intake of bioactive substances compared to established reference standards or recommendations based on physiological needs. *Note: Bioactive substances are not included as part of the Dietary Reference Intakes, and therefore there are no established minimum requirements or Tolerable Upper Intake Levels. However, RDs can assess whether estimated intakes are adequate or excessive using the patient/client goal or nutrition prescription for comparison.* *Working definition of bioactive substances—physiologically active components of foods that may offer health benefits beyond traditional macro- or micro-nutrient requirements. There is not scientific consensus about a definition for bioactive substances/components.*	233-234

Nutrition Diagnosis Terms and Definitions

Nutrition Diagnostic Term	Term Number	Definition	Reference Sheet Page Numbers
Excessive bioactive substance intake	NI-4.2	Higher intake of bioactive substances compared to established reference standards or recommendations based on physiological needs. *Note: Working definition of bioactive substances—physiologically active components of foods that may offer health benefits beyond traditional macro- or micronutrient requirements. There is not scientific consensus about a definition for bioactive substances/components.*	235-236
Excessive alcohol intake	NI-4.3	Intake more than the suggested limits for alcohol.	237-238
Class: Nutrient (5)		Actual or estimated intake of specific nutrient groups or single nutrients as compared with desired levels.	
Increased nutrient needs (specify)	NI-5.1	Increased need for a specific nutrient compared to established reference standards or recommendations based on physiological needs	239-240
Malnutrition	NI-5.2	Inadequate intake of protein and/or energy over prolonged periods of time resulting in loss of fat stores and/or muscle wasting.	241-242
Inadequate protein-energy intake	NI-5.3	Inadequate intake of protein and/or energy compared to established reference standards or recommendations based on physiological needs of short or recent duration. *Note: Whenever possible, nutrient intake data should be considered in combination with clinical, biochemical, anthropometric information, medical diagnosis, clinical status, and/or other factors as well as diet to provide a valid assessment of nutritional status based on a totality of the evidence. (Dietary Reference Intakes. Applications in Dietary Assessment. Institute of Medicine. Washington, D.C.: National Academy Press; 2000.)*	243-244
Decreased nutrient needs (specify)	NI-5.4	Decreased need for a specific nutrient compared to established reference standards or recommendations based on physiological needs.	245-246
Imbalance of nutrients	NI-5.5	An undesirable combination of nutrients, such that the amount of one nutrient interferes with or alters absorption and/or utilization of another nutrient.	247-248

Nutrition Diagnosis Terms and Definitions

Nutrition Diagnostic Term	Term Number	Definition	Reference Sheet Page Numbers
Subclass: Fat and Cholesterol (5.6)			
Inadequate fat intake	NI-5.6.1	Lower fat intake compared to established reference standards or recommendations based on physiological needs. *Note: May not be an appropriate nutrition diagnosis when recommendation is for weight loss or during end-of-life care. Whenever possible, nutrient intake data should be considered in combination with clinical, biochemical, anthropometric information, medical diagnosis, clinical status, and/or other factors as well as diet to provide a valid assessment of nutritional status based on a totality of the evidence.* (Dietary Reference Intakes. Applications in Dietary Assessment. *Institute of Medicine. Washington, D.C.: National Academy Press; 2000.)*	249-250
Excessive fat intake	NI-5.6.2	Higher fat intake compared to established reference standards or recommendations based on physiological needs.	251-252
Inappropriate intake of fats (specify)	NI-5.6.3	Intake of wrong type or quality of fats compared to established reference standards or recommendations based on physiological needs.	253-254
Subclass: Protein (5.7)			
Inadequate protein intake	NI-5.7.1	Lower intake of protein compared to established reference standards or recommendations based on physiological needs. *Note: Whenever possible, nutrient intake data should be considered in combination with clinical, biochemical, anthropometric information, medical diagnosis, clinical status, and/or other factors as well as diet to provide a valid assessment of nutritional status based on a totality of the evidence.* (Dietary Reference Intakes. Applications in Dietary Assessment. *Institute of Medicine. Washington, D.C.: National Academy Press; 2000.)*	255-256
Excessive protein intake	NI-5.7.2	Intake more than the recommended level of protein compared to established reference standards or recommendations based on physiological needs.	257-258
Inappropriate intake of amino acids (specify)	NI-5.7.3	Intake that is more or less than recommended level and/or type of amino acids compared to established reference standards or recommendations based on physiological needs	259-260

Diagnosis

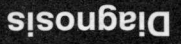

Nutrition Diagnosis Terms and Definitions

Nutrition Diagnostic Term	Term Number	Definition	Reference Sheet Page Numbers
Subclass: Carbohydrate and Fiber (5.8)			
Inadequate carbohydrate intake	NI-5.8.1	Lower intake of carbohydrate compared to established reference standards or recommendations based on physiological needs. *Note: Whenever possible, nutrient intake data should be considered in combination with clinical, biochemical, anthropometric information, medical diagnosis, clinical status, and/or other factors as well as diet to provide a valid assessment of nutritional status based on a totality of the evidence.* (Dietary Reference Intakes. Applications in Dietary Assessment. *Institute of Medicine. Washington, D.C.: National Academy Press; 2000.)*	261-262
Excessive carbohydrate intake	NI-5.8.2	Intake more than the recommended level and type of carbohydrate compared to established reference standards or recommendations based on physiological needs.	263-264
Inappropriate intake of types of carbohydrate (specify)	NI-5.8.3	Intake or the type or amount of carbohydrate that is more or less than the established reference standards or recommendations based on physiological needs.	265-266
Inconsistent carbohydrate intake	NI-5.8.4	Inconsistent timing of carbohydrate intake throughout the day, day to day, or a pattern of carbohydrate intake that is not consistent with recommended pattern based on physiological needs.	267-268
Inadequate fiber intake	NI-5.8.5	Lower intake of fiber compared to established reference standards or recommendations based on physiological needs. *Note: Whenever possible, nutrient intake data should be considered in combination with clinical, biochemical, anthropometric information, medical diagnosis, clinical status, and/or other factors as well as diet to provide a valid assessment of nutritional status based on a totality of the evidence.* (Dietary Reference Intakes. Applications in Dietary Assessment. *Institute of Medicine. Washington, D.C.: National Academy Press; 2000.)*	269-270
Excessive fiber intake	NI-5.8.6	Higher intake of fiber compared to recommendations based on patient/client condition.	271-272

Nutrition Diagnosis Terms and Definitions

Nutrition Diagnostic Term	Term Number	Definition	Reference Sheet Page Numbers
Subclass: Vitamin (5.9)			
Inadequate vitamin intake (specify)	NI-5.9.1	Lower intake of one or more vitamins compared to established reference standards or recommendations based on physiological needs. *Note: Whenever possible, nutrient intake data should be considered in combination with clinical, biochemical, anthropometric information, medical diagnosis, clinical status, and/or other factors as well as diet to provide a valid assessment of nutritional status based on a totality of the evidence. (Dietary Reference Intakes. Applications in Dietary Assessment. Institute of Medicine. Washington, D.C.: National Academy Press; 2000.)*	273-275
Excessive vitamin intake (specify)	NI-5.9.2	Higher intake of one or more vitamins compared to established reference standards or recommendations based on physiological needs.	276-277
Subclass: Mineral (5.10)			
Inadequate mineral intake (specify)	NI-5.10.1	Lower intake of one or more minerals compared to established reference standards or recommendations based on physiological needs. *Note: Whenever possible, nutrient intake data should be considered in combination with clinical, biochemical, anthropometric information, medical diagnosis, clinical status, and/or other factors as well as diet to provide a valid assessment of nutritional status based on a totality of the evidence. (Dietary Reference Intakes. Applications in Dietary Assessment. Institute of Medicine. Washington, D.C.: National Academy Press; 2000.)*	278-280
Excessive mineral intake (specify)	NI-5.10.2	Higher intake of one or more minerals compared to established reference standards or recommendations based on physiological needs.	281-282
DOMAIN: CLINICAL	NC	Nutritional findings/problems identified that relate to medical or physical conditions.	
Class: Functional (1)		Change in physical or mechanical functioning that interferes with or prevents desired nutritional consequences.	
Swallowing difficulty	NC-1.1	Impaired or difficult movement of food and liquid within the oral cavity to the stomach.	283-284
Biting/Chewing (masticatory) difficulty	NC-1.2	Impaired ability to bite or chew food in preparation for swallowing.	285-287

Diagnosis

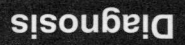

Nutrition Diagnosis Terms and Definitions

Nutrition Diagnostic Term	Term Number	Definition	Reference Sheet Page Numbers
Breastfeeding difficulty	NC-1.3	Inability to sustain nutrition through breastfeeding.	288-289
Altered GI function	NC-1.4	Changes in ability to digest or absorb nutrients.	290-291
Class: Biochemical (2)		Change in capacity to metabolize nutrients as a result of medications, surgery, or as indicated by altered lab values.	
Impaired nutrient utilization	NC-2.1	Changes in ability to absorb or metabolize nutrients and bioactive substances.	292-293
Altered nutrition-related laboratory values (specify)	NC-2.2	Changes due to body composition, medications, body system changes or genetics, or changes in ability to eliminate byproducts of digestive and metabolic processes.	294-295
Food-medication interaction	NC-2.3	Undesirable/harmful interaction(s) between food and over-the-counter (OTC) medications, prescribed medications, herbals, botanicals, and/or dietary supplements that diminishes, enhances, or alters effect of nutrients and/or medications.	296-297
Class: Weight (3)		Chronic weight or changed weight status when compared with usual or desired body weight.	
Underweight	NC-3.1	Low body weight compared to established reference standards or recommendations.	298-300
Involuntary weight loss	NC-3.2	Modified the definition: Decrease in body weight that is not planned or desired. *Note: May not be an appropriate nutrition diagnosis when changes in body weight are due to fluid.*	301-302
Overweight/obesity	NC-3.3	Increased adiposity compared to established reference standards or recommendations, ranging from overweight to morbid obesity.	303-304
Involuntary weight gain	NC-3.4	Weight gain more than that which is desired or planned.	305-306

Nutrition Diagnosis Terms and Definitions

Nutrition Diagnostic Term	Term Number	Definition	Reference Sheet Page Numbers
DOMAIN: BEHAVIORAL-ENVIRONMENTAL	NB	Nutritional findings/problems identified that relate to knowledge, attitudes/beliefs, physical environment, access to food, or food safety.	
Class: Knowledge and Beliefs (1)		Actual knowledge and beliefs as reported, observed, or documented.	
Food- and nutrition-related knowledge deficit	NB-1.1	Incomplete or inaccurate knowledge about food, nutrition, or nutrition-related information and guidelines, e.g., nutrient requirements, consequences of food behaviors, life stage requirements, nutrition recommendations, diseases and conditions, physiological function, or products	307-308
Harmful beliefs/attitudes about food or nutrition-related topics USE WITH CAUTION TO BE SENSITIVE TO PATIENT CONCERNS	NB-1.2	Beliefs/attitudes and practices about food, nutrition, and nutrition-related topics that are incompatible with sound nutrition principles, nutrition care, or disease/condition (excluding disordered eating patterns and eating disorders).	309-310
Not ready for diet/lifestyle change	NB-1.3	Lack of perceived value of nutrition-related behavior change compared to costs (consequences or effort required to make changes); conflict with personal value system; antecedent to behavior change.	311-312
Self-monitoring deficit	NB-1.4	Lack of data recording to track personal progress.	313-314
Disordered eating pattern	NB-1.5	Beliefs, attitudes, thoughts, and behaviors related to food, eating, and weight management, including classic eating disorders as well as less severe, similar conditions that negatively impact health.	315-317
Limited adherence to nutrition-related recommendations	NB-1.6	Lack of nutrition-related changes as per intervention agreed upon by client or population.	318-319
Undesirable food choices	NB-1.7	Food and/or beverage choices that are inconsistent with DRIs, US Dietary Guidelines, or MyPyramid, or with targets defined in the nutrition prescription or Nutrition Care Process.	320-321

Nutrition Diagnosis Terms and Definitions

Nutrition Diagnostic Term	Term Number	Definition	Reference Sheet Page Numbers
Class: Physical Activity and Function (2)		Actual physical activity, self-care, and quality-of-life problems as reported, observed, or documented.	
Physical inactivity	NB-2.1	Low level of activity or sedentary behavior to the extent that it reduces energy expenditure and impacts health.	322-323
Excessive physical activity	NB-2.2	Involuntary or voluntary physical activity or movement that interferes with energy needs, growth, or exceeds that which is necessary to achieve optimal health.	324-325
Inability or lack of desire to manage self-care	NB-2.3	Lack of capacity or unwillingness to implement methods to support healthful food- and nutrition-related behavior.	326-327
Impaired ability to prepare foods/meals	NB-2.4	Cognitive or physical impairment that prevents preparation of foods/fluids.	328-329
Poor nutrition quality of life (NQOL)	NB-2.5	Diminished patient/client perception of quality of life in response to nutrition problems and recommendations.	330-331
Self feeding difficulty	NB-2.6	Impaired actions to place food or beverages in mouth.	332-333
Class: Food Safety and Access (3)		Actual problems with food access or food safety.	
Intake of unsafe food	NB-3.1	Intake of food and/or fluids intentionally or unintentionally contaminated with toxins, poisonous products, infectious agents, microbial agents, additives, allergens, and/or agents of bioterrorism.	334-335
Limited access to food	NB-3.2	Diminished ability to acquire a sufficient quantity and variety of healthful food based upon the U.S. Dietary Guidelines or MyPyramid. Limitation to food because of concerns about weight or aging.	336-337

Increased Energy Expenditure (NI-1.2)

Definition

Resting metabolic rate (RMR) more than predicted requirements due to body composition, medications, endocrine, neurologic, or genetic changes.

Note: RMR is the sum of metabolic processes of active cell mass related to the maintenance of normal body functions and regulatory balance during rest.

Etiology (Cause/Contributing Risk Factors)

Factors gathered during the nutrition assessment process that contribute to the existence or the maintenance of pathophysiological, psychosocial, situational, developmental, cultural, and/or environmental problems:

- Physiological causes increasing nutrient needs due to anabolism, growth, maintenance of body temperature
- Voluntary or involuntary physical activity/movement

Signs/Symptoms (Defining Characteristics)

A typical cluster of subjective and objective signs and symptoms gathered during the nutrition assessment process that provide evidence that a problem exists; quantify the problem and describe its severity.

Nutrition Assessment Category	Potential Indicators of this Nutrition Diagnosis (one or more must be present)
Biochemical Data, Medical Tests and Procedures	
Anthropometric Measurements	• Unintentional weight loss of ≥ 10% in 6 months, ≥ 5% in 1 month (adults and pediatrics) and > 2% in 1 week (pediatrics) • Evidence of need for accelerated or catch-up growth or weight gain in children; absence of normal growth • Increased proportion of lean body mass
Nutrition-Focused Physical Findings	• Fever • Measured RMR > estimated or expected RMR
Food/Nutrition-Related History	• Increased physical activity, e.g., endurance athlete • Medications that increase energy expenditure
Client History	• Conditions associated with a diagnosis or treatment, e.g., Parkinson's disease, cerebral palsy, Alzheimer's disease, cystic fibrosis, chronic obstructive pulmonary disease (COPD)

References

1. Frankenfield D, Roth-Yousey L, Compher C. Comparison of predictive equations to measured resting metabolic rate in healthy nonobese and obese individuals, a systematic review. *J Am Diet Assoc.* 2005;105:775-789.

Updated: 2009 Edition

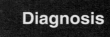

Diagnosis

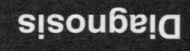

Intake Domain – Energy Balance

Inadequate* Energy Intake (NI-1.4)

Definition

Energy intake that is less than energy expenditure, established reference standards, or recommendations based on physiological needs.

Note: May not be an appropriate nutrition diagnosis when the goal is weight loss, during end-of-life care, upon initiation of EN/PN, or acute stressed state (e.g., surgery, organ failure).

Whenever possible, nutrient intake data should be considered in combination with clinical, biochemical, anthropometric information, medical diagnosis, clinical status, and/or other factors as well as diet to provide a valid assessment of nutritional status based on a totality of the evidence. (Dietary Reference Intakes. Applications in Dietary Assessment. Institute of Medicine. Washington, D.C.: National Academy Press; 2000.)

Etiology (Cause/Contributing Risk Factors)

Factors gathered during the nutrition assessment process that contribute to the existence or the maintenance of pathophysiological, psychosocial, situational, developmental, cultural, and/or environmental problems:

- Pathologic or physiological causes that result in increased energy requirements or decreased ability to consume sufficient energy, e.g., increased nutrient needs due to prolonged catabolic illness
- Lack of access to food or artificial nutrition, e.g., economic constraints, restricting food given to elderly and/or children
- Cultural practices that affect ability to access food
- Food- and nutrition-related knowledge deficit concerning energy intake
- Psychological causes such as depression and disordered eating

Signs/Symptoms (Defining Characteristics)

A typical cluster of subjective and objective signs and symptoms gathered during the nutrition assessment process that provide evidence that a problem exists; quantify the problem and describe its severity.

Nutrition Assessment Category	Potential Indicators of this Nutrition Diagnosis (one or more must be present)
Biochemical Data, Medical Tests and Procedures	
Anthropometric Measurements	• Failure to gain or maintain appropriate weight
Nutrition-Focused Physical Findings	• Poor dentition

*If a synonym, or alternate word with the same meaning, for the term "inadequate" is helpful or needed, an approved alternate is the word "suboptimal."

Inadequate* Energy Intake (NI-1.4)

Food/Nutrition-Related History	Reports or observations of: • Estimated energy intake from diet less than needs based on estimated or measured resting metabolic rate • Restriction or omission of energy-dense foods from diet • Food avoidance and/or lack of interest in food • Inability to independently consume foods/fluids (diminished joint mobility of wrist, hand, or digits) • Estimated parenteral or enteral nutrition intake insufficient to meet needs based on estimated or measured resting metabolic rate • Excessive consumption of alcohol or other drugs that reduce hunger • Medications that affect appetite
Client History	• Conditions associated with diagnosis or treatment, e.g., mental illness, eating disorders, dementia, alcoholism, substance abuse, and acute or chronic pain management

References

1   National Academy of Sciences, Institute of Medicine. *Dietary Reference Intakes for Energy, Carbohydrate, Fiber, Fat, Fatty Acids*, Cholesterol, Protein, and Amino Acids. Washington, DC: National Academy Press; 2002.

Updated: 2009 Edition

If a synonym, or alternate word with the same meaning, for the term "inadequate" is helpful or needed, an approved alternate is the word "suboptimal."

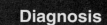

Diagnosis

Excessive Energy Intake (NI-1.5)

Definition

Energy intake that exceeds energy expenditure, established reference standards, or recommendations based on physiological needs.

Note: May not be appropriate nutrition diagnosis when weight gain is desired.

Etiology (Cause/Contributing Risk Factors)

Factors gathered during the nutrition assessment process that contribute to the existence or the maintenance of pathophysiological, psychosocial, situational, developmental, cultural, and/or environmental problems:

- Harmful beliefs/attitudes about food, nutrition, and nutrition-related topics
- Food-and nutrition-related knowledge deficit concerning energy intake
- Lack of or limited access to healthful food choices, e.g., healthful food choices not provided as an option by caregiver or parent, homeless
- Lack of value for behavior change, competing values
- Medications that increase appetite, e.g., steroids, antidepressants
- Overfeeding of parenteral/enteral nutrition (PN/EN)
- Calories unaccounted for from IV infusion and/or medications
- Unwilling or disinterested in reducing energy intake
- Failure to adjust for lifestyle changes and decreased metabolism (e.g., aging)
- Resolution of prior hypermetabolism without reduction in intake

Signs/Symptoms (Defining Characteristics)

A typical cluster of subjective and objective signs and symptoms gathered during the nutrition assessment process that provide evidence that a problem exists; quantify the problem and describe its severity.

Nutrition Assessment Category	Potential Indicators of this Nutrition Diagnosis (one or more must be present)
Biochemical Data, Medical Tests and Procedures	• Abnormal liver function tests after prolonged exposure (3-6 weeks) • Respiratory quotient >1.0
Anthropometric Measurements	• Body fat percentage > 25% for men and > 32% for women • BMI > 25 (adults), BMI > 95th percentile (pediatrics) • Weight gain

Excessive Energy Intake (NI-1.5)

Nutrition-Focused Physical Findings	• Increased body adiposity • Increased respiratory rate
Food/Nutrition-Related History	Reports or observations of: • Intake of high caloric density or large portions of foods/beverages • EN/PN more than estimated or measured (e.g., indirect calorimetry) energy expenditure
Client History	

References

1. McClave SA, Lowen CC, Kleber MJ, McConnell JW, Jung LY, Goldsmith LJ. Clinical use of the respiratory quotient obtained from indirect calorimetry. *JPEN J Parenter Enteral Nutr*. 2003;27:21-26.

2. McClave SA, Lowen CC, Kleber MJ, Nicholson JF, Jimmerson SC, McConnell JW, Jung LY. Are patients fed appropriately according to their caloric requirements? *JPEN J Parenter Enteral Nutr*. 1998;22:375-381.

3. Overweight and Obesity: Health Consequences. www.surgeongeneral.gov/topics/obesity/calltoaction/fact_consequences.htm. Accessed August 28, 2004.

Updated: 2008 Edition

Diagnosis

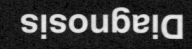

Intake Domain – Oral or Nutrition Support Intake

Inadequate* Oral Food/Beverage Intake (NI-2.1)

Definition

Oral food/beverage intake that is less than established reference standards or recommendations based on physiological needs.

> *Note: May not be an appropriate nutrition diagnosis when the goal is weight loss, during end-of-life care, upon initiation of feeding, or during combined oral/EN/PN therapy.*
>
> *Whenever possible, nutrient intake data should be considered in combination with clinical, biochemical, anthropometric information, medical diagnosis, clinical status, and/or other factors as well as diet to provide a valid assessment of nutritional status based on a totality of the evidence.* (Dietary Reference Intakes. Applications in Dietary Assessment. *Institute of Medicine. Washington, D.C.: National Academy Press; 2000.*)

Etiology (Cause/Contributing Risk Factors)

Factors gathered during the nutrition assessment process that contribute to the existence or the maintenance of pathophysiological, psychosocial, situational, developmental, cultural, and/or environmental problems:

- Physiological causes increasing nutrient needs due to prolonged catabolic illness
- Lack of or limited access to food, e.g., economic constraints, restricting food given to elderly and/or children
- Cultural practices that affect ability to access food
- Food- and nutrition-related knowledge deficit concerning appropriate oral food/beverage intake
- Psychological causes such as depression and disordered eating

Signs/Symptoms (Defining Characteristics)

A typical cluster of subjective and objective signs and symptoms gathered during the nutrition assessment process that provide evidence that a problem exists; quantify the problem and describe its severity.

Nutrition Assessment Category	Potential Indicators of this Nutrition Diagnosis (one or more must be present)
Biochemical Data, Medical Tests and Procedures	
Anthropometric Measurements	• Weight loss, insufficient growth velocity
Nutrition-Focused Physical Findings	• Dry skin, mucous membranes, poor skin turgor • Anorexia, nausea, or vomiting • Change in appetite or taste

If a synonym, or alternate word with the same meaning, for the term "inadequate" is helpful or needed, an approved alternate is the word "suboptimal."

Inadequate* Oral Food/Beverage Intake (NI-2.1)

Food/Nutrition-Related History	Reports or observations of: • Estimates of insufficient intake of energy or high-quality protein from diet when compared to requirements • Economic constraints that limit food availability • Excessive consumption of alcohol or other drugs that reduce hunger • Medications that cause anorexia
Client History	• Conditions associated with a diagnosis or treatment of catabolic illness such as AIDS, tuberculosis, anorexia nervosa, sepsis or infection from recent surgery, depression, acute or chronic pain • Protein and/or nutrient malabsorption

References

1. National Academy of Sciences, Institute of Medicine. *Dietary Reference Intakes for Energy, Carbohydrate, Fiber, Fat, Fatty Acids, Cholesterol, Protein, and Amino Acids*. Washington, DC: National Academy Press; 2002.
2. National Academy of Sciences, Institute of Medicine. *Dietary Reference Intakes for Water, Potassium, Sodium, Chloride, and Sulfate*. Washington, DC: National Academy Press; 2002.

Updated: 2009 Edition

If a synonym, or alternate word with the same meaning, for the term "inadequate" is helpful or needed, an approved alternate is the word "suboptimal."

Diagnosis

Intake Domain – Oral or Nutrition Support Intake

Excessive Oral Food/Beverage Intake (NI-2.2)

Definition

Oral food/beverage intake that exceeds estimated energy needs, established reference standards, or recommendations based on physiological needs.

Note: May not be an appropriate nutrition diagnosis when weight gain is desired.

Etiology (Cause/Contributing Risk Factors)

Factors gathered during the nutrition assessment process that contribute to the existence or the maintenance of pathophysiological, psychosocial, situational, developmental, cultural, and/or environmental problems:

- Harmful beliefs/attitudes about food, nutrition, and nutrition-related topics
- Food- and nutrition-related knowledge deficit concerning appropriate oral food/beverage intake
- Lack of or limited access to healthful food choices, e.g., healthful food choices not provided as an option by caregiver or parent, homeless
- Lack of value for behavior change, competing values
- Inability to limit or refuse offered foods
- Lack of food planning, purchasing, and preparation skills
- Loss of appetite awareness
- Medications that increase appetite, e.g., steroids, antidepressants
- Mental illness, depression
- Unwilling or disinterested in reducing intake

Signs/Symptoms (Defining Characteristics)

A typical cluster of subjective and objective signs and symptoms gathered during the nutrition assessment process that provide evidence that a problem exists; quantify the problem and describe its severity.

Nutrition Assessment Category	Potential Indicators of this Nutrition Diagnosis (one or more must be present)
Biochemical Data, Medical Tests and Procedures	
Anthropometric Measurements	• Weight gain not attributed to fluid retention or normal growth
Nutrition-Focused Physical Findings	

Excessive Oral Food/Beverage Intake (NI-2.2)

Food/Nutrition-Related History	Reports or observations of: • Intake of high caloric-density foods/beverages (juice, soda, or alcohol) at meals and/or snacks • Intake of large portions of foods/beverages, food groups, or specific food items • Estimated intake that exceeds estimated or measured energy needs • Highly variable estimated daily energy intake • Binge eating patterns • Frequent, excessive fast food or restaurant intake
Client History	• Conditions associated with a diagnosis or treatment, e.g., obesity, overweight, or metabolic syndrome, depression, anxiety disorder

References

1. Overweight and Obesity: Health Consequences. www.surgeongeneral.gov/topics/obesity/calltoaction/fact_consequences.htm. Accessed August 28, 2004. Position of the American Dietetic Association: Weight management. *J Am Diet Assoc*. 2002;102:1145-1155.

2. Position of the American Dietetic Association: Total diet approach to communicating food and nutrition information. *J Am Diet Assoc*. 2007;107:1224-1232.

3. Position of the American Dietetic Association: The role of dietetics professionals in health promotion and disease prevention. *J Am Diet Assoc*. 2006;106:1875-1884.

Updated: 2008 Edition

Diagnosis

Intake Domain – Oral or Nutrition Support Intake

Inadequate* Intake from Enteral/Parenteral (EN/PN) Nutrition (NI-2.3)

Definition

Enteral or parenteral infusion that provides fewer calories or nutrients compared to established reference standards or recommendations based on physiological needs.

> *Note: May not be an appropriate nutrition diagnosis when recommendation is for weight loss, during end-of-life care, upon initiation of feeding, or during acute stressed states (e.g., surgery, organ failure).*
>
> *Whenever possible, nutrient intake data should be considered in combination with clinical, biochemical, anthropometric information, medical diagnosis, clinical status, and/or other factors as well as diet to provide a valid assessment of nutritional status based on a totality of the evidence. (*Dietary Reference Intakes. Applications in Dietary Assessment. *Institute of Medicine. Washington, D.C.: National Academy Press; 2000.)*

Etiology (Cause/Contributing Risk Factors)

Factors gathered during the nutrition assessment process that contribute to the existence or the maintenance of pathophysiological, psychosocial, situational, developmental, cultural, and/or environmental problems:

- Altered absorption or metabolism of nutrients, e.g., medications
- Food- and nutrition-related knowledge deficit concerning appropriate formula/formulation given for EN/PN
- Lack of, compromised, or incorrect access for delivering EN/PN
- Physiological causes increasing nutrient needs due to accelerated growth, wound healing, chronic infection, multiple fractures
- Intolerance of EN/PN
- Infusion volume not reached or schedule for infusion interrupted

Signs/Symptoms (Defining Characteristics)

A typical cluster of subjective and objective signs and symptoms gathered during the nutrition assessment process that provide evidence that a problem exists; quantify the problem and describe its severity.

Nutrition Assessment Category	Potential Indicators of this Nutrition Diagnosis (one or more must be present)
Biochemical Data, Medical Tests and Procedures	• Metabolic cart/indirect calorimetry measurement, e.g., respiratory quotient < 0.7 • Vitamin/mineral abnormalities: 　▪ Calcium < 9.2 mg/dL (2.3 mmol/L) 　▪ Vitamin K—abnormal international normalized ratio (INR) 　▪ Copper < 70 μg/dL (11 μmol/L) 　▪ Zinc < 78 μg/dL (12 μmol/L) 　▪ Iron < 50 μg/dL(nmol/L); iron-binding capacity < 250 μg/dL (44.8 μmol/L)

*If a synonym, or alternate word with the same meaning, for the term "inadequate" is helpful or needed, an approved alternate is the word "suboptimal."

Inadequate* Intake from Enteral/Parenteral (EN/PN) Nutrition (NI-2.3)

Anthropometric Measurements	• Growth failure, based on National Center for Health Statistics (NCHS) growth standards and fetal growth failure • Insufficient maternal weight gain • Lack of planned weight gain • Unintentional weight loss of ≥ 5% in 1 month or ≥ 10% in 6 months (not attributed to fluid) in adults • Any weight loss in infants or children • Underweight (BMI < 18.5)
Nutrition-Focused Physical Findings	• Clinical evidence of vitamin/mineral deficiency (e.g., hair loss, bleeding gums, pale nail beds, neurologic changes) • Evidence of dehydration, e.g., dry mucous membranes, poor skin turgor • Loss of skin integrity, delayed wound healing, or pressure ulcers • Loss of muscle mass and/or subcutaneous fat • Nausea, vomiting, diarrhea
Food/Nutrition-Related History	Reports or observations of: • Inadequate EN/PN volume compared to estimated or measured (indirect calorimetry) requirements • Feeding tube or venous access in wrong position or removed • Altered capacity for desired levels of physical activity or exercise, easy fatigue with increased activity
Client History	• Conditions associated with a diagnosis or treatment, e.g., intestinal resection, Crohn's disease, HIV/AIDS, burns, pre-term birth, malnutrition

*If a synonym, or alternate word with the same meaning, for the term "inadequate" is helpful or needed, an approved alternate is the word "suboptimal."

Diagnosis

Intake Domain – Oral or Nutrition Support Intake

Inadequate* Intake from Enteral/Parenteral (EN/PN) Nutrition (NI-2.3)

References

1. McClave SA, Spain DA, Skolnick JL, Lowen CC, Kieber MJ, Wickerham PS, Vogt JR, Looney SW. Achievement of steady state optimizes results when performing indirect calorimetry. *JPEN J Parenter Enteral Nutr*. 2003;27:16-20.

2. McClave SA, Lowen CC, Kleber MJ, McConnell JW, Jung LY, Goldsmith LJ. Clinical use of the respiratory quotient obtained from indirect calorimetry. *JPEN J Parenter Enteral Nutr*. 2003;27:21-26.

3. McClave SA, Snider HL. Clinical use of gastric residual volumes as a monitor for patients on enteral tube feeding. *JPEN J Parenter Enteral Nutr*. 2002;26(Suppl):S43-S48; discussion S49-S50.

4. McClave SA, DeMeo MT, DeLegge MH, DiSario JA, Heyland DK, Maloney JP, Metheny NA, Moore FA, Scolapio JS, Spain DA, Zaloga GP. North American Summit on Aspiration in the Critically Ill Patient: consensus statement. *JPEN J Parenter Enteral Nutr*. 2002;26(Suppl):S80-S85.

5. McClave SA, McClain CJ, Snider HL. Should indirect calorimetry be used as part of nutritional assessment? *J Clin Gastroenterol*. 2001;33:14-19.

6. McClave SA, Sexton LK, Spain DA, Adams JL, Owens NA, Sullins MB, Blandford BS, Snider HL. Enteral tube feeding in the intensive care unit: factors impeding adequate delivery. *Crit Care Med*. 1999;27:1252-1256.

7. McClave SA, Lowen CC, Kleber MJ, Nicholson JF, Jimmerson SC, McConnell JW, Jung LY. Are patients fed appropriately according to their caloric requirements? *JPEN J Parenter Enteral Nutr*. 1998;22:375-381.

8. Spain DA, McClave SA, Sexton LK, Adams JL, Blanford BS, Sullins ME, Owens NA, Snider HL. Infusion protocol improves delivery of enteral tube feeding in the critical care unit. *JPEN J Parenter Enteral Nutr*. 1999;23:288-292.

Updated: 2009 Edition

If a synonym, or alternate word with the same meaning, for the term "inadequate" is helpful or needed, an approved alternate is the word "suboptimal."

Excessive Intake from Enteral or Parenteral Nutrition (NI-2.4)

Definition

Enteral or parenteral infusion that provides more calories or nutrients compared to established reference standards or recommendations based on physiological needs.

Etiology (Cause/Contributing Risk Factors)

Factors gathered during the nutrition assessment process that contribute to the existence or the maintenance of pathophysiological, psychosocial, situational, developmental, cultural, and/or environmental problems:

- Physiological causes, e.g., decreased needs related to low activity levels with critical illness or organ failure
- Food- and nutrition-related knowledge deficit concerning appropriate amount of EN/PN

Signs/Symptoms (Defining Characteristics)

A typical cluster of subjective and objective signs and symptoms gathered during the nutrition assessment process that provide evidence that a problem exists; quantify the problem and describe its severity.

Nutrition Assessment Category	Potential Indicators of this Nutrition Diagnosis (one or more must be present)
Biochemical Data, Medical Tests and Procedures	• Elevated BUN:creatinine ratio (protein) • Hyperglycemia (carbohydrate) • Hypercapnia • Elevated liver enzymes
Anthropometric Measurements	• Weight gain in excess of lean tissue accretion
Nutrition-Focused Physical Findings	• Edema with excess fluid administration
Food/Nutrition-Related History	Reports or observations of: • Estimated intake from enteral or parenteral nutrients that is consistently more than recommended intake for carbohydrate, protein, and fat (e.g., 36 kcal/kg for well, active adults, 25 kcal/kg or as measured by indirect calorimetry for critically ill adults, 0.8 g/kg protein for well adults, 1.5 g/kg protein for critically ill adults, 4 mg/kg/minute of dextrose for critically ill adults, 1.2 g/kg lipid for adults, or 3 g/kg for children)* • Use of drugs that reduce requirements or impair metabolism of energy, protein, fat, or fluid. • Unrealistic expectations of weight gain or ideal weight
Client History	

* When entering weight (e.g.., gram) information into the medical record, use institution– or Joint Commission–approved abbreviation list.

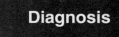

Diagnosis

Intake Domain – Oral or Nutrition Support Intake

Excessive Intake from Enteral or Parenteral Nutrition (NI-2.4)

References

1. National Academy of Sciences, Institute of Medicine. *Dietary Reference Intakes for Energy, Carbohydrate, Fiber, Fat, Fatty Acids, Cholesterol, Protein, and Amino Acids*. Washington, DC: National Academy Press, 2002.

2. National Academy of Sciences, Institute of Medicine. *Dietary Reference Intakes for Water, Potassium, Sodium, Chloride, and Sulfate*. Washington, DC: National Academy Press, 2004.

3. Aarsland A, Chinkes D, Wolfe RR. Hepatic and whole-body fat synthesis in humans during carbohydrate overfeeding. *Am J Clin Nutr*. 1997;65:1774-1782.

4. McClave SA, Lowen CC, Kleber MJ, Nicholson JF, Jimmerson SC, McConnell JW, Jung LY. Are patients fed appropriately according to their caloric requirements? *JPEN J Parenter Enteral Nutr*. 1998;22:375-381.

5. McClave SA, Lowen CC, Kleber MJ, McConnell JW, Jung LY, Goldsmith LJ. Clinical use of the respiratory quotient obtained from indirect calorimetry. *JPEN J Parenter Enteral Nutr*. 2003;27:21-26.

6. Wolfe RR, O'Donnell TF Jr, Stone MD, Richmand DA, Burke JF. Investigation of factors determining the optimal glucose infusion rate in total parenteral nutrition. *Metabolism*. 1980;29:892-900.

7. Jensen GL, Mascioli EA, Seidner DL, Istfan NW, Domnitch AM, Selleck K, Babayan VK, Blackburn GL, Bistrian BR. Parenteral infusion of long- and medium-chain triglycerides and reticulothelial system function in man. *JPEN J Parenter Enteral Nutr*. 1990;14:467-471.

8. Joint Commission Official "Do not use" list of abbreviations. Available: http://www.jointcommission.org/PatientSafety/DoNotUseList. Accessed May 2007.

Inappropriate Infusion of Enteral or Parenteral Nutrition (NI-2.5)

Use with caution–only after discussion with other health team members

Definition

Enteral or parenteral infusion that provides either fewer or more calories and/or nutrients or is of the wrong composition or type, parenteral or enteral nutrition that is not warranted because the patient/client is able to tolerate an enteral intake, or is unsafe because of the potential for sepsis or other complications.

Etiology (Cause/Contributing Risk Factors)

Factors gathered during the nutrition assessment process that contribute to the existence or the maintenance of pathophysiological, psychosocial, situational, developmental, cultural, and/or environmental problems:

- Physiological causes, e.g., improvement in patient/client status, allowing return to total or partial oral diet; changes in the course of disease resulting in changes in nutrient requirements
- Food and nutrition-related knowledge deficit concerning EN/PN product
- End-of-life care if patient/client or family do not desire nutrition support

Signs/Symptoms (Defining Characteristics)

A typical cluster of subjective and objective signs and symptoms gathered during the nutrition assessment process that provide evidence that a problem exists; quantify the problem and describe its severity.

Nutrition Assessment Category	Potential Indicators of this Nutrition Diagnosis (one or more must be present)
Biochemical Data, Medical Tests and Procedures	• Abnormal liver function tests in patient/client on long-term (more than 3-6 weeks) nutrition support • Abnormal levels of markers specific for various nutrients, e.g., hyperphosphatemia in patient/client receiving feedings with a high phosphorus content, hypokalemia in patient/client receiving feedings with low potassium content
Anthropometric Measurements	• Weight gain in excess of lean tissue accretion • Weight loss
Nutrition-Focused Physical Findings	• Edema with excess fluid administration • Loss of subcutaneous fat and muscle stores • Nausea, vomiting, diarrhea, high gastric residual volume

Diagnosis

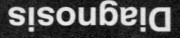

Intake Domain – Oral or Nutrition Support Intake

Inappropriate Infusion of Enteral or Parenteral Nutrition (NI-2.5)

Food/Nutrition-Related History	Reports or observations of:
	• Estimated intake from enteral or parenteral nutrients that is consistently more or less than recommended intake for carbohydrate, protein, and/or fat– especially related to patient/client's ability to consume an oral diet that meets needs at this point in time
	• Estimated intake of other nutrients that is consistently more or less than recommended
	• History of enteral or parenteral nutrition intolerance
Client History	• Complications such as fatty liver in the absence of other causes

References

1. Aarsland A, Chinkes D, Wolfe RR. Hepatic and whole-body fat synthesis in humans during carbohydrate overfeeding. *Am J Clin Nutr.* 1997;65:1774-1782.

2. McClave SA, Lowen CC, Kleber MJ, Nicholson JF, Jimmerson SC, McConnell JW, Jung LY. Are patients fed appropriately according to their caloric requirements? *JPEN J Parenter Enteral Nutr.* 1998;22:375-381.

3. McClave SA, Lowen CC, Kleber MJ, McConnell JW, Jung LY, Goldsmith LJ. Clinical use of the respiratory quotient obtained from indirect calorimetry. JPEN J Parenter Enteral Nutr. 2003;27:21-26.

4. National Academy of Sciences, Institute of Medicine. *Dietary Reference Intakes for Energy, Carbohydrate, Fiber, Fat, Fatty Acids, Cholesterol, Protein, and Amino Acids*. Washington, DC: National Academy Press; 2002.

5. National Academy of Sciences, Institute of Medicine. *Dietary Reference Intakes for Water, Potassium, Sodium, Chloride, and Sulfate*, Washington DC: National Academy Press; 2004.

6. National Academy of Sciences, Institute of Medicine. *Dietary Reference Intakes for Calcium, Phosphorus, Magnesium, Vitamin D, and Fluoride*. Washington, DC: National Academy Press; 1997.

7. National Academy of Sciences, Institute of Medicine. *Dietary Reference Intakes for Vitamin C, Vitamin E, Selenium, and Carotenoids*. Washington, DC: National Academy Press; 2000.

8. Wolfe RR, O'Donnell TF, Jr., Stone MD, Richmand DA, Burke JF. Investigation of factors determining the optimal glucose infusion rate in total parenteral nutrition. *Metabolism.* 1980;29:892-900.

Inadequate* Fluid Intake (NI-3.1)

Definition

Lower intake of fluid-containing foods or substances compared to established reference standards or recommendations based on physiological needs.

> Note: Whenever possible, nutrient intake data should be considered in combination with clinical, biochemical, anthropometric information, medical diagnosis, clinical status, and/or other factors as well as diet to provide a valid assessment of nutritional status based on a totality of the evidence. (Dietary Reference Intakes. Applications in Dietary Assessment. Institute of Medicine. Washington, D.C.: National Academy Press; 2000.)

Etiology (Cause/Contributing Risk Factors)

Factors gathered during the nutrition assessment process that contribute to the existence or the maintenance of pathophysiological, psychosocial, situational, developmental, cultural, and/or environmental problems:

- Physiological causes increasing fluid needs due to climate/temperature change, increased exercise or conditions leading to increased fluid losses, fever causing increased insensible losses, decreased thirst sensation, or use of drugs that reduce thirst
- Lack of or limited access to fluid, e.g., economic constraints, unable to access fluid independently such as elderly or children
- Cultural practices that affect the ability to access fluid
- Food- and nutrition-related knowledge deficit concerning appropriate fluid intake
- Psychological causes, e.g., depression or disordered eating
- Impaired cognitive ability, including learning disabilities, neurological or sensory impairment, and/or dementia

Signs/Symptoms (Defining Characteristics)

A typical cluster of subjective and objective signs and symptoms gathered during the nutrition assessment process that provide evidence that a problem exists; quantify the problem and describe its severity.

Nutrition Assessment Category	Potential Indicators of this Nutrition Diagnosis (one or more must be present)
Biochemical Data, Medical Tests and Procedures	• Plasma or serum osmolality greater than 290 mOsm/kg • ↑ BUN, ↑ Na • Urine output <30 mL/hr
Anthropometric Measurements	• Acute weight loss

*If a synonym, or alternate word with the same meaning, for the term "inadequate" is helpful or needed, an approved alternate is the word "suboptimal."

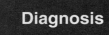

Diagnosis

Intake Domain – Fluid Intake

Inadequate* Fluid Intake (NI-3.1)

Nutrition-Focused Physical Findings	• Dry skin and mucous membranes, poor skin turgor • Thirst • Difficulty swallowing
Food/Nutrition-Related History	Reports or observations of: • Estimated intake of fluid less than requirements (e.g., per body surface area for pediatrics) • Use of drugs that reduce thirst
Client History	• Conditions associated with a diagnosis or treatment, e.g., Alzheimer's disease or other dementia resulting in decreased recognition of thirst, diarrhea

References

1. National Academy of Sciences, Institute of Medicine. *Dietary Reference Intakes for Water, Potassium, Sodium, Chloride, and Sulfate*, Washington, DC: National Academy Press; 2004.

2. Grandjean AC, Campbell, SM. *Hydration: Fluids for Life*. Monograph Series. Washington DC: International Life Sciences Institute North America; 2004.

3. Grandjean AC, Reimers KJ, Buyckx ME. Hydration: Issues for the 21st Century. *Nutr Rev.* 2003;61:261-271.

Updated: 2009 Edition

If a synonym, or alternate word with the same meaning, for the term "inadequate" is helpful or needed, an approved alternate is the word "suboptimal."

Excessive Fluid Intake (NI-3.2)

Definition

Higher intake of fluid compared to established reference standards or recommendations based on physiological needs.

Etiology (Cause/Contributing Risk Factors)

Factors gathered during the nutrition assessment process that contribute to the existence or the maintenance of pathophysiological, psychosocial, situational, developmental, cultural, and/or environmental problems:

- Physiological causes, e.g., kidney, liver, cardiac, endocrine, neurological, and/or pulmonary dysfunction; diminished water and sodium losses due to changes in exercise or climate, syndrome of inappropriate antidiuretic hormone (SIADH)
- Food- and nutrition-related knowledge deficit concerning appropriate fluid intake
- Psychological causes such as depression and disordered eating

Signs/Symptoms (Defining Characteristics)

A typical cluster of subjective and objective signs and symptoms gathered during the nutrition assessment process that provide evidence that a problem exists; quantify the problem and describe its severity.

Nutrition Assessment Category	Potential Indicators of this Nutrition Diagnosis (one or more must be present)
Biochemical Data, Medical Tests and Procedures	• Lowered plasma osmolarity (270-280 mOsm/kg), only if positive fluid balance is in excess of positive sodium balance • Decreased serum sodium in SIADH
Anthropometric Measurements	• Weight gain
Nutrition-Focused Physical Findings	• Edema in the skin of the legs, sacral area, or diffusely; weeping of fluids from lower legs • Ascites • Pulmonary edema as evidenced by shortness of breath; orthopnea; crackles or rales • Nausea, vomiting, anorexia, headache, muscle spasms, convulsions • Shortness of breath or dyspnea with exertion or at rest • Providing medications in large amounts of fluid • Use of drugs that impair fluid excretion

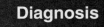

Diagnosis

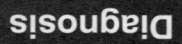

Intake Domain – Fluid Intake

Excessive Fluid Intake (NI-3.2)

Food/Nutrition-Related History	Reports or observations of: • Estimated intake of fluid more than requirements (e.g., per body surface area for pediatrics) • Estimated salt intake in excess of recommendations
Client History	• Conditions associated with a diagnosis or treatment, e.g., end-stage renal disease, nephrotic syndrome, heart failure, or liver disease • Coma (SIADH)

References

1. National Academy of Sciences, Institute of Medicine. *Dietary Reference Intakes for Water, Potassium, Sodium, Chloride, and Sulfate*, Washington DC. National Academy Press; 2004.
2. Schirer, R.W. ed. *Renal and Electrolyte Disorders*. Philadelphia, PA: Lipincott Williams and Willkins; 2003.
3. SIADH: http://www.nlmnih.gov/medlineplus/ency/article/000394.htm. Accessed May 30, 2006.

Updated: 2008 Edition

Inadequate* Bioactive Substance Intake (NI-4.1)

Definition

Lower intake of bioactive substances compared to established reference standards or recommendations based on physiological needs.

> *Note: Bioactive substances are not included as part of the Dietary Reference Intakes, and therefore there are no established minimum requirements or Tolerable Upper Intake Levels. However, RDs can assess whether estimated intakes are adequate or excessive using the patient/client goal or nutrition prescription for comparison.*
>
> *Working definition of bioactive substances—physiologically active components of foods that may offer health benefits beyond traditional macro- or micronutrient requirements. There is not scientific consensus about a definition for bioactive substances/components.*

Etiology (Cause/Contributing Risk Factors)

Factors gathered during the nutrition assessment process that contribute to the existence or the maintenance of pathophysiological, psychosocial, situational, developmental, cultural, and/or environmental problems:

Food- and nutrition-related knowledge deficit concerning recommended bioactive substance intake

Lack of or limited access to food that contains a bioactive substance

Alteration in gastrointestinal tract structure and/or function

Signs/Symptoms (Defining Characteristics)

A typical cluster of subjective and objective signs and symptoms gathered during the nutrition assessment process that provide evidence that a problem exists; quantify the problem and describe its severity.

Nutrition Assessment Category	Potential Indicators of this Nutrition Diagnosis (one or more must be present)
Biochemical Data, Medical Tests and Procedures	
Anthropometric Measurements	
Nutrition-Focused Physical Findings	

If a synonym, or alternate word with the same meaning, for the term "inadequate" is helpful or needed, an approved alternate is the word "suboptimal."

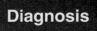

Diagnosis

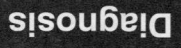

Intake Domain – Bioactive Substances

Inadequate* Bioactive Substance Intake (NI-4.1)

Food/Nutrition-Related History	Reports or observations of: • Estimated intake of plant foods containing the following lower than recommended: • Soluble fiber, e.g., psyllium ($\downarrow$ total and LDL cholesterol) • Soy protein ($\downarrow$ total and LDL cholesterol) • β-glucan, e.g., whole oat products ($\downarrow$ total and LDL cholesterol) • Plant sterol and stanol esters, e.g., fortified margarines ($\downarrow$ total and LDL cholesterol)
Client History	• Conditions associated with a diagnosis or treatment, e.g., cardiovascular disease, elevated cholesterol

References

1. Position of the American Dietetic Association: Functional foods. *J Am Diet Assoc*. 2004;104:814-826.

Updated: 2009 Edition

If a synonym, or alternate word with the same meaning, for the term "inadequate" is helpful or needed, an approved alternate is the word "suboptimal."

Excessive Bioactive Substance Intake (NI-4.2)

Definition

Higher intake of bioactive substances compared to established reference standards or recommendations based on physiological needs.

Note: Working definition of bioactive substances—physiologically active components of foods that may offer health benefits beyond traditional macro- or micronutrient requirements. There is not scientific consensus about a definition for bioactive substances/components.

Etiology (Cause/Contributing Risk Factors)

Factors gathered during the nutrition assessment process that contribute to the existence or the maintenance of pathophysiological, psychosocial, situational, developmental, cultural, and/or environmental problems:

- Food- and nutrition-related knowledge deficit concerning recommended bioactive substance intake
- Contamination, misname, mislabel, misuse, recent brand change, recent dose increase, recent formulation change of substance consumed
- Frequent intake of foods containing bioactive substances
- Alteration in gastrointestinal tract structure and/or function

Signs/Symptoms (Defining Characteristics)

A typical cluster of subjective and objective signs and symptoms gathered during the nutrition assessment process that provide evidence that a problem exists; quantify the problem and describe its severity.

Nutrition Assessment Category	Potential Indicators of this Nutrition Diagnosis (one or more must be present)
Biochemical Data, Medical Tests and Procedures	• Lab values indicating excessive intake of the specific substance, such as rapid decrease in cholesterol from intake of stanol or sterol esters and a statin drug and related dietary changes or medications • Increased hepatic enzyme reflecting hepatocellular damage
Anthropometric Measurements	• Weight loss as a result of malabsorption or maldigestion
Nutrition-Focused Physical Findings	• Constipation or diarrhea related to estimated intake higher than recommended • Neurologic changes, e.g., anxiety, mental status changes • Cardiovascular changes, e.g., heart rate, blood pressure • Discomfort or pain associated with intake of foods rich in bioactive substances, e.g., soluble fiber, β-glucan, soy protein

Diagnosis

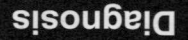

Intake Domain – Bioactive Substances

Excessive Bioactive Substance Intake (NI-4.2)

Food/Nutrition-Related History	Reports or observations of: • High intake of plant foods containing: • Soy protein ($\downarrow$ total and LDL cholesterol) • β-glucan, e.g., whole oat products ($\downarrow$ total and LDL cholesterol) • Plant sterol and stanol esters, e.g., fortified margarines ($\downarrow$ total and LDL cholesterol) or other foods based on dietary substance, concentrate, metabolite, constituent, extract, or combination • Substances that interfere with digestion or absorption of foodstuffs • Ready access to available foods/products with bioactive substance, e.g., as from dietary supplement vendors • Attempts to use supplements or bioactive substances for weight loss, to treat constipation, or to prevent or cure chronic or acute disease
Client History	• Conditions associated with a diagnosis or treatment, e.g., cardiovascular disease, elevated cholesterol, hypertension • Cardiovascular changes, e.g., EKG changes

References

1. National Academy of Sciences, Institute of Medicine. *Dietary Supplements: A framework for evaluating safety*. Washington, DC: National Academy Press; 2004.
2. Position of the American Dietetic Association: Functional foods. *J Am Diet Assoc*. 2004;104:814-826.

Updated: 2009 Edition

Excessive Alcohol Intake (NI-4.3)

Definition

Intake more than the suggested limits for alcohol.

Etiology (Cause/Contributing Risk Factors)

Factors gathered during the nutrition assessment process that contribute to the existence or the maintenance of pathophysiological, psychosocial, situational, developmental, cultural, and/or environmental problems:

- Harmful beliefs/attitudes about food, nutrition, and nutrition-related topics
- Food- and nutrition-related knowledge deficit concerning appropriate alcohol intake
- Lack of value for behavior change, competing values
- Alcohol addiction

Signs/Symptoms (Defining Characteristics)

A typical cluster of subjective and objective signs and symptoms gathered during the nutrition assessment process that provide evidence that a problem exists; quantify the problem and describe its severity.

Nutrition Assessment Category	Potential Indicators of this Nutrition Diagnosis (one or more must be present)
Biochemical Data, Medical Tests and Procedures	• Elevated aspartate aminotransferase (AST), gamma-glutamyl transferase (GGT), carbohydrate-deficient transferrin, mean corpuscular volume, blood alcohol levels
Anthropometric Measurements	
Nutrition-Focused Physical Findings	
Food/Nutrition-Related History	Reports or observations of: • Intake of > 2 drinks*/day (men) • Intake of > 1 drink*/day (women) • Binge drinking • Consumption of any alcohol when contraindicated, e.g., during pregnancy *1 drink = 5 oz wine, 12 oz beer, 1.5 oz distilled alcohol*

Diagnosis

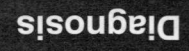

Intake Domain – Bioactive Substances

Excessive Alcohol Intake (NI-4.3)

Client History	• Conditions associated with a diagnosis or treatment, e.g., severe hypertriglyceridemia, elevated blood pressure, depression, liver disease, pancreatitis
	• New medical diagnosis or change in existing diagnosis or condition
	• History of estimated alcohol intake in excess of recommended
	• Giving birth to an infant with fetal alcohol syndrome

References

1. Position of the American Dietetic Association: The role of dietetics professionals in health promotion and disease prevention. *J Am Diet Assoc.* 2006;106:1875-1884.

Updated: 2009 Edition

Increased Nutrient Needs (specify) (NI-5.1)

Definition

Increased need for a specific nutrient compared to established reference standards or recommendations based on physiological needs.

Etiology (Cause/Contributing Risk Factors)

Factors gathered during the nutrition assessment process that contribute to the existence or the maintenance of pathophysiological, psychosocial, situational, developmental, cultural, and/or environmental problems:

- Altered absorption or metabolism of nutrient, e.g., from medications
- Compromise of organs related to GI function, e.g., pancreas, liver
- Decreased functional length of intestine, e.g., short-bowel syndrome
- Decreased or compromised function of intestine, e.g., celiac disease, Crohn's disease
- Food- and nutrition-related knowledge deficit concerning sufficient nutrient intake
- Increased demand for nutrient, e.g., accelerated growth, wound healing, chronic infection

Signs/Symptoms (Defining Characteristics)

A typical cluster of subjective and objective signs and symptoms gathered during the nutrition assessment process that provide evidence that a problem exists; quantify the problem and describe its severity.

Nutrition Assessment Category	Potential Indicators of this Nutrition Diagnosis (one or more must be present)
Biochemical Data, Medical Tests and Procedures	• Decreased total cholesterol < 160 mg/dL, albumin, prealbumin, C-reactive protein, indicating increased stress and increased metabolic needs • Electrolyte/mineral (e.g., potassium, magnesium, phosphorus) abnormalities • Urinary or fecal losses of specific or related nutrient (e.g., fecal fat, d-xylose test) • Vitamin and/or mineral deficiency
Anthropometric Measurements	• Growth failure, based on National Center for Health Statistics (NCHS) growth standards and fetal growth failure • Unintentional weight loss of ≥5% in 1 month or ≥10% in 6 months • Underweight (BMI < 18.5)
Nutrition-Focused Physical Findings	• Clinical evidence of vitamin/mineral deficiency (e.g., hair loss, bleeding gums, pale nail beds) • Loss of skin integrity, delayed wound healing, or pressure ulcers • Loss of muscle mass, subcutaneous fat

Diagnosis

Intake Domain – Nutrient

Increased Nutrient Needs (specify) (NI-5.1)

Food/Nutrition-Related History	Reports or observations of: • Estimated intake of foods/supplements containing needed nutrient less than estimated requirements • Intake of foods that do not contain sufficient quantities of available nutrient (e.g., overprocessed, overcooked, or stored improperly) • Food- and nutrition-related knowledge deficit (e.g., lack of information, incorrect information or noncompliance with intake of needed nutrient) • Medications affecting absorption or metabolism of needed nutrient
Client History	• Conditions associated with a diagnosis or treatment, e.g., intestinal resection, Crohn's disease, HIV/AIDS, burns, pre-term birth, malnutrition

References

1. Beyer P. Gastrointestinal disorders: Roles of nutrition and the dietetics practitioner. *J Am Diet Assoc*. 1998;98:272-277.
2. Position of the American Dietetic Association and Dietitians of Canada: Nutrition intervention in the care of persons with human immunodeficiency virus infection. *J Am Diet Assoc*. 2004;104:1425-1441.

Updated: 2008 Edition

Malnutrition (NI-5.2)

Definition

Inadequate intake of protein and/or energy over prolonged periods of time resulting in loss of fat stores and/or muscle wasting.

Etiology (Cause/Contributing Risk Factors)

Factors gathered during the nutrition assessment process that contribute to the existence or the maintenance of pathophysiological, psychosocial, situational, developmental, cultural, and/or environmental problems:

- Physiological causes increasing nutrient needs due to prolonged catabolic illness
- Alteration in gastrointestinal tract structure and/or function
- Lack of or limited access to food, e.g., economic constraints, restricting food given to elderly and/or children
- Cultural practices that affect the ability to access food
- Food- and nutrition-related knowledge deficit concerning amount of energy and amount and type of dietary protein
- Psychological causes, e.g., depression or eating disorders

Signs/Symptoms (Defining Characteristics)

A typical cluster of subjective and objective signs and symptoms gathered during the nutrition assessment process that provide evidence that a problem exists; quantify the problem and describe its severity.

Nutrition Assessment Category	Potential Indicators of this Nutrition Diagnosis (one or more must be present)
Biochemical Data, Medical Tests and Procedures	*
Anthropometric Measurements	• BMI < 18.5 indicates underweight; BMI for older adults (older than 65 years) < 23 • Failure to thrive, e.g., failure to attain desirable growth rates • Inadequate maternal weight gain • Weight loss, adults, of > 10% in 6 months, > 5% in 1 month • Growth, pediatrics, not gaining weight as expected and/or a shift downward in their growth percentiles, crossing two or more percentiles on their growth charts. • Underweight with muscle wasting

In the past, hepatic transport protein measures (e.g. albumin and prealbumin) were used as indicators of malnutrition. The sensitivity of these as nutrition indicators has been questioned. An ADA evidence-analysis project is evaluating the body of science.

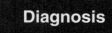
Diagnosis

Intake Domain – Nutrient

Malnutrition (NI-5.2)

Nutrition-Focused Physical Findings	• Uncomplicated malnutrition: Thin, wasted appearance; severe muscle wasting; minimal body fat; sparse, thin, dry, easily pluckable hair; dry, thin skin; obvious bony prominences, temporal wasting; lowered body temperature, blood pressure, heart rate; changes in hair or nails consistent with insufficient protein intake
	• Disease/trauma related malnutrition: Thin to normal appearance, with peripheral edema, ascites, or anasarca; edema of the lower extremities; some muscle wasting with retention of some body fat; dyspigmentation of hair (flag sign) and skin
	• Delayed wound healing
Food/Nutrition-Related History	Reports or observations of:
	• Estimated energy intake from diet less than estimated or measured RMR
	• Estimated intake of high-quality protein less than estimated requirements
	• Food avoidance and/or lack of interest in food
	• Excessive consumption of alcohol or other drugs that reduce appetite
Client History	• Chronic or acute disease or trauma, geographic location and socioeconomic status associated with altered nutrient intake of indigenous phenomenon
	• Severe protein and/or nutrient malabsorption (e.g., extensive bowel resection)
	• Enlarged fatty liver

References

1. American Medical Association. AMA ICD-9-CM 2007: *Physician, International Classification of Diseases: Clinical Modification*, 9th Revised Ed. Chicago, IL: American Medical Association Press; 2006.
2. Centers for Disease Control and Prevention website: http://www.cdc.gov/nccdphp/dnpa/bmi/bmi-adult.htm. Accessed October 5, 2004.
3. Fuhrman MP, Charney P, Mueller CM. Hepatic proteins and nutrition assessment. *J Am Diet Assoc*. 2004;104:1258-1264.
4. Jelliffe DB, Jelliffe EF. Causation of kwashiorkor: Toward a multifactoral consensus. *Pediatrics*. 1992;90:110-113.
5. Ranhoff AH, Gjoen AU, Mowe M. Screening for malnutrition in elderly acute medical patients: the usefulness of MNA-SF. *J Nutr Health Aging*. Jul-Aug 2005;9:221-225.
6. Seres DS, Resurrection, LB. Kwashiorkor: Dysmetabolism versus malnutrition. *Nutr Clin Pract*. 2003;18:297-301.
7. Wellcome Trust Working Party. Classification of infantile malnutrition. *Lancet*. 1970;2:302-303.

Updated: 2009 Edition

Inadequate* Protein–Energy Intake (NI-5.3)

Definition

Inadequate intake of protein and/or energy compared to established reference standards or recommendations based on physiological needs of short or recent duration.

> *Note: Whenever possible, nutrient intake data should be considered in combination with clinical, biochemical, anthropometric information, medical diagnosis, clinical status, and/or other factors as well as diet to provide a valid assessment of nutritional status based on a totality of the evidence. (Dietary Reference Intakes. Applications in Dietary Assessment. Institute of Medicine. Washington, D.C.: National Academy Press; 2000.)*

Etiology (Cause/Contributing Risk Factors)

Factors gathered during the nutrition assessment process that contribute to the existence or the maintenance of pathophysiological, psychosocial, situational, developmental, cultural, and/or environmental problems:

- Physiological causes increasing nutrient needs due to catabolic illness, malabsorption
- Lack of or limited access to food, e.g., economic constraints, restricting food given or food selected
- Cultural practices that affect ability to access food
- Food- and nutrition-related knowledge deficit concerning appropriate amount and type of dietary fat and/or protein
- Psychological causes such as depression and disordered eating

Signs/Symptoms (Defining Characteristics)

A typical cluster of subjective and objective signs and symptoms gathered during the nutrition assessment process that provide evidence that a problem exists; quantify the problem and describe its severity.

Nutrition Assessment Category	Potential Indicators of this Nutrition Diagnosis (one or more must be present)
Biochemical Data, Medical Tests and Procedures	• Normal albumin (in the setting of normal liver function despite decreased protein-energy intake)
Anthropometric Measurements	• Inadequate maternal weight gain (mild but not severe) • Weight loss of 5%-7% during past 3 months in adults, any weight loss in children • Normal or slightly underweight • Growth failure in children
Nutrition-Focused Physical Findings	• Slow wound healing in pressure ulcer or surgical patient/client

If a synonym, or alternate word with the same meaning, for the term "inadequate" is helpful or needed, an approved alternate is the word "suboptimal."

Diagnosis

Intake Domain – Nutrient

Inadequate* Protein–Energy Intake (NI-5.3)

Food/Nutrition-Related History	Reports or observations of:
	• Estimated energy intake from diet less than estimated or measured RMR or recommended levels
	• Restriction or omission of food groups such as dairy or meat group foods (protein); bread or milk group foods (energy)
	• Recent food avoidance and/or lack of interest in food
	• Lack of ability to prepare meals
	• Excessive consumption of alcohol or other drugs that reduce hunger
	• Hunger in the face of inadequate access to food supply
Client History	• Conditions associated with a diagnosis or treatment of mild protein-energy malnutrition, recent illness, e.g., pulmonary or cardiac failure, flu, infection, surgery
	• Nutrient malabsorption (e.g., bariatric surgery, diarrhea, steatorrhea)
	• Lack of funds for purchase of appropriate foods

References

1. Centers for Disease Control and Prevention website: http://www.cdc.gov/nccdphp/dnpa/bmi/bmi-adult.htm. Accessed October 5, 2004.
2. Fuhrman MP, Charney P, Mueller CM. Hepatic proteins and nutrition assessment. *J Am Diet Assoc*. 2004;104:1258-1264.
3. American Medical Association. *AMA ICD-9-CM 2007: Physician, International Classification of Diseases: Clinical Modification*, 9th Revised Ed. Chicago, IL: American Medical Association Press; 2006.

Updated: 2009 Edition

*If a synonym, or alternate word with the same meaning, for the term "inadequate" is helpful or needed, an approved alternate is the word "suboptimal."

Decreased Nutrient Needs (specify) (NI-5.4)

Definition

Decreased need for a specific nutrient compared to established reference standards or recommendations based on physiological needs.

Etiology (Cause/Contributing Risk Factors)

Factors gathered during the nutrition assessment process that contribute to the existence or the maintenance of pathophysiological, psychosocial, situational, developmental, cultural, and/or environmental problems:

- Renal dysfunction
- Liver dysfunction
- Altered cholesterol metabolism/regulation
- Heart failure
- Food intolerances, e.g., irritable bowel syndrome

Signs/Symptoms (Defining Characteristics)

A typical cluster of subjective and objective signs and symptoms gathered during the nutrition assessment process that provide evidence that a problem exists; quantify the problem and describe its severity.

Nutrition Assessment Category	Potential Indicators of this Nutrition Diagnosis (one or more must be present)
Biochemical Data, Medical Tests and Procedures	- Total cholesterol > 200 mg/dL (5.2 mmol/L), LDL cholesterol > 100 mg/dL (2.59 mmol/L), HDL cholesterol < 40 mg/dL (1.036 mmol/L), triglycerides > 150 mg/dL (1.695 mmol/L) - Phosphorus > 5.5 mg/dL (1.78 mmol/L) - Glomerular filtration rate (GFR) < 90 mL/min/1.73 m^2 - Elevated BUN, creatinine, potassium - Liver function tests indicating severe liver disease
Anthropometric Measurements	- Interdialytic weight gain greater than expected
Nutrition-Focused Physical Findings	- Edema/fluid retention
Food/Nutrition-Related History	Reports or observations of: - Estimated intake higher than recommended for fat, phosphorus, sodium, protein, fiber
Client History	- Conditions associated with a diagnosis or treatment that require a specific type and/or amount of nutrient, e.g., cardiovascular disease (fat), early renal disease (protein, phos), ESRD (phos, sodium, potassium, fluid), advanced liver disease (protein), heart failure (sodium, fluid), irritable bowel disease/Crohn's flare up (fiber) - Diagnosis of hypertension, confusion related to liver disease

245

Diagnosis

Intake Domain – Nutrient

Decreased Nutrient Needs (specify) (NI-5.4)

References

1. Aparicio M, Chauveau P, Combe C. Low protein diets and outcomes of renal patients. *J Nephro*l. 2001;14:433-439.

2. Beto JA, Bansal VK. Medical nutrition therapy in chronic kidney failure: Integrating clinical practice guidelines. *J Am Diet Assoc*. 2004;104:404-409.

3. Cupisti A, Morelli E, D'Alessandro C, Lupetti S, Barsotti G. Phosphate control in chronic uremia: don't forget diet. *J Nephrol*. 2003;16:29-33.

4. Durose CL, Holdsworth M, Watson V, Przygrodzka F. Knowledge of dietary restrictions and the medical consequences of noncompliance by patients on hemodialysis are not predictive of dietary compliance. *J Am Diet Assoc*. 2004;104:35-41.

5. Floch MH, Narayan R. Diet in the irritable bowel syndrome. *Clin Gastroenterol*. 2002;35:S45-S52.

6. Kato J, Kobune M, Nakamura T, Kurojwa G, Takada K, Takimoto R, Sato Y, Fujikawa K, Takahashi M, Takayama T, Ikeda T, Niitsu Y. Normalization of elevated hepatic 8-hydroxy-2'-deoxyguanosine levels in chronic hepatitis C patients by phlebotomy and low iron diet. *Cancer Res*. 2001;61:8697-8702.

7. Lee SH, Molassiotis A. Dietary and fluid compliance in Chinese hemodialysis patients. *Int J Nurs Stud*. 2002;39:695-704.

8. Poduval RD, Wolgemuth C, Ferrell J, Hammes MS. Hyperphosphatemia in dialysis patients: is there a role for focused counseling? *J Ren Nutr*. 2003;13:219-223.

9. Tandon N, Thakur V, Guptan RK, Sarin SK. Beneficial influence of an indigenous low-iron diet on serum indicators of iron status in patients with chronic liver disease. *Br J Nutr*. 2000;83:235-239.

10. Zrinyi M, Juhasz M, Balla J, Katona E, Ben T, Kakuk G, Pall D. Dietary self-efficacy: determinant of compliance behaviours and biochemical outcomes in haemodialysis patients. *Nephrol Dial Transplant*. 2003;19:1869-1873.

Imbalance of Nutrients (NI-5.5)

Definition

An undesirable combination of nutrients, such that the amount of one nutrient interferes with or alters absorption and/or utilization of another nutrient.

Etiology (Cause/Contributing Risk Factors)

Factors gathered during the nutrition assessment process that contribute to the existence or the maintenance of pathophysiological, psychosocial, situational, developmental, cultural, and/or environmental problems:

- Consumption of high-dose nutrient supplements
- Food- and nutrition-related knowledge deficit concerning nutrient interactions
- Harmful beliefs/attitudes about food, nutrition, and nutrition-related information
- Food faddism
- Insufficient electrolyte replacement when initiating feeding (PN/EN, including oral)

Signs/Symptoms (Defining Characteristics)

A typical cluster of subjective and objective signs and symptoms gathered during the nutrition assessment process that provide evidence that a problem exists; quantify the problem and describe its severity.

Nutrition Assessment Category	Potential Indicators of this Nutrition Diagnosis (one or more must be present)
Biochemical Data, Medical Tests and Procedures	• Severe hypophosphatemia (in the presence of ↑ carbohydrate) • Severe hypokalemia (in the presence of ↑ protein) • Severe hypomagnesemia (in the presence of ↑carbohydrate) • Refeeding syndrome
Anthropometric Data	
Nutrition-Focused Physical Findings	• Diarrhea or constipation (iron supplements) • Epigastric pain, nausea, vomiting, diarrhea (zinc supplements)

247

Diagnosis

Intake Domain – Nutrient

Imbalance of Nutrients (NI-5.5)

Food/Nutrition-Related History	Reports or observations of: • Estimated intake of iron supplements (↓ zinc absorption) higher than recommended • Estimated intake of zinc supplements (↓ copper status) higher than recommended • Estimated intake of manganese (↓ iron status) higher than recommended
Client History	

References

1. National Academy of Sciences, Institute of Medicine. *Dietary Reference Intakes for Vitamin A, Vitamin K, Arsenic, Boron, Chromium, Copper, Iodine, Iron, Manganese, Molybdenum, Nickel, Silicon, Vanadium, Zinc*. Washington, DC: National Academy Press; 2001.

2. National Academy of Sciences, Institute of Medicine. *Dietary Reference Intakes for Calcium, Phosphorus, Magnesium, Vitamin D, and Fluoride*. Washington, DC: National Academy Press; 1997.

Updated: 2008 Edition

Inadequate* Fat Intake (NI-5.6.1)

Definition

Lower fat intake compared to established reference standards or recommendations based on physiological needs.

> *Note: May not be an appropriate nutrition diagnosis when the goal is weight loss or during end-of-life care.*
>
> *Whenever possible, nutrient intake data should be considered in combination with clinical, biochemical, anthropometric information, medical diagnosis, clinical status, and/or other factors as well as diet to provide a valid assessment of nutritional status based on a totality of the evidence.* (Dietary Reference Intakes. Applications in Dietary Assessment. *Institute of Medicine. ashington, D.C.: National Academy Press; 2000).*

Etiology (Cause/Contributing Risk Factors)

Factors gathered during the nutrition assessment process that contribute to the existence or the maintenance of pathophysiological, psychosocial, situational, developmental, cultural, and/or environmental problems:

- Alteration in gastrointestinal tract structure and/or function
- Inappropriate food choices, e.g., economic constraints, restricting food given to elderly and/or children, specific food choices
- Cultural practices that affect ability to make appropriate food choices
- Food- and nutrition-related knowledge deficit concerning appropriate amount of dietary fat
- Psychological causes such as depression and disordered eating

Signs/Symptoms (Defining Characteristics)

A typical cluster of subjective and objective signs and symptoms gathered during the nutrition assessment process that provide evidence that a problem exists; quantify the problem and describe its severity.

Nutrition Assessment Category	Potential Indicators of this Nutrition Diagnosis (one or more must be present)
Biochemical Data, Medical Tests and Procedures	• Triene: tetraene ratio > 0.2
Anthropometric Measurements	• Impaired growth • Weight loss if insufficient calories consumed
Nutrition-Focused Physical Findings	• Scaly skin and dermatitis consistent with essential fatty acid deficiency
Food/Nutrition-Related History	Reports or observations of: • Estimated intake of essential fatty acids less than 10% of energy (primarily associated with PN)

If a synonym, or alternate word with the same meaning, for the term "inadequate" is helpful or needed, an approved alternate is the word "suboptimal."

Diagnosis

Intake Domain – Fat and Cholesterol

Inadequate* Fat Intake (NI-5.6.1)

Client History	• Conditions associated with a diagnosis or treatment, e.g., prolonged catabolic illness (e.g., AIDS, tuberculosis, anorexia nervosa, sepsis or severe infection from recent surgery)
	• Severe fat malabsorption with bowel resection, pancreatic insufficiency, or hepatic disease accompanied by steatorrhea

References

1. National Academy of Science, Institute of Medicine. *Dietary Reference Intakes for Energy, Carbohydrate, Fiber, Fat, Fatty Acids, Cholesterol, Protein, and Amino Acids.* Washington, DC: National Academy Press; 2002.

Updated: 2009 Edition

If a synonym, or alternate word with the same meaning, for the term "inadequate" is helpful or needed, an approved alternate is the word "suboptimal."

Excessive Fat Intake (NI-5.6.2)

Definition

Higher fat intake compared to established reference standards or recommendations based on physiological needs.

Etiology (Cause/Contributing Risk Factors)

Factors gathered during the nutrition assessment process that contribute to the existence or the maintenance of pathophysiological, psychosocial, situational, developmental, cultural, and/or environmental problems:

- Food- and nutrition-related knowledge deficit concerning appropriate amount of dietary fat
- Harmful beliefs/attitudes about food, nutrition, and nutrition-related topics
- Lack of or limited access to healthful food choices, e.g., healthful food choices not provided as an option by caregiver or parent, homeless
- Changes in taste and appetite or preference
- Lack of value for behavior change, competing values

Signs/Symptoms (Defining Characteristics)

A typical cluster of subjective and objective signs and symptoms gathered during the nutrition assessment process that provide evidence that a problem exists; quantify the problem and describe its severity.

Nutrition Assessment Category	Potential Indicators of this Nutrition Diagnosis (one or more must be present)
Biochemical Data, Medical Tests and Procedures	• Cholesterol > 200 mg/dL (5.2 mmol/L), LDL cholesterol > 100 mg/dL (2.59 mmol/L), HDL cholesterol < 40 mg/dL (1.036 mmol/L), triglycerides > 150 mg/dL (1.695 mmol/L) • Elevated serum amylase and/or lipase • Elevated LFTs, T. Bili • Fecal fat > 7g/24 hours
Anthropometric Measurements	
Nutrition-Focused Physical Findings	• Evidence of xanthomas • Diarrhea, cramping, steatorrhea, epigastric pain

Diagnosis

Intake Domain – Fat and Cholesterol

Excessive Fat Intake (NI-5.6.2)

Food/Nutrition-Related History	Reports or observations of: • Frequent or large portions of high-fat foods • Frequent food preparation with added fat • Frequent consumption of high risk lipids (i.e., saturated fat, trans fat, cholesterol) • Report of foods containing fat more than diet prescription • Medication, e.g., pancreatic enzymes, cholesterol- or other lipid-lowering medications
Client History	• Conditions associated with a diagnosis or treatment, e.g., hyperlipidemia, cystic fibrosis, angina, artherosclerosis, pancreatic, liver, and biliary diseases, post-transplantation • Family history of hyperlipidemia, atherosclerosis, or pancreatitis

References

1. National Academy of Sciences, Institute of Medicine. *Dietary Reference Intakes for Energy, Carbohydrate, Fiber, Fat, Fatty Acids, Cholesterol, Protein, and Amino Acids*. Washington, DC: National Academy Press; 2002.

2. Position of the American Dietetic Association. Weight management. *J Am Diet Assoc*. 2002;102:1145-1155.

3. Position of the American Dietetic Association. Total diet approach to communicating food and nutrition information. *J Am Diet Assoc*. 2007;107:1224-1232.

4. Position of the American Dietetic Association. The role of dietetics professionals in health promotion and disease prevention. *J Am Diet Assoc*. 2006;106:1875-1884.

Updated: 2008 Edition

Inappropriate Intake of Fats (specify) (NI-5.6.3)

Definition

Intake of wrong type or quality of fats compared to established reference standards or recommendations based on physiological needs.

Etiology (Cause/Contributing Risk Factors)

Factors gathered during the nutrition assessment process that contribute to the existence or the maintenance of pathophysiological, psychosocial, situational, developmental, cultural, and/or environmental problems:

- Food- and nutrition-related knowledge deficit concerning type of fat (e.g., fats added to food, formula/breastmilk)
- Harmful beliefs/attitudes about food, nutrition, and nutrition-related topics
- Lack of or limited access to healthful food choices, e.g., healthful food choices not provided as an option by caregiver or parent, homeless
- Changes in taste and appetite or preference
- Lack of value for behavior change, competing values

Signs/Symptoms (Defining Characteristics)

A typical cluster of subjective and objective signs and symptoms gathered during the nutrition assessment process that provide evidence that a problem exists; quantify the problem and describe its severity.

Nutrition Assessment Category	Potential Indicators of this Nutrition Diagnosis (one or more must be present)
Biochemical Data, Medical Tests and Procedures	• Cholesterol > 200 mg/dL (5.2 mmol/L), LDL cholesterol > 100 mg/dL (2.59 mmol/L), HDL cholesterol < 40 mg/dL (1.036 mmol/L), triglycerides > 150 mg/dL (1.695 mmol/L) • Elevated serum amylase and/or lipase • Elevated LFTs, T. Bili, C-reactive protein
Anthropometric Measurements	
Nutrition-Focused Physical Findings	• Evidence of dermatitis • Diarrhea, cramping, steatorrhea, epigastric pain

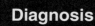
Diagnosis

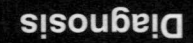

Intake Domain – Fat and Cholesterol

Inappropriate Intake of Fats (specify) (NI-5.6.3)

Food/Nutrition-Related History	Reports or observations of:
	• Frequent food preparation with added fat that is not of desired type for condition
	• Frequent consumption of fats that are undesirable for condition (e.g., saturated fat, trans fat, cholesterol, n-6 fatty acids)
	• Estimated intake of monounsaturated, polyunsaturated, n-3 fatty acids, or DHA/ARA less than recommended or in suboptimal ratio
Client History	• Conditions associated with a diagnosis or treatment of diabetes, cardiac diseases, obesity, liver or biliary disorders
	• Family history of diabetes-related heart disease, hyperlipidemia, atherosclerosis, or pancreatitis

References

1. de Lorgeril M, Salen P, Martin J-L, Monjaud I, Delaye J, Mamelle N. Mediterranean diet, traditional risk factors, and the rate of cardiovascular complications after myocardial infarction. Final report of the Lyon Diet Heart Study. *Circulation.* 1999; 99:779-785.

2. Franz MJ, Bantle JP, Beebe CA, Brunzell JD, Chiasson J-L, Garg A, Holzmeister LA, Hoogwerf B, Mayer-Davis E, Mooradian AD, Purnell JQ, Wheeler M. Technical review. Evidence-based nutrition principles and recommendations for the treatment and prevention of diabetes and related complications. *Diabetes Care.* 2002;202:148-198.

3. Knoops KTB, de Grott LCPGM, Kromhout D, Perrin A-E, Varela M-V, Menotti A, van Staveren WA. Mediterranean diet, lifestyle factors, and 10-year mortality in elderly European men and women. *JAMA.* 2004;292:1433-1439,

4. Kris-Etherton PM, Harris WS, Appel LJ, for the Nutrition Committee. AHA scientific statement. Fish consumption, fish oil, omega-3 fatty acids, and cardiovascular disease. *Circulation.* 2002;106:2747-2757.

5. National Academy of Sciences, Institute of Medicine. *Dietary Reference Intakes for Energy, Carbohydrate, Fiber, Fat, Fatty Acids, Cholesterol, Protein, and Amino Acids.* Washington, DC: National Academy Press; 2002.

6. Panagiotakos DB, Pitsavos C, Polychronopoulos E, Chrysohoou C, Zampelas A, Trichopoulou A. Can a Mediterranean diet moderate the development and clinical progression of coronary heart disease? A systematic review. *Med Sci Monit.* 2004;10:RA193-RA198.

7. Position of the American Dietetic Association. Weight management. *J Am Diet Assoc.* 2002;102:1145-1155.

8. Position of the American Dietetic Association. Total diet approach to communicating food and nutrition information. *J Am Diet Assoc.* 2007;107:1224-1232.

9. Position of the American Dietetic Association. The role of dietetics professionals in health promotion and disease prevention. *J Am Diet Assoc.* 2006;106:1875-1884.

10. Zhao G, Etherton TD, Martin KR, West SG, Gilles PJ, Kris-Etherton PM. Dietary alpha-linolenic acid reduces inflammatory and lipid cardiovascular risk factors in hypercholesterolemic men and women. *J Nutr.* 2004;134:2991-2997.

Updated: 2009 Edition

Inadequate* Protein Intake (NI-5.7.1)

Definition

Lower intake of protein compared to established reference standards or recommendations based on physiological needs.

> *Note: Whenever possible, nutrient intake data should be considered in combination with clinical, biochemical, anthropometric information, medical diagnosis, clinical status, and/or other factors as well as diet to provide a valid assessment of nutritional status based on a totality of the evidence. (Dietary Reference Intakes. Applications in Dietary Assessment. Institute of Medicine. Washington, D.C.: National Academy Press; 2000.)*

Etiology (Cause/Contributing Risk Factors)

Factors gathered during the nutrition assessment process that contribute to the existence or the maintenance of pathophysiological, psychosocial, situational, developmental, cultural, and/or environmental problems:

- Physiological causes increasing nutrient needs due to prolonged catabolic illness, malabsorption, age, or condition
- Lack of or limited access to food, e.g., economic constraints, restricting food given to elderly and/or children
- Cultural practices that affect the ability to access food
- Food- and nutrition-related knowledge deficit concerning amount of protein
- Psychological causes such as depression and disordered eating

Signs/Symptoms (Defining Characteristics)

A typical cluster of subjective and objective signs and symptoms gathered during the nutrition assessment process that provide evidence that a problem exists; quantify the problem and describe its severity.

Nutrition Assessment Category	Potential Indicators of this Nutrition Diagnosis (one or more must be present)
Biochemical Data, Medical Tests and Procedures	
Anthropometric Measurements	
Nutrition-Focused Physical Findings	• Edema, failure to thrive (infants/children), poor musculature, dull skin, thin and fragile hair

If a synonym, or alternate word with the same meaning, for the term "inadequate" is helpful or needed, an approved alternate is the word "suboptimal."

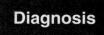
Diagnosis

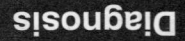

Intake Domain – Protein

Inadequate* Protein Intake (NI-5.7.1)

Food/Nutrition-Related History	Reports or observation of: • Estimated intake of protein insufficient to meet requirements • Cultural or religious practices that limit protein intake • Economic constraints that limit food availability • Prolonged adherence to a very–low-protein weight-loss diet
Client History	• Conditions associated with a diagnosis or treatment, e.g., severe protein malabsorption such as bowel resection

References

1. National Academy of Sciences, Institute of Medicine. *Dietary Reference Intakes for Energy, Carbohydrate, Fiber, Fat, Fatty Acids, Cholesterol, Protein, and Amino Acids.* Washington DC: National Academy Press; 2002.

Updated: 2009 Edition

If a synonym, or alternate word with the same meaning, for the term "inadequate" is helpful or needed, an approved alternate is the word "suboptimal."

Excessive Protein Intake (NI-5.7.2)

Definition

Intake more than the recommended level of protein compared to established reference standards or recommendations based on physiological needs.

Etiology (Cause/Contributing Risk Factors)

Factors gathered during the nutrition assessment process that contribute to the existence or the maintenance of pathophysiological, psychosocial, situational, developmental, cultural, and/or environmental problems:

- Liver dysfunction
- Renal dysfunction
- Harmful beliefs/attitudes about food, nutrition, and nutrition-related topics
- Lack of, or limited access to specialized protein products
- Metabolic abnormality
- Food faddism

Signs/Symptoms (Defining Characteristics)

A typical cluster of subjective and objective signs and symptoms gathered during the nutrition assessment process that provide evidence that a problem exists; quantify the problem and describe its severity.

Nutrition Assessment Category	Potential Indicators of this Nutrition Diagnosis (one or more must be present)
Biochemical Data, Medical Tests and Procedures	• Altered laboratory values, e.g., ↑ BUN, ↓ glomerular filtration rate (altered renal status)
Anthropometric Measurements	• Growth stunting or failure based on National Center for Health Statistics growth charts (metabolic disorders)
Nutrition-Focused Physical Findings	
Food/Nutrition-Related History	Reports or observations of: • Estimated total protein intake higher than recommended, e.g., early renal disease, advanced liver disease with confusion • Inappropriate supplementation
Client History	• Conditions associated with a diagnosis or treatment, e.g., early renal disease or advanced liver disease with confusion

257

Diagnosis

Intake Domain – Protein

Excessive Protein Intake (NI-5.7.2)

References

1. Position of the American Dietetic Association. Food and nutrition misinformation. *J Am Diet Assoc*. 2006;106:601-607.

2. Beto JA, Bansal VK. Medical nutrition therapy in chronic kidney failure: Integrating clinical practice guidelines. *J Am Diet Assoc*. 2004;104:404-409.

3. Brandle E, Sieberth HG, Hautmann RE. Effect of chronic dietary protein intake on the renal function in healthy subjects. *Eur J Clin Nutr*. 1996;50:734-740.

4. Frassetto LA, Todd KM, Morris RC Jr, Sebastian A. Estimation of net endogenous noncarbonic acid production in humans from diet, potassium and protein contents. *Am J Clin Nutr*. 1998;68:576-583.

5. Friedman N, ed. *Absorption and Utilization of Amino Acids*, Vol. I. Boca Raton, FL: CRC Press; 1989: 229-242.

6. Hoogeveen EK, Kostense PJ, Jager A, Heine RJ, Jakobs C, Bouter LM, Donker AJ, Stehower CD. Serum homocysteine level and protein intake are related to risk of microalbuminuria: the Hoorn study. *Kidney Int*. 1998;54:203-209.

7. Rudman D, DiFulco TJ, Galambos JT, Smith RB 3rd, Salam AA, Warren WD. Maximum rate of excretion and synthesis of urea in normal and cirrhotic subjects. *J Clin Invest*. 1973;52:2241-2249.

Inappropriate Intake of Amino Acids (specify) (NI-5.7.3)

Definition

Intake that is more or less than recommended level and/or type of amino acids compared to established reference standards or recommendations based on physiological needs.

Etiology (Cause/Contributing Risk Factors)

Factors gathered during the nutrition assessment process that contribute to the existence or the maintenance of pathophysiological, psychosocial, situational, developmental, cultural, and/or environmental problems:

- Liver dysfunction
- Renal dysfunction
- Harmful beliefs/attitudes about food, nutrition, and nutrition-related topics
- Misused specialized protein products
- Metabolic abnormality
- Food faddism
- Inborn errors of metabolism

Signs/Symptoms (Defining Characteristics)

A typical cluster of subjective and objective signs and symptoms gathered during the nutrition assessment process that provide evidence that a problem exists; quantify the problem and describe its severity.

Nutrition Assessment Category	Potential Indicators of this Nutrition Diagnosis (one or more must be present)
Biochemical Data, Medical Tests and Procedures	• Altered laboratory values, e.g., ↑ BUN, ↓ glomerular filtration rate (altered renal status) • Elevated specific amino acids (inborn errors of metabolism) • Elevated homocysteine or ammonia
Anthropometric Measurements	
Nutrition-Focused Physical Findings	• Physical or neurological changes (inborn errors of metabolism)

Diagnosis

Intake Domain – Protein

Inappropriate Intake of Amino Acids (specify) (NI-5.7.3)

Food/Nutrition-Related History	Reports or observation of:
	• Estimated amino acid intake higher than recommended, e.g., early renal disease, advanced liver disease, inborn error of metabolism
	• Estimated intake of certain types of amino acids higher than recommended for prescribed parenteral and enteral nutrition therapy
	• Inappropriate amino acid or protein supplementation, as for athletes
	• Estimated amino acid intake higher than recommended, e.g., excess phenylalanine intake
Client History	• Conditions associated with a diagnosis or treatment of illness that requires EN/PN therapy
	• History of inborn error of metabolism
	• Uremia, azotemia (renal patients)

References

1. Beto JA, Bansal VK. Medical nutrition therapy in chronic kidney failure: Integrating clinical practice guidelines. *J Am Diet Assoc*. 2004;104:404-409.
2. Brandle E, Sieberth HG, Hautmann RE. Effect of chronic dietary protein intake on the renal function in healthy subjects. *Eur J Clin Nutr*. 1996;50 :734-740.
3. Cohn RM, Roth KS. Hyperammonia, bane of the brain. *Clin Pediatr*. 2004;43:683.
4. Frassetto LA, Todd KM, Morris RC Jr, Sebastian A. Estimation of net endogenous noncarbonic acid production in humans from diet, potassium and protein contents. *Am J Clin Nutr*. 1998;68:576-583.
5. Friedman N, ed. *Absorption and Utilization of Amino Acids*, Vol. I. Boca Raton, FL: CRC Press; 1989:229-242.
6. Hoogeveen EK, Kostense PJ, Jager A, Heine RJ, Jakobs C, Bouter LM, Donker AJ, Stehower CD. Serum homocysteine level and protein intake are related to risk of microalbuminuria: the Hoorn study. *Kidney Int*. 1998;54:203-209.
7. Position of the American Dietetic Association: Food and nutrition misinformation. *J Am Diet Assoc*. 2006;106:601-607.
8. Rudman D, DiFulco TJ, Galambos JT, Smith RB 3rd, Salam AA, Warren WD. Maximal rate of excretion and synthesis of urea in normal and cirrhotic subjects. *J Clin Invest*. 1973;52:2241-2249.

Updated: 2009 Edition

Inadequate* Carbohydrate Intake (NI-5.8.1)

Definition

Lower intake of carbohydrate compared to established reference standards or recommendations based on physiological needs.

> *Note: Whenever possible, nutrient intake data should be considered in combination with clinical, biochemical, anthropometric information, medical diagnosis, clinical status, and/or other factors as well as diet to provide a valid assessment of nutritional status based on a totality of the evidence.* (Dietary Reference Intakes. Applications in Dietary Assessment. Institute of Medicine. Washington, D.C.: National Academy Press; 2000.)

Etiology (Cause/Contributing Risk Factors)

Factors gathered during the nutrition assessment process that contribute to the existence or the maintenance of pathophysiological, psychosocial, situational, developmental, cultural, and/or environmental problems:

- Physiological causes, e.g., increased energy needs due to increased activity level or metabolic change, malabsorption
- Lack of or limited access to food, e.g., economic constraints, restricting food given to elderly and/or children
- Cultural practices that affect the ability to access food
- Food- and nutrition-related knowledge deficit concerning appropriate amount of dietary carbohydrate
- Psychological causes such as depression and disordered eating

Signs/Symptoms (Defining Characteristics)

A typical cluster of subjective and objective signs and symptoms gathered during the nutrition assessment process that provide evidence that a problem exists; quantify the problem and describe its severity.

Nutrition Assessment Category	Potential Indicators of this Nutrition Diagnosis (one or more must be present)
Biochemical Data, Medical Tests and Procedures	
Anthropometric Measurements	
Nutrition-Focused Physical Findings	• Ketone smell on breath
Food/Nutrition-Related History	Reports or observation of: • Estimated carbohydrate intake less than recommended amounts • Inability to independently consume foods/fluids, e.g., diminished mobility in hand, wrist, or digits

If a synonym, or alternate word with the same meaning, for the term "inadequate" is helpful or needed, an approved alternate is the word "suboptimal."

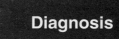

Diagnosis

Intake Domain – Carbohydrate and Fiber

Inadequate* Carbohydrate Intake (NI-5.8.1)

Client History	• Conditions associated with a diagnosis or treatment, e.g., pancreatic insufficiency, hepatic disease, celiac disease, seizure disorder, or carbohydrate malabsorption

References

1. National Academy of Sciences, Institute of Medicine. *Dietary Reference Intakes for Energy, Carbohydrate, Fiber, Fat, Fatty Acids, Cholesterol, Protein, and Amino Acids.* Washington, DC: National Academy Press; 2002.

Updated: 2009 Edition

*If a synonym, or alternate word with the same meaning, for the term "inadequate" is helpful or needed, an approved alternate is the word "suboptimal."

Excessive Carbohydrate Intake (NI-5.8.2)

Definition

Intake more than the recommended level and type of carbohydrate compared to established reference standards or recommendations based on physiological needs.

Etiology (Cause/Contributing Risk Factors)

Factors gathered during the nutrition assessment process that contribute to the existence or the maintenance of pathophysiological, psychosocial, situational, developmental, cultural, and/or environmental problems:

- Physiological causes requiring modified carbohydrate intake, e.g., diabetes mellitus, lactase deficiency, sucrase-isomaltase deficiency, aldolase-B deficiency
- Cultural practices that affect the ability to reduce carbohydrate intake
- Food- and nutrition-related knowledge deficit concerning appropriate amount of carbohydrate intake
- Food and nutrition compliance limitations, e.g., lack of willingness or failure to modify carbohydrate intake in response to recommendations from a dietitian or physician
- Psychological causes such as depression and disordered eating

Signs/Symptoms (Defining Characteristics)

A typical cluster of subjective and objective signs and symptoms gathered during the nutrition assessment process that provide evidence that a problem exists; quantify the problem and describe its severity.

Nutrition Assessment Category	Potential Indicators of this Nutrition Diagnosis (one or more must be present)
Biochemical Data, Medical Tests and Procedures	• Hyperglycemia (fasting blood sugar > 126 mg/dL) • Hemoglobin A1C > 6% • Abnormal oral glucose tolerance test (2-hour post load glucose > 200 mg/dL)
Anthropometric Measurements	
Nutrition-Focused Physical Findings	• Dental caries • Diarrhea in response to carbohydrate feeding

Diagnosis

Excessive Carbohydrate Intake (NI-5.8.2)

Food/Nutrition-Related History	Reports or observation of: • Cultural or religious practices that do not support modification of dietary carbohydrate intake • Estimated carbohydrate intake that is consistently more than recommended amounts • Chronic use of medications that cause hyperglycemia, e.g., steroids
Client History	• Conditions associated with a diagnosis or treatment, e.g., diabetes mellitus, inborn errors of carbohydrate metabolism, lactase deficiency, severe infection, sepsis, or obesity • Pancreatic insufficiency resulting in reduced insulin production • Economic constraints that limit availability of appropriate foods

References

1. Bowman BA, Russell RM. *Present Knowledge in Nutrition*. 8th Ed. Washington, DC: ILSI Press; 2001.

2. Clement S, Braithwaite SS, Magee MF, Ahmann A, Smith EP, Schafer RG, Hirsch IB, American Diabetes Association Diabetes in Hospitals Writing Committee. Management of diabetes in hospitals. *Diabetes Care*. 2004;27:553-592.

3. National Academy of Sciences, Institute of Medicine. *Dietary Reference Intakes for Energy, Carbohydrate, Fiber, Fat, Fatty Acids, Cholesterol, Protein, and Amino Acids*. Washington, DC: National Academy Press; 2002.

4. The Expert Committee on the Diagnosis and Classification of Diabetes Mellitus. Diagnosis and classification of diabetes mellitus. *Diabetes Care*. 2004;27:S5-S10.

Inappropriate Intake of Types of Carbohydrates (specify) (NI-5.8.3)

Definition
Intake of the type or amount of carbohydrate that is more or less than the established reference standards or recommendations based on physiological needs.

Etiology (Cause/Contributing Risk Factors)
Factors gathered during the nutrition assessment process that contribute to the existence or the maintenance of pathophysiological, psychosocial, situational, developmental, cultural, and/or environmental problems:

- Physiological causes requiring careful use of modified carbohydrate, e.g., diabetes mellitus, metabolic syndrome, hypoglycemia, celiac disease, allergies, obesity
- Cultural practices that affect the ability to regulate types of carbohydrate consumed
- Food- and nutrition-related knowledge deficit concerning appropriate amount or types of carbohydrate
- Food and nutrition compliance limitations, e.g., lack of willingness or failure to modify carbohydrate intake in response to recommendations from a dietitian, physician, or caregiver
- Psychological causes such as depression and disordered eating

Signs/Symptoms (Defining Characteristics)
A typical cluster of subjective and objective signs and symptoms gathered during the nutrition assessment process that provide evidence that a problem exists; quantify the problem and describe its severity.

Nutrition Assessment Category	Potential Indicators of this Nutrition Diagnosis (one or more must be present)
Biochemical Data, Medical Tests and Procedures	• Hypoglycemia or hyperglycemia documented on regular basis when compared with goal of maintaining glucose levels at or less than 140 mg/dL throughout the day
Anthropometric Measurements	
Nutrition-Focused Physical Findings	• Diarrhea in response to high intake of refined carbohydrates
Food/Nutrition-Related History	Reports or observations of: • Carbohydrate intake that is different from recommended types • Limited knowledge of carbohydrate composition of foods or of carbohydrate metabolism • Chronic use of medications that cause altered glucose levels, e.g., steroids, antidepressants, antipsychotics
Client History	• Conditions associated with a diagnosis or treatment, e.g., diabetes mellitus, obesity, metabolic syndrome, hypoglycemia • Allergic reactions to certain carbohydrate foods or food groups • Economic constraints that limit availability of appropriate foods

Diagnosis

Intake Domain – Carbohydrate and Fiber

Inappropriate Intake of Types of Carbohydrates (specify) (NI-5.8.3)

References

1. Bowman BA, Russell RM. *Present Knowledge in Nutrition*. 8th Ed. Washington, DC: ILSI Press, 2001.

2. Clement S, Braithwaite SS, Magee MF, Ahmann A, Smith EP, Schafer RG, Hirsch IB, American Diabetes Association Diabetes in Hospitals Writing Committee. Management of diabetes in hospitals. *Diabetes Care*. 2004;27:553-592.

3. Franz MJ, Bantle JP, Beebe CA, Brunzell JD, Chiasson J-L, Garg A, Holzmeister LA, Hoogwerf B, Mayer-Davis E, Mooradian AD, Purnell JQ, Wheeler M. Technical review. Evidence-based nutrition principles and recommendations for the treatment and prevention of diabetes and related complications. *Diabetes Care*. 2002;202:148-198.

4. Sheard NF, Clark NG, Brand-Miller JC, Franz MJ, Pi-Sunyer FX, Mayer-Davis E, Kulkarni K, Geil P. A statement by the American Diabetes Association. Dietary carbohydrate (amount and type) in the prevention and management of diabetes. *Diabetes Care*. 2004;27:2266-2271.

5. Gross LS, Li L, Ford ES, Liu S. Increased consumption of refined carbohydrates and epidemic or type 2 diabetes in the United States: an ecologic assessment. *Am J Clin Nutr*. 2004;79:774-779.

6. French S, Lin B-H, Gutherie JF. National trends in soft drink consumption among children and adolescents age 6 to17 years: prevalence, amounts, and sources, 1977/1978 to 1994/1998. *J Am Diet Assoc*. 2003;103L1326-1331,

7. National Academy of Sciences, Institute of Medicine. *Dietary Reference Intakes for Energy, Carbohydrate, Fiber, Fat, Fatty Acids, Cholesterol, Protein, and Amino Acids*. Washington, DC: National Academy Press; 2002.

8. Teff KL, Elliott SS, Tschöp M, Kieffer TJ, Rader D, Heiman M, Townsend RR, Keim NL, D'Alessio D, Havel PJ. Dietary fructose reduces circulating insulin and leptin, attenuates postprandial suppression of ghrelin, and increases triglycerides in women. *J Clin Endocrinol Metab*. 2004;89:2963-2972.

9. The Expert Committee on the Diagnosis and Classification of Diabetes Mellitus. Diagnosis and classification of diabetes mellitus. *Diabetes Care*. 2004;27:S5-S10.

Inconsistent Carbohydrate Intake (NI-5.8.4)

Definition

Inconsistent timing of carbohydrate intake throughout the day, day to day, or a pattern of carbohydrate intake that is not consistent with recommended pattern based on physiological or medication needs.

Etiology (Cause/Contributing Risk Factors)

Factors gathered during the nutrition assessment process that contribute to the existence or the maintenance of pathophysiological, psychosocial, situational, developmental, cultural, and/or environmental problems:

- Physiological causes requiring careful timing and consistency in the amount of carbohydrate, e.g., diabetes mellitus, hypoglycemia, PN/EN delivery
- Cultural practices that affect the ability to regulate timing of carbohydrate consumption
- Food- and nutrition-related knowledge deficit concerning appropriate timing of carbohydrate intake
- Food and nutrition compliance limitations, e.g., lack of willingness or failure to modify carbohydrate timing in response to recommendations from a dietitian, physician, or caregiver
- Psychological causes such as depression and disordered eating

Signs/Symptoms (Defining Characteristics)

A typical cluster of subjective and objective signs and symptoms gathered during the nutrition assessment process that provide evidence that a problem exists; quantify the problem and describe its severity.

Nutrition Assessment Category	Potential Indicators of this Nutrition Diagnosis (one or more must be present)
Biochemical Data, Medical Tests and Procedures	• Hypoglycemia or hyperglycemia documented on regular basis associated with inconsistent carbohydrate intake • Wide variations in blood glucose levels
Anthropometric Measurements	
Nutrition-Focused Physical Findings	
Food/Nutrition-Related History	Reports or observations of: • Estimated carbohydrate intake that is different from recommended types or ingested on an irregular basis • Use of insulin or insulin secretagogues • Chronic use of medications that cause altered glucose levels, e.g., steroids, antidepressants, antipsychotics
Client History	• Conditions associated with a diagnosis or treatment, e.g., diabetes mellitus, obesity, metabolic syndrome, hypoglycemia • Economic constraints that limit availability of appropriate foods

Diagnosis

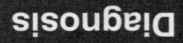

Intake Domain – Carbohydrate and Fiber

Inconsistent Carbohydrate Intake (NI-5.8.4)

References

1. Bowman BA, Russell RM. *Present Knowledge in Nutrition*. 8th Ed. Washington, DC: ILSI Press; 2001.

2. Clement S, Braithwaite SS, Magee MF, Ahmann A, Smith EP, Schafer RG, Hirsch IB, American Diabetes Association Diabetes in Hospitals Writing Committee. Management of diabetes in hospitals. *Diabetes Care*. 2004;27:553-592.

3. Cryer PE, Davis SN, Shamoon H. Technical review. Hypoglycemia in diabetes. *Diabetes Care*. 2003;26L1902-1912.

4. Franz MJ, Bantle JP, Beebe CA, Brunzell JD, Chiasson J-L, Garg A, Holzmeister LA, Hoogwerf B, Mayer-Davis E, Mooradian AD, Purnell JQ, Wheeler M. Technical review. Evidence-based nutrition principles and recommendations for the treatment and prevention of diabetes and related complications. *Diabetes Care*. 2002;202:148-198.

5. National Academy of Sciences, Institute of Medicine. *Dietary Reference Intakes for Energy, Carbohydrate, Fiber, Fat, Fatty Acids, Cholesterol, Protein, and Amino Acids*. Washington, DC: National Academy Press; 2002.

6. Rabasa-Lhoret R, Garon J, Langelier H, Poisson D, Chiasson J-L. The effects of meal carbohydrate content on insulin requirements in type 1 patients with diabetes treated intensively with the basal bolus (ultralente-regular) insulin regimen. *Diabetes Care*. 1999;22:667-673.

7. Savoca MR, Miller CK, Ludwig DA. Food habits are related to glycemic control among people with type 2 diabetes mellitus. *J Am Diet Assoc*. 2004;104:560-566.

8. The Expert Committee on the Diagnosis and Classification of Diabetes Mellitus. Diagnosis and classification of diabetes mellitus. *Diabetes Care*. 2004;27:S5-S10.

9. Wolever TMS, Hamad S, Chiasson J-L, Josse RG, Leiter LA, Rodger NW, Ross SA, Ryan EA. Day-to-day consistency in amount and source of carbohydrate intake associated with improved glucose control in type 1 diabetes. *J Am Coll Nutr*. 1999; 18:242-247.

Updated: 2009 Edition

Inadequate* Fiber Intake (NI-5.8.5)

Definition
Lower intake of fiber compared to established reference standards or recommendations based on physiological needs.

> Note: Whenever possible, nutrient intake data should be considered in combination with clinical, biochemical, anthropometric information, medical diagnosis, clinical status, and/or other factors as well as diet to provide a valid assessment of nutritional status based on a totality of the evidence. (Dietary Reference Intakes. Applications in Dietary Assessment. Institute of Medicine. Washington, D.C.: National Academy Press; 2000.)

Etiology (Cause/Contributing Risk Factors)
Factors gathered during the nutrition assessment process that contribute to the existence or the maintenance of pathophysiological, psychosocial, situational, developmental, cultural, and/or environmental problems:

- Lack of or limited access to fiber-containing foods/fluids
- Food- and nutrition-related knowledge deficit concerning desirable quantities of fiber
- Psychological causes such as depression and disordered eating
- Prolonged adherence to a low-fiber or low-residue diet
- Difficulty chewing or swallowing high-fiber foods
- Economic constraints that limit availability of appropriate foods
- Inability or unwillingness to purchase or consume fiber-containing foods
- Inappropriate food preparation practices, e.g., reliance on overprocessed, overcooked foods

Signs/Symptoms (Defining Characteristics)
A typical cluster of subjective and objective signs and symptoms gathered during the nutrition assessment process that provide evidence that a problem exists; quantify the problem and describe its severity.

Nutrition Assessment Category	Potential Indicators of this Nutrition Diagnosis (one or more must be present)
Biochemical Data, Medical Tests and Procedures	
Anthropometric Measurements	
Nutrition-Focused Physical Findings	• Inadequate fecal bulk

*If a synonym, or alternate word with the same meaning, for the term "inadequate" is helpful or needed, an approved alternate is the word "suboptimal."

Diagnosis

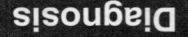

Intake Domain – Carbohydrate and Fiber

Inadequate* Fiber Intake (NI-5.8.5)

Food/Nutrition-Related History	Reports or observations of: • Estimated intake of fiber that is insufficient when compared to recommended amounts (38 g/day for men and 25 g/day for women)
Client History	• Conditions associated with a diagnosis or treatment, e.g., ulcer disease, inflammatory bowel disease, or short-bowel syndrome treated with a low-fiber diet

References

1. DiPalma JA. Current treatment options for chronic constipation. *Rev Gastroenterol Disord*. 2004;2:S34-S42.
2. Higgins PD, Johanson JF. Epidemiology of constipation in North America: a systematic review. *Am J Gastroenterol*. 2004;99:750-759.
3. Lembo A, Camilieri M. Chronic constipation. *New Engl J Med*. 2003;349:360-368.
4. National Academy of Sciences, Institute of Medicine. *Dietary Reference Intakes for Energy, Carbohydrate, Fiber, Fat, Fatty Acids, Cholesterol, Protein, and Amino Acids*. Washington, DC: National Academy Press; 2002.
5. Talley NJ. Definition, epidemiology, and impact of chronic constipation. *Rev Gastroenterol Disord*. 2004;2:S3-S10.

Updated: 2009 Edition

If a synonym, or alternate word with the same meaning, for the term "inadequate" is helpful or needed, an approved alternate is the word "suboptimal."

Excessive Fiber Intake (NI-5.8.6)

Definition
Higher intake of fiber compared to recommendations based on patient/client condition.

Etiology (Cause/Contributing Risk Factors)
Factors gathered during the nutrition assessment process that contribute to the existence or the maintenance of pathophysiological, psychosocial, situational, developmental, cultural, and/or environmental problems:

- Food- and nutrition-related knowledge deficit concerning desirable quantities of fiber
- Harmful beliefs or attitudes about food- or nutrition-related topics, e.g., obsession with bowel frequency and habits
- Lack of knowledge about appropriate fiber intake for condition
- Food preparation or eating patterns that involve only high-fiber foods to the exclusion of other nutrient-dense foods

Signs/Symptoms (Defining Characteristics)
A typical cluster of subjective and objective signs and symptoms gathered during the nutrition assessment process that provide evidence that a problem exists; quantify the problem and describe its severity.

Nutrition Assessment Category	Potential Indicators of this Nutrition Diagnosis (one or more must be present)
Biochemical Data, Medical Tests and Procedures	
Anthropometric Measurements	
Nutrition-Focused Physical Findings	• Nausea, vomiting, excessive flatulence, diarrhea, abdominal cramping, high stool volume or frequency that causes discomfort to the individual
Food/Nutrition-Related History	Reports or observations of: • Estimated fiber intake higher than tolerated or generally recommended for current medical condition
Client History	• Conditions associated with a diagnosis or treatment, e.g., ulcer disease, irritable bowel syndrome, inflammatory bowel disease, short-bowel syndrome, diverticulitis, obstructive constipation, prolapsing hemorrhoids, gastrointestinal stricture, eating disorders, or mental illness with obsessive-compulsive tendencies • Obstruction, phytobezoar

Diagnosis

Intake Domain – Carbohydrate and Fiber

Excessive Fiber Intake (NI-5.8.6)

References

1. DiPalma JA. Current treatment options for chronic constipation. *Rev Gastroenterol Disord*. 2004;2:S34-S42.

2. Higgins PD, Johanson JF. Epidemiology of constipation in North America: a systematic review. *Am J Gastroenterol*. 2004;99:750-759.

3. Lembo A, Camilieri M. Chronic constipation. *New Engl J Med*. 2003;349:360-368.

4. National Academy of Sciences, Institute of Medicine. *Dietary Reference Intakes for Energy, Carbohydrate, Fiber, Fat, Fatty Acids, Cholesterol, Protein, and Amino Acids*. Washington, DC: National Academy Press; 2002.

5. Position of the American Dietetic Association: Health implications of dietary fiber. *J Am Diet Assoc*. 2002;102:993-1000.

6. Talley NJ. Definition, epidemiology, and impact of chronic constipation. *Rev Gastroenterol Disord*. 2004;2:S3-S10.

7. van den Berg H, van der Gaag M, Hendriks H. Influence of lifestyle on vitamin bioavailability. *Int J Vitam Nutr Res*. 2002;72:53-55.

8. Wald A. Irritable bowel syndrome. *Curr Treat Options Gastroenterol*. 1999;2:13-19.

Updated: 2008 Edition

Inadequate* Vitamin Intake (specify) (NI-5.9.1)

Definition

Lower intake of one or more vitamins compared to established reference standards or recommendations based on physiological needs.

> Note: Whenever possible, nutrient intake data should be considered in combination with clinical, biochemical, anthropometric information, medical diagnosis, clinical status, and/or other factors as well as diet to provide a valid assessment of nutritional status based on a totality of the evidence. (Dietary Reference Intakes. Applications in Dietary Assessment. Institute of Medicine. Washington, D.C.: National Academy Press; 2000.)

Etiology (Cause/Contributing Risk Factors)

Factors gathered during the nutrition assessment process that contribute to the existence or the maintenance of pathophysiological, psychosocial, situational, developmental, cultural, and/or environmental problems:

- Physiological causes increasing nutrient needs due to prolonged catabolic illness, disease state, malabsorption, or medications
- Lack of or limited access to food, e.g., economic constraints, restricting food given to elderly and/or children
- Cultural practices that affect ability to access food
- Food- and nutrition-related knowledge deficit concerning food and supplemental sources of vitamins
- Psychological causes, e.g., depression or eating disorders

*If a synonym, or alternate word with the same meaning, for the term "inadequate" is helpful or needed, an approved alternate is the word "suboptimal."

Diagnosis

Inadequate* Vitamin Intake (specify) (NI-5.9.1)

Signs/Symptoms (Defining Characteristics)

A typical cluster of subjective and objective signs and symptoms gathered during the nutrition assessment process that provide evidence that a problem exists; quantify the problem and describe its severity.

Nutrition Assessment Category	Potential Indicators of this Nutrition Diagnosis (one or more must be present)
Biochemical Data, Medical Tests and Procedures	• Vitamin A: serum retinol < 10 µg/dL (0.35 µmol/L) • Vitamin C: plasma concentrations < 0.2 mg/dL (11.4 µmol/L) • Vitamin D: ionized calcium < 3.9 mg/dL (0.98 mmol/L) with elevated parathyroid hormone, normal serum calcium, and serum phosphorus < 2.6 mg/dL (0.84 mmol/L) • Vitamin E: plasma alpha-tocopherol < 18 µmol/g (41.8 µmol/L) • Vitamin K: elevated prothrombin time; altered INR (without anticoagulation therapy) • Thiamin: erythrocyte transketolase activity > 1.20 µg/mL/h • Riboflavin: erythrocyte glutathione reductase > 1.2 IU/g hemoglobin • Niacin: N'methyl-nicotinamide excretion < 5.8 µmol/day • Vitamin B-6: plasma pryrdoxal 5'phosphate <5 ng/mL (20 nmol/L) • Vitamin B-12: serum concentration < 24.4 ng/dL (180 pmol/L); elevated homocysteine • Folic acid—serum concentration < 0.3 µg/dL (7 nmol/L); red cell folate < 315 nmol/L
Anthropometric Measurements	
Nutrition-Focused Physical Findings	• Vitamin A: night blindness, Bitot's spots, xerophthalmia, follicular hyperkeratosis • Vitamin C: follicular hyperkeratosis, petichiae, ecchymosis, coiled hairs, inflamed and bleeding gums, perifollicular hemorrhages, joint effusions, arthralgia, and impaired wound healing • Vitamin D: widening at ends of long bones • Riboflavin: sore throat, hyperemia, edema of pharyngeal and oral mucous membranes, cheilosis, angular stomatitis, glossitis, magenta tongue, seborrheic dermatitis, and normochromic, normocytic anemia with pure erythrocyte cytoplasia of the bone marrow • Niacin: symmetrical, pigmented rash on areas exposed to sunlight; bright red tongue • Vitamin B-6: seborrheic dermatitis, stomatitis, cheilosis, glossitis, confusion, depression • Vitamin B-12: tingling and numbness in extremities, diminished vibratory and position sense, motor disturbances including gait disturbances

*If a synonym, or alternate word with the same meaning, for the term "inadequate" is helpful or needed, an approved alternate is the word "suboptimal."

Inadequate* Vitamin Intake (specify) (NI-5.9.1)

Food/Nutrition-Related History	Reports or observations of: • Estimated intake of foods containing specific vitamins less than requirements or recommended level • Excessive intake of foods that do not contain available vitamins, e.g., over processed, overcooked, or improperly stored foods • Prolonged use of substances known to increase vitamin requirements or reduce vitamin absorption • Lack of interest in foods
Client History	• Conditions associated with a diagnosis or treatment, e.g., malabsorption as a result of celiac disease, short-bowel syndrome, or inflammatory bowel • Certain environmental conditions, e.g., infants exclusively fed breast milk with limited exposure to sunlight (Vitamin D) • Rachitic rosary in children, rickets, osteomalacia • Pellegra • Vitamin/mineral deficiency

References

1. National Academy of Sciences, Institute of Medicine. *Dietary Reference Intakes for Vitamin A, Vitamin K, Arsenic, Boron, Chromium, Copper, Iodine, Iron, Manganese, Molybdenum, Nickel, Silicon, Vanadium, and Zinc*. Washington, DC: National Academy Press; 2000.

2. National Academy of Sciences, Institute of Medicine. *Dietary Reference Intakes for Thiamin, Riboflavin, Niacin, Vitamin B6, Folate, Vitamin B12, Pantothenic Acid, Biotin, and Choline*. Washington, DC: National Academy Press; 2000.

3. National Academy of Sciences, Institute of Medicine. *Dietary Reference Intakes for Vitamin C, Vitamin E, Selenium, and Carotenoids*. Washington, DC: National Academy Press; 2000.

4. National Academy of Sciences, Institute of Medicine. *Dietary Reference Intakes for Calcium, Phosphorus, Magnesium, Vitamin D, and Fluoride*. Washington, DC: National Academy Press; 1997.

Updated: 2009 Edition

If a synonym, or alternate word with the same meaning, for the term "inadequate" is helpful or needed, an approved alternate is the word "suboptimal."

Diagnosis

Intake Domain – Vitamin

Excessive Vitamin Intake (specify) (NI-5.9.2)

Definition

Higher intake of one or more vitamins compared to established reference standards or recommendations based on physiological needs.

Etiology (Cause/Contributing Risk Factors)

Factors gathered during the nutrition assessment process that contribute to the existence or the maintenance of pathophysiological, psychosocial, situational, developmental, cultural, and/or environmental problems:

- Physiological causes decreasing nutrient needs due to prolonged immobility or chronic renal disease
- Access to foods and supplements in excess of needs, e.g., cultural or religious practices; inappropriate food and supplements given to pregnant women, elderly, or children
- Food- and nutrition-related knowledge deficit concerning food and supplemental sources of vitamins
- Psychological causes, e.g., depression or eating disorders
- Accidental overdose from oral and supplemental forms, enteral or parenteral sources

Signs/Symptoms (Defining Characteristics)

A typical cluster of subjective and objective signs and symptoms gathered during the nutrition assessment process that provide evidence that a problem exists; quantify the problem and describe its severity.

Nutrition Assessment Category	Potential Indicators of this Nutrition Diagnosis (one or more must be present)
Biochemical Data, Medical Tests and Procedures	• Vitamin D: ionized calcium > 5.4 mg/dL (1.35 mmol/L) with elevated parathyroid hormone, normal serum calcium, and serum phosphorus > 2.6 mg/dL (0.84 mmol/L) • Vitamin K: slowed prothrombin time or altered INR • Niacin: N'methyl-nicotinamide excretion > 7.3 μmol/day • Vitamin B-6: plasma pryrdoxal 5'phosphate > 15.7 ng/mL (94 noml/L) • Vitamin A: serum retinol concentration > 60 μg/dL (2.09 μmol/L)
Anthropometric Measurements	• Vitamin D: growth retardation

Excessive Vitamin Intake (specify) (NI-5.9.2)

Nutrition-Focused Physical Findings	• Vitamin A: changes in the skin and mucous membranes; dry lips (cheilitis); early—dryness of the nasal mucosa and eyes; later—dryness, erythema, scaling and peeling of the skin, hair loss, and nail fragility. Headache, nausea, and vomiting. Infants may have bulging fontanelle; children may develop bone alterations. • Vitamin D: elevated serum calcium (hypercalcemia) and phosphorus (hyperphosphatemia) levels; calcification of soft tissues (calcinosis), including the kidney, lungs, heart, and even the tympanic membrane of the ear, which can result in deafness. Headache and nausea. Infants given excessive amounts of vitamin D may have gastrointestinal upset, bone fragility. • Vitamin K: hemolytic anemia in adults or severe jaundice in infants have been noted on rare occasions • Niacin: histamine release, which causes flushing, aggravation of asthma, or liver disease
Food/Nutrition-Related History	Reports or observations of: • Estimated intake reflects excessive intake of foods and supplements containing vitamins as compared to estimated requirements, including fortified cereals, meal replacements, vitamin-mineral supplements, other dietary supplements (e.g., fish liver oils or capsules), tube feeding, and/or parenteral solutions • Estimated intake > Tolerable Upper Limit (UL) for vitamin A (as retinol ester, not as β-carotene) is 600 µg/d for infants and toddlers; 900 µg/d for children 4-8 y, 1700 µg/d for children 9-13 y, 2800 for children 14-18 y, and 3000 µg/d for adults • Estimated intake more than UL for vitamin D is 25 µg/d for infants and 50 µg/d for children and adults • Estimated intake of Niacin: clinical, high-dose niacinamide (NA), 1-2 g, three times per day, can have side effects
Client History	• Conditions associated with a diagnosis or treatment, e.g., chronic liver or kidney diseases, heart failure, cancer

References

1. Allen LH, Haskell M. Estimating the potential for vitamin A toxicity in women and young children. *J Nutr*. 2002;132:S2907-S2919.

2. Croquet V, Pilette C, Lespine A, Vuillemin E, Rousselet MC, Oberti F, Saint Andre JP, Periquet B, Francois S, Ifrah N, Cales P. Hepatic hyper-vitaminosis A: importance of retinyl ester level determination. E*ur J Gastroenterol Hepatol*. 2000;12:361-364.

3. Krasinski SD, Russell RM, Otradovec CL, Sadowski JA, Hartz SC, Jacob RA, McGandy RB. Relationship of vitamin A and vitamin E intake to fasting plasma retinol, retinol-binding protein, retinyl esters, carotene, alpha-tocopherol, and cholesterol among elderly people and young adults: increased plasma retinyl esters among vitamin A-supplement users. *Am J Clin Nutr*. 1989;49:112-120.

4. National Academy of Sciences, Institute of Medicine. *Dietary Reference Intakes for Vitamin A, Vitamin K, Arsenic, Boron, Chromium, Copper, Iodine, Iron, Manganese, Molybdenum, Nickel, Silicon, Vanadium, and Zinc*. Washington, DC: National Academy Press; 2000.

5. National Academy of Sciences, Institute of Medicine. *Dietary Reference Intakes for Thiamine, Riboflavin, Niacin, Vitamin B6, Folate, Vitamin B12, Pantothenic Acid, Biotin, and Choline*. Washington, DC: National Academy Press; 2000.

6. National Academy of Sciences, Institute of Medicine. *Dietary Reference Intakes for Vitamin C, Vitamin E, Selenium, and Carotenoids*. Washington, DC: National Academy Press; 2000.

7. Russell RM. New views on RDAs for older adults. *J Am Diet Assoc*. 1997;97:515-518.

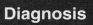

Diagnosis

Intake Domain – Mineral

Inadequate* Mineral Intake (specify) (NI-5.10.1)

Definition

Lower intake of one or more minerals compared to established reference standards or recommendations based on physiological needs.

> *Note: Whenever possible, nutrient intake data should be considered in combination with clinical, biochemical, anthropometric information, medical diagnosis, clinical status, and/or other factors as well as diet to provide a valid assessment of nutritional status based on a totality of the evidence. (Dietary Reference Intakes. Applications in Dietary Assessment. Institute of Medicine. Washington, D.C.: National Academy Press; 2000.)*

Etiology (Cause/Contributing Risk Factors)

Factors gathered during the nutrition assessment process that contribute to the existence or the maintenance of pathophysiological, psychosocial, situational, developmental, cultural, and/or environmental problems:

- Physiological causes increasing nutrient needs due to prolonged catabolic illness, malabsorption, hyperexcretion, nutrient/drug and nutrient/nutrient interaction, growth and maturation
- Lack of or limited access to food, e.g., economic constraints, restricting food given to elderly and/or children
- Cultural practices that affect ability to access food
- Food- and nutrition-related knowledge deficit concerning food and supplemental sources of minerals
- Misdiagnosis of lactose intolerance/lactase deficiency; perception of conflicting nutrition messages from health professionals; inappropriate reliance on supplements
- Psychological causes, e.g., depression or eating disorders
- Environmental causes, e.g., inadequately tested nutrient bioavailability of fortified foods, beverages, and supplements; inappropriate marketing of fortified foods/beverages/supplements as a substitute for natural food source of nutrient(s)

*If a synonym, or alternate word with the same meaning, for the term "inadequate" is helpful or needed, an approved alternate is the word "suboptimal."

Inadequate* Mineral Intake (specify) (NI-5.10.1)

Signs/Symptoms (Defining Characteristics)

A typical cluster of subjective and objective signs and symptoms gathered during the nutrition assessment process that provide evidence that a problem exists; quantify the problem and describe its severity.

Nutrition Assessment Category	Potential Indicators of this Nutrition Diagnosis (one or more must be present)
Biochemical Data, Medical Tests and Procedures	• Calcium: bone mineral content (BMC) below the young adult mean. Hypocalciuria, serum 25(OH)D < 32 ng/mL • Phosphorus < 2.6 mg/dL (0.84 mmol/L) • Magnesium <1.8 mg/dL (0.7 mmol/L) • Iron: hemoglobin < 13 g/L (2 mmol/L) (males); < 12 g/L (1.86 mmol/L) (females) • Iodine: urinary excretion < 100 µg/L (788 nmol/L) • Copper, serum copper < 64 µg/dL (10 µmol/L)
Anthropometric Measurements	• Height loss
Nutrition-Focused Physical Findings	• Calcium: hypertension
Food/Nutrition-Related History	Reports or observations of: • Estimated mineral intake from diet less than recommended intake • Food avoidance and/or elimination of whole food group(s) from diet • Lack of interest in food • Inappropriate food choices and/or chronic dieting behavior
Client History	• Conditions associated with a diagnosis or treatment, e.g., malabsorption as a result of celiac disease, short bowel syndrome, inflammatory bowel disease, or post-menopausal women without estrogen supplementation and increased calcium need • Polycystic ovary syndrome, premenstrual syndrome, kidney stones, colon polyps • Other significant medical diagnoses and therapies • Geographic latitude and history of Ultraviolet-B exposure/use of sunscreen • Change in living environment/independence • Calcium: obesity • Vitamin/mineral deficiency

*If a synonym, or alternate word with the same meaning, for the term "inadequate" is helpful or needed, an approved alternate is the word "suboptimal."

Diagnosis

Intake Domain – Mineral

Inadequate* Mineral Intake (specify) (NI-5.10.1)

References

1. Appel LJ, Moore TJ, Obarzanek E, Vollmer WM, Svetkey LP, Sacks FM, Bray GA, Vogt TM, Cutler JA, Windhauser MM, Lin P-H, Karanja N. A clinical trial of the effects of dietary patterns on blood pressure. *N Engl J Med*. 1997;336:1117-1124.

2. Heaney RP. Role of dietary sodium in osteoporosis. *J Am Coll Nutr*. 25(3 suppl):S271-S276. 2006.

3. Heaney RP. Nutrients, interactions, and foods. The Importance of Source. In Burckhardt P, Dawson-Hughes B, Heaney RP, Eds. *Nutritional Aspects of Osteoporosis* 2nd Ed. San Diego, CA: Elsevier, 2004:61-76.

4. Heaney RP. Nutrients, interactions, and foods. Serum 25-hydroxy-vitamin D and the health of the calcium economy. In Burckhardt P, Dawson-Hughes B, Heaney RP, Eds. *Nutritional Aspects of Osteoporosis* 2nd Ed. San Diego, CA: Elsevier, 2004:227-244.

5. Heaney RP, Rafferty K, Bierman J. Not all calcium-fortified beverages are equal. *Nutr Today*. 2005;40:39-41.

6. Heaney RP, Dowell MS, Hale CA, Bendich A. Calcium absorption varies within the reference range for serum 25-hydroxyvitamin D. *J Am Coll Nutr*. 2003;22:142-146.

7. Heaney RP, Dowell MS, Rafferty K, Bierman J. Bioavailability of the calcium in fortified soy imitation milk, with some observations on method. *Am J Clin Nutr*. 2000;71:1166-1169.

8. Holick MF. Functions of vitamin D: importance for prevention of common cancers, Type I diabetes and heart Disease. *Nutritional Aspects of Osteoporosis*, 2nd Edition. Burckhardt P, Dawson-Hughes B, Heaney RP, eds. San Diego, CA: Elsevier Inc.;2004:181-201

9. Massey LK, Whiting SJ. Dietary salt, urinary calcium, and bone loss. J Bone Miner Res. 1996; 11:731-736.

10. Suaraz FL, Savaiano D, Arbisi P, Levitt MD. Tolerance to the daily ingestion of two cups of milk by individuals claiming lactose intolerance. *Am J Clin Nutr*. 1997;65:1502-1506.

11. Thys- Jacobs S, Donovan D, Papadopoulos A, Sarrel P. Bilezikian JP. Vitamin D and calcium dysregulation in the polycystic ovarian syndrome. *Steroids*.1999; 64:430-435.

12. Thys-Jacobs S, Starkey P, Bernstein D, Tian J. Calcium carbonate and the premenstrual syndrome: Effects on premenstrual and menstrual symptomatology. *Am J Obstet Gynecol*. 1998;179:444-452.

13. Zemel MB, Thompson W, Milstead A, Morris K, Campbell P. Calcium and dairy acceleration of weight and fat loss during energy restriction in obese adults. *Obesity Res*. 2004;12:582-590.

Updated: Edition 2009

If a synonym, or alternate word with the same meaning, for the term "inadequate" is helpful or needed, an approved alternate is the word "suboptimal."

Excessive Mineral Intake (specify) (NI-5.10.2)

Definition
Higher intake of one or more minerals compared to established reference standards or recommendations based on physiological needs.

Etiology (Cause/Contributing Risk Factors)
Factors gathered during the nutrition assessment process that contribute to the existence or the maintenance of pathophysiological, psychosocial, situational, developmental, cultural, and/or environmental problems:

- Food- and nutrition-related knowledge deficit concerning food and supplemental sources of minerals
- Harmful beliefs/attitudes about food, nutrition, and nutrition-related topics
- Food faddism
- Accidental oversupplementation
- Overconsumption of a limited variety of foods
- Lack of knowledge about management of diagnosed genetic disorder altering mineral homeostasis [hemochromatosis (iron), Wilson's disease (copper)]
- Lack of knowledge about management of diagnosed disease state requiring mineral restriction [cholestatic liver disease (copper and manganese), renal insufficiency (phosphorus, magnesium, potassium)]

Signs/Symptoms (Defining Characteristics)
A typical cluster of subjective and objective signs and symptoms gathered during the nutrition assessment process that provide evidence that a problem exists; quantify the problem and describe its severity.

Nutrition Assessment Category	Potential Indicators of this Nutrition Diagnosis (one or more must be present)
Biochemical Data, Medical Tests and Procedures	Changes in appropriate laboratory values, such as: • ↑ TSH (iodine supplementation) • ↓ HDL (zinc supplementation) • ↑ Serum ferritin and transferrin saturation (iron overload) • Hyperphosphatemia • Hypermagnesemia • Copper deficiency anemia (zinc)
Anthropometric Measurements	

Diagnosis

Intake Domain – Mineral

Excessive Mineral Intake (specify) (NI-5.10.2)

Nutrition-Focused Physical Findings	• Hair and nail changes (selenium) • Anorexia (zinc supplementation) • GI disturbances (iron, magnesium, copper, zinc, selenium)
Food/Nutrition-Related History	Reports or observations of: • Estimated intake of foods or supplements containing high amounts of mineral compared to DRIs
Client History	• Liver damage (copper, iron), enamel or skeletal fluorosis (fluoride)

References

1. Bowman BA, Russell RM, eds. *Present Knowledge in Nutrition.* 8th Ed. Washington, DC: ILSI Press; 2001.
2. National Academy of Sciences, Institute of Medicine. *Dietary Reference Intakes for Vitamin A, Vitamin K, Arsenic, Boron, Chromium, Copper, Iodine, Iron, Manganese, Molybdenum, Nickel, Silicon, Vanadium, Zinc.* Washington, DC: National Academy Press; 2001.
3. National Academy of Sciences, Institute of Medicine. *Dietary Reference Intakes for Calcium, Phosphorus, Magnesium, Vitamin D, and Fluoride.* Washington, DC: National Academy Press; 1997.
4. Position of the American Dietetic Association: Food and nutrition misinformation. *J Am Diet Assoc.* 2006;106:601-607.

Swallowing Difficulty (NC-1.1)

Definition

Impaired or difficult movement of food and liquid within the oral cavity to the stomach

Etiology (Cause/Contributing Risk Factors)

Factors gathered during the nutrition assessment process that contribute to the existence or the maintenance of pathophysiological, psychosocial, situational, developmental, cultural, and/or environmental problems:

- Mechanical causes, e.g., inflammation, surgery, stricture, or oral, pharyngeal and esophageal tumors, mechanical ventilation
- Motor causes, e.g., neurological or muscular disorders, such as cerebral palsy, stroke, multiple sclerosis, scleroderma, or prematurity, altered suck, swallow, breathe patterns

Signs/Symptoms (Defining Characteristics)

A typical cluster of subjective and objective signs and symptoms gathered during the nutrition assessment process that provide evidence that a problem exists; quantify the problem and describe its severity.

Nutrition Assessment Category	Potential Indicators of this Nutrition Diagnosis (one or more must be present)
Biochemical Data, Medical Tests and Procedures	• Radiological findings, e.g., abnormal swallow study
Anthropometric Measurements	
Nutrition-Focused Physical Findings	• Evidence of dehydration, e.g., dry mucous membranes, poor skin turgor • Non-normal findings in cranial nerves and (CN VII) muscles of facial expression, (Nerve IX) gag reflex, swallow (Nerve X) and tongue range of motions (Nerve XII), cough reflex, drooling, facial weakness and ability to perform and wet and dry swallow • Coughing, choking, prolonged chewing, pouching of food, regurgitation, facial expression changes during eating, drooling, noisy wet upper airway sounds, feeling of "food getting stuck," pain while swallowing

Diagnosis

Clinical Domain – Functional

Swallowing Difficulty (NC-1.1)

Food/Nutrition-Related History	Reports or observations of: • Prolonged feeding time • Decreased estimated food intake • Avoidance of foods • Mealtime resistance
Client History	• Conditions associated with a diagnosis or treatment, e.g., dysphagia, achalasia • Repeated upper respiratory infections and or pneumonia

References

1. Braunwald E, Fauci AS, Kasper DL, Hauser SL, Longo DL, Jameson JL, ed. *Harrison's Principles of Internal Medicine*, 15th Edition. New York, NY: McGraw-Hill; 2001.

2. Brody R, Touger-Decker R, O'Sullivan-Maillet J. The effectiveness of dysphagia screening by an RD on the determination of dysphagia risk. *J Am Diet Assoc.* 2000;100:1029-1037.

3. Huhmann M, Touger-Decker R, Byham-Gray L, O'Sullivan-Maillet J, Von Hagen S. Comparison of dysphagia screening by a registered dietitian in acute stroke patients to speech language pathologist's evaluation. *Topics in Clinical Nutrition.* 2004;19:239-249.

4. Groher ME. *Dysphagia Diagnosis and Management*, 3rd ed. Boston: Butterworth-Heinemann 1997.

Updated: 2009 Edition

Biting/Chewing (Masticatory) Difficulty (NC-1.2)

Definition

Impaired ability to bite or chew food in preparation for swallowing.

Etiology (Cause/Contributing Risk Factors)

Factors gathered during the nutrition assessment process that contribute to the existence or the maintenance of pathophysiological, psychosocial, situational, developmental, cultural, and/or environmental problems:

- Craniofacial malformations
- Oral surgery
- Neuromuscular dysfunction
- Partial or complete edentulism
- Soft tissue disease (primary or oral manifestations of a systemic disease)
- Xerostomia

Signs/Symptoms (Defining Characteristics)

A typical cluster of subjective and objective signs and symptoms gathered during the nutrition assessment process that provide evidence that a problem exists; quantify the problem and describe its severity.

Nutrition Assessment Category	Potential Indicators of this Nutrition Diagnosis (one or more must be present)
Biochemical Data, Medical Tests and Procedures	
Anthropometric Measurements	
Nutrition-Focused Physical Findings	• Partial or complete edentulism • Alterations in cranial nerve function (V, VII, IX, X, XII) • Dry mouth • Oral lesions interfering with eating ability • Impaired tongue movement • Ill-fitting dentures or broken dentures

Diagnosis

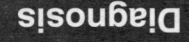

Clinical Domain – Functional

Biting/Chewing (Masticatory) Difficulty (NC-1.2)

Food/Nutrition-Related History	Reports or observations of: • Decreased estimated food intake • Alterations in estimated food intake from usual • Decreased estimated intake or avoidance of food difficult to form into a bolus, e.g., nuts, whole pieces of meat, poultry, fish, fruits, vegetables • Avoidance of foods of age-appropriate texture • Spitting food out or prolonged feeding time
Client History	• Conditions associated with a diagnosis or treatment, e.g., alcoholism; Alzheimer's; head, neck or pharyngeal cancer; cerebral palsy; cleft lip/palate; oral soft tissue infections (e.g., candidiasis, leukoplakia); lack of developmental readiness; oral manifestations of systemic disease (e.g., rheumatoid arthritis, lupus, Crohn's disease, penphigus vulgaris, HIV, diabetes) • Recent major oral surgery • Wired jaw • Chemotherapy with oral side effects • Radiation therapy to oral cavity

References

1. Bailey R, Ledikwe JH, Smiciklas-Wright H, Mitchell DC, Jensen GL. Persistent oral health problems associated with comorbidity and impaired diet quality in older adults. *J Am Diet Assoc.* 2004;104:1273-1276.

2. Chernoff R, ed. Oral health in the elderly. *Geriatric Nutrition.* Gaithersburg, MD: Aspen Publishers; 1999.

3. Dormenval V, Mojon P, Budtz-Jorgensen E. Association between self-assessed masticatory ability, nutritional status and salivary flow rate in hospitalized elderly. *Oral Diseases.* 1999;5:32-38.

4. Hildebrand GH, Dominguez BL, Schork MA, Loesche WJ. Functional units, chewing, swallowing and food avoidance among the elderly. *J Prosthet Dent.* 1997;77:585-595.

5. Hirano H, Ishiyama N, Watanabe I, Nasu I. Masticatory ability in relation to oral status and general health in aging. *J Nutr Health Aging.* 1999;3:48-52.

6. Huhmann M, Touger-Decker R, Byham-Gray L, O'Sullivan-Maillet J, Von Hagen S. Comparison of dysphagia screening by a registered dietitian in acute stroke patients to speech language pathologist's evaluation. *Top Clin Nutr.* 2004;19:239-249.

7. Kademani D, Glick M. Oral ulcerations in individuals infected with human immunodeficiency virus: clinical presentations, diagnosis, management and relevance to disease progression. *Quintessence International.* 1998;29:1103-1108.

8. Keller HH, Ostbye T, Bright-See E. Predictors of dietary intake in Ontario seniors. *Can J Public Health.* 1997;88:303-309.

9. Krall E, Hayes C, Garcia R. How dentition status and masticatory function affect nutrient intake. *J Am Dent Assoc.* 1998;129:1261-1269.

10. Joshipura K, Willett WC, Douglass CW. The impact of edentulousness on food and nutrient intake. *J Am Dent Assoc.* 1996;127:459-467.

11. Mackle T, Touger-Decker R, O'Sullivan Maillet J, Holland, B. Registered Dietitians' use of physical assessment parameters in practice. *J Am Diet Assoc.* 2004;103:1632-1638.

12. Mobley C, Saunders M. Oral health screening guidelines for nondental healthcare providers. *J Am Diet Assoc.* 1997;97:S123-S126.

Biting/Chewing (Masticatory) Difficulty (NC-1.2)

References, cont'd

13. Morse D. Oral and pharyngeal cancer. In: Touger-Decker R, Sirois D, Mobley C (eds). *Nutrition and oral medicine*. Totowa, N.J.: Humana Press; 2005; 205-222.

14. Moynihan P, Butler T, Thomason J, Jepson N. Nutrient intake in partially dentate patients: the effect of prosthetic rehabilitation. *J Dent*. 2000;28:557-563.

15. Position of the American Dietetic Association: Oral health and nutrition. *J Am Diet Assoc*. 2007;107:1418-1428.

16. Sayhoun NR Lin CL, Krall E. Nutritional status of the older adult is associated with dentition status. *J Am Diet Assoc*. 2003;103:61-66.

17. Sheiham A, Steele JG. The impact of oral health on stated ability to eat certain foods; finding from the national diet and nutrition survey of older people in Great Britain. *Gerodontology*. 1999;16:11-20.

18. Ship J, Duffy V, Jones J, Langmore S. Geriatric oral health and its impact on eating. *J Am Geriatr Soc*. 1996;44:456-464.

19. Touger-Decker R. Clinical and laboratory assessment of nutrition status. *Dent Clin North Am*. 2003;47:259-278.

20. Touger-Decker R, Sirois D, Mobley C (eds). *Nutrition and oral medicine*. Totowa, N.J.: Humana Press; 2005.

21. Walls AW, Steele JG, Sheiham A, Marcenes W, Moynihan PJ. Oral health and nutrition in older people. *J Public Health Dent*. 2000;60:304-307.

Updated: 2008 Edition

Diagnosis

Breastfeeding Difficulty (NC-1.3)

Definition

Inability to sustain infant nutrition through breastfeeding.

Etiology (Cause/Contributing Risk Factors)

Factors gathered during the nutrition assessment process that contribute to the existence or the maintenance of pathophysiological, psychosocial, situational, developmental, cultural, and/or environmental problems:

Infant:

- Difficulty latching on, e.g., tight frenulum
- Poor sucking ability
- Oral pain
- Malnutrition/malabsorption
- Lethargy, sleepiness
- Irritability
- Swallowing difficulty

Mother:

- Painful breasts, nipples
- Breast or nipple abnormality
- Mastitis
- Perception of or actual inadequate milk supply
- Lack of social or environmental support
- Cultural practices that affect the ability to breastfeed

Signs/Symptoms (Defining Characteristics)

A typical cluster of subjective and objective signs and symptoms gathered during the nutrition assessment process that provide evidence that a problem exists; quantify the problem and describe its severity.

Nutrition Assessment Category	Potential Indicators of this Nutrition Diagnosis (one or more must be present)
Biochemical Data, Medical Tests and Procedures	• Laboratory evidence of dehydration (infant) • Fewer than six wet diapers in 24 hours (infant)
Anthropometric Measurements	• Any weight loss or poor weight gain (infant)
Nutrition-Focused Physical Findings	• Frenulum abnormality (infant) • Vomiting or diarrhea (infant) • Hunger, lack of satiety after feeding (infant)

Breastfeeding Difficulty (NC-1.3)

Food/Nutrition-Related History	Reports or observations of (infant): • Coughing • Crying, latching on and off, pounding on breasts • Decreased feeding frequency/duration, early cessation of feeding, and/or feeding resistance • Lethargy Reports or observations of (mother): • Small amount of milk when pumping • Lack of confidence in ability to breastfeed • Doesn't hear infant swallowing • Concerns regarding mother's choice to breastfeed/lack of support • Insufficient knowledge of breastfeeding or infant hunger/satiety signals • Lack of facilities or accommodations at place of employment or in community for breastfeeding
Client History	• Conditions associated with a diagnosis or treatment (infant), e.g., cleft lip/palate, thrush, premature birth, malabsorption, infection • Conditions associated with a diagnosis or treatment (mother), e.g., mastitis, candidiasis, engorgement, history of breast surgery

References

1. Barron SP, Lane HW, Hannan TE, Struempler B, Williams JC. Factors influencing duration of breast feeding among low-income women. *J Am Diet Assoc*. 1988;88:1557-1561.

2. Bryant C, Coreil J, D'Angelo SL, Bailey DFC, Lazarov MA. A strategy for promoting breastfeeding among economically disadvantaged women and adolescents. *NAACOGs Clin Issu Perinat Womens Health Nurs*. 1992;3:723-730.

3. Bentley ME, Caulfield LE, Gross SM, Bronner Y, Jensen J, Kessler LA, Paige DM. Sources of influence on intention to breastfeed among African-American women at entry to WIC. *J Hum Lact*. 1999;15:27-34.

4. Moreland JC, Lloyd L, Braun SB, Heins JN. A new teaching model to prolong breastfeeding among Latinos. *J Hum Lact*. 2000;16:337-341.

5. Position of the American Dietetic Association: Promoting and supporting breastfeeding. *J Am Diet Assoc*. 2005;105:1810-818.

6. Wooldrige MS, Fischer C. Colic, "overfeeding" and symptoms of lactose malabsorption in the breast-fed baby. *Lancet*. 1988;2:382-384.

Updated: 2009 Edition

Diagnosis

Clinical Domain – Functional

Altered Gastrointestinal (GI) Function (NC-1.4)

Definition

Changes in ability to digest or absorb nutrients

Etiology (Cause/Contributing Risk Factors)

Factors gathered during the nutrition assessment process that contribute to the existence or the maintenance of pathophysiological, psychosocial, situational, developmental, cultural, and/or environmental problems:

- Alteration in gastrointestinal tract structure and/or function
- Changes in the GI tract motility, e.g., gastroparesis
- Compromised function of related GI organs, e.g., pancreas, liver
- Decreased functional length of the GI tract, e.g., short-bowel syndrome

Signs/Symptoms (Defining Characteristics)

A typical cluster of subjective and objective signs and symptoms gathered during the nutrition assessment process that provide evidence that a problem exists; quantify the problem and describe its severity.

Nutrition Assessment Category	Potential Indicators of this Nutrition Diagnosis (one or more must be present)
Biochemical Data, Medical Tests and Procedures	• Abnormal digestive enzyme and fecal fat studies • Abnormal hydrogen breath test, d-xylose test, stool culture, and gastric emptying and/or small bowel transit time • Endoscopic or colonoscopic examination results, biopsy results
Anthropometric Measurements	
Nutrition-Focused Physical Findings	• Abdominal distension • Increased (or sometimes decreased) bowel sounds • Wasting due to malnutrition in severe cases • Anorexia, nausea, vomiting, diarrhea, steatorrhea, constipation, abdominal pain
Food/Nutrition-Related History	Reports or observations of: • Avoidance or limitation of estimated total intake or intake of specific foods/food groups due to GI symptoms, e.g., bloating, cramping, pain, diarrhea, steatorrhea (greasy, floating, foul-smelling stools) especially following ingestion of food

Altered Gastrointestinal (GI) Function (NC-1.4)

Client History	• Conditions associated with a diagnosis or treatment, e.g., malabsorption, maldigestion, steatorrhea, constipation, diverticulitis, Crohn's disease, inflammatory bowel disease, cystic fibrosis, celiac disease, irritable bowel syndrome, infection
	• Surgical procedures, e.g., esophagectomy, dilatation, gastrectomy, vagotomy, gastric bypass, bowel resections

References

1. Braunwald E, Fauci AS, Kasper DL, Hauser SL, Longo DL, Jameson JL, ed. *Harrison's Principles of Internal Medicine*. 15th Edition. New York, NY: McGraw-Hill; 2001.

Updated: 2009 Edition

Diagnosis

Clinical Domain – Biochemical

Impaired Nutrient Utilization (NC-2.1)

Definition
Changes in ability to absorb or metabolize nutrients and bioactive substances.

Etiology (Cause/Contributing Risk Factors)
Factors gathered during the nutrition assessment process that contribute to the existence or the maintenance of pathophysiological, psychosocial, situational, developmental, cultural, and/or environmental problems:

- Alteration in gastrointestinal tract structure and/or function
- Compromised function of related GI organs, e.g., pancreas, liver
- Decreased functional length of the GI tract
- Metabolic disorders

Signs/Symptoms (Defining Characteristics)
A typical cluster of subjective and objective signs and symptoms gathered during the nutrition assessment process that provide evidence that a problem exists; quantify the problem and describe its severity.

Nutrition Assessment Category	Potential Indicators of this Nutrition Diagnosis (one or more must be present)
Biochemical Data, Medical Tests and Procedures	• Abnormal digestive enzyme and fecal fat studies • Abnormal hydrogen breath test, d-xylose test • Abnormal tests for inborn errors of metabolism • Endoscopic or colonoscopic examination results, biopsy results
Anthropometric Measurements	• Weight loss of ≥ 5% in one month, ≥ 10% in six months • Growth stunting or failure
Nutrition-Focused Physical Findings	• Abdominal distension, bloating, cramping, pain, diarrhea, steatorrhea (greasy, floating, foul-smelling stools) especially following ingestion of food • Increased or decreased bowel sounds • Evidence of vitamin and/or mineral deficiency, e.g., glossitis, cheilosis, mouth lesions

Impaired Nutrient Utilization (NC-2.1)

Food/Nutrition-Related History	Reports or observations of: • Avoidance or limitation of estimated total intake or intake of specific foods/food groups due to GI symptoms,
Client History	• Conditions associated with a diagnosis or treatment, e.g., malabsorption, maldigestion, cystic fibrosis, celiac disease, Crohn's disease, infection, radiation therapy, inborn errors of metabolism • Surgical procedures, e.g., gastric bypass, bowel resection

References

1. Beyer P. Gastrointestinal disorders: Roles of nutrition and the dietetics practitioner. *J Am Diet Assoc*. 1998;98:272-277.
2. Position of the American Dietetic Association: Health implications of dietary fiber. *J Am Diet Assoc*. 2002;102:993-1000.

Diagnosis

Clinical Domain – Biochemical

Altered Nutrition-Related Laboratory Values (specify) (NC-2.2)

Definition
Changes due to body composition, medications, body system changes or genetics, or changes in ability to eliminate byproducts of digestive and metabolic processes.

Etiology (Cause/Contributing Risk Factors)
Factors gathered during the nutrition assessment process that contribute to the existence or the maintenance of pathophysiological, psychosocial, situational, developmental, cultural, and/or environmental problems:

- Kidney, liver, cardiac, endocrine, neurologic, and/or pulmonary dysfunction
- Prematurity
- Other organ dysfunction that leads to biochemical changes

Signs/Symptoms (Defining Characteristics)
A typical cluster of subjective and objective signs and symptoms gathered during the nutrition assessment process that provide evidence that a problem exists; quantify the problem and describe its severity.

Nutrition Assessment Category	Potential Indicators of this Nutrition Diagnosis (one or more must be present)
Biochemical Data, Medical Tests and Procedures	• Increased AST, ALT, T. bili, serum ammonia (liver disorders) • Abnormal BUN, Cr, K, phosphorus, glomerular filtration rate (GFR) (kidney disorders) • Altered pO_2 and pCO_2 (pulmonary disorders) • Abnormal serum lipids • Abnormal plasma glucose and/or HgbA1c levels • Inadequate blood glucose control • Other findings of acute or chronic disorders that are abnormal and of nutritional origin or consequence
Anthropometric Measurements	• Rapid weight changes • Other anthropometric measures that are altered
Nutrition-Focused Physical Findings	• Jaundice, edema, ascites, pruritis (liver disorders) • Edema, shortness of breath (cardiac disorders) • Blue nail beds, clubbing (pulmonary disorders) • Anorexia, nausea, vomiting

Altered Nutrition-Related Laboratory Values (specify) (NC-2.2)

Food/Nutrition-Related History	Reports or observations of:
	• Estimated intake of foods high in or overall excess intake of protein, potassium, phosphorus, sodium, fluid
	• Estimated intake of micronutrients less than recommendations
	• Food- and nutrition-related knowledge deficit, e.g., lack of information, incorrect information, or noncompliance with modified diet
Client History	• Conditions associated with a diagnosis or treatment, e.g., renal or liver disease, alcoholism, cardiopulmonary disorders, diabetes

References

1. Beto JA, Bansal VK. Medical nutrition therapy in chronic kidney failure: integrating clinical practice guidelines. *J Am Diet Assoc*. 2004;104:404-409.

2. Davern II TJ, Scharschmidt BF. Biochemical liver tests. In Feldman M, Scharschmidt BF, Sleisenger MH (eds): *Sleisenger and Fordtran's Gasrointestinal and Liver Disease*, ed 6, vol 2, Philadelphia, PA: WB Saunders; 1998: 1112-1122.

3. Durose CL, Holdsworth M, Watson V, Przygrodzka F. Knowledge of dietary restrictions and the medical consequences of noncompliance by patients on hemodialysis are not predictive of dietary compliance. *J Am Diet Assoc*. 2004;104:35-41.

4. Kassiske BL, Lakatua JD, Ma JZ, Louis TA. A meta-analysis of the effects of dietary protein restriction on the rate of decline in renal function. *Am J Kidney Dis*. 1998;31;954-961.

5. Knight EL, Stampfer MJ, Hankinson SE, Spiegelman D, Curhan GC. The impact of protein intake on renal function decline in women with normal renal function or mild renal insufficiency. *Ann Intern Med*. 2003;138:460-467.

6. Nakao T, Matsumoto, Okada T, Kanazawa Y, Yoshino M, Nagaoka Y, Takeguchi F. Nutritional management of dialysis patients: balancing among nutrient intake, dialysis dose, and nutritional status. *Am J Kidney Dis*. 2003;41:S133-S136.

7. National Kidney Foundation, Inc. Part 5. Evaluation of laboratory measurements for clinical assessment of kidney disease. *Am J Kidney Dis*. 2002;39:S76-S92.

8. National Kidney Foundation, Inc. Guideline 9. Association of level of GFR with nutritional status. *Am J Kidney Dis*. 2002;39:S128-S142.

Updated: 2009 Edition

Diagnosis

Clinical Domain – Biochemical

Food–Medication Interaction (NC-2.3)

Definition
Undesirable/harmful interaction(s) between food and over-the-counter (OTC) medications, prescribed medications, herbals, botanicals, and/or dietary supplements that diminishes, enhances, or alters effect of nutrients and/or medications.

Etiology (Cause/Contributing Risk Factors)
Factors gathered during the nutrition assessment process that contribute to the existence or the maintenance of pathophysiological, psychosocial, situational, developmental, cultural, and/or environmental problems:

- Combined ingestion or administration of medication and food that results in undesirable/harmful interaction

Signs/Symptoms (Defining Characteristics)
A typical cluster of subjective and objective signs and symptoms gathered during the nutrition assessment process that provide evidence that a problem exists; quantify the problem and describe its severity.

Nutrition Assessment Category	Potential Indicators of this Nutrition Diagnosis (one or more must be present)
Biochemical Data, Medical Tests and Procedures	• Alterations of biochemical tests based on medication affect and patient/client condition
Anthropometric Measurements	• Alterations of anthropometric measurements based on medication effect and patient/client conditions, e.g., weight gain and corticosteroids
Nutrition-Focused Physical Findings	• Changes in appetite or taste

Food–Medication Interaction (NC-2.3)

Food/Nutrition-Related History	Reports or observations of:
	• Intake that is problematic or inconsistent with OTC, prescribed drugs, herbals, botanicals, and dietary supplements, such as:
	▪ fish oils and prolonged bleeding
	▪ coumadin, vitamin K–rich foods
	▪ high-fat diet while on cholesterol-lowering medications
	▪ iron supplements, constipation and low-fiber diet
	• Intake that does not support replacement or mitigation of OTC, prescribed drugs, herbals, botanicals, and dietary supplements effects such as potassium-wasting diuretics
	• Multiple drugs (OTC, prescribed drugs, herbals, botanicals, and dietary supplements) that are known to have food–medication interactions
	• Medications that require nutrient supplementation that can not be accomplished via food intake, e.g., isoniazid and vitamin B-6
Client History	

References

1. Position of the American Dietetic Association: Integration of nutrition and pharmacotherapy. *J Am Diet Assoc*. 2003;103:1363-1370.

Diagnosis

Clinical Domain – Weight

Underweight (NC-3.1)

Definition

Low body weight compared to established reference standards or recommendations.

Etiology (Cause/Contributing Risk Factors)

Factors gathered during the nutrition assessment process that contribute to the existence or the maintenance of pathophysiological, psychosocial, situational, developmental, cultural, and/or environmental problems:

- Disordered eating pattern
- Excessive physical activity
- Harmful beliefs/attitudes about food, nutrition, and nutrition-related topics
- Inadequate energy intake
- Increased energy needs
- Lack of or limited access to food
- Small for gestational age, intrauterine growth retardation/restriction and/or lack of progress/appropriate weight gain per day

Signs/Symptoms (Defining Characteristics)

A typical cluster of subjective and objective signs and symptoms gathered during the nutrition assessment process that provide evidence that a problem exists; quantify the problem and describe its severity.

Nutrition Assessment Category	Potential Indicators of this Nutrition Diagnosis (one or more must be present)
Biochemical Data, Medical Tests and Procedures	• Measured resting metabolic rate (RMR) measurement higher than expected and/or estimated RMR

Underweight (NC-3.1)

Anthropometric Measurements	• Decreased skinfold thickness and mid-arm muscle circumference
	• BMI < 18.5 (adults)
	• BMI for older adults (older than 65 years) < 23
	• Birth to 2 years
	  ▪ Weight for age < 5th percentile
	  ▪ Weight for length < 5th percentile (Note: this is for the recumbent length growth chart, which only goes to 36 months. Once a child's height is measured while standing, use the 2-20 year chart for BMI.)
	  ▪ Length for age < 5th percentile
	  ▪ Head circumference < 5th percentile
	• Age 2-20 years
	  ▪ Weight for stature < 5th percentile (Note: this is for standing height, but BMI is probably a better indicator. This is only applicable for children up to 53 inches and requires a different growth chart that is readily available; some WIC programs use it.)
	  ▪ BMI < 5th percentile (for children 2-20)
	  ▪ Weight for age/ Length for age < 5th percentile

Nutrition-Focused Physical Findings	• Decreased muscle mass, muscle wasting (gluteal and temporal) • Hunger
Food/Nutrition-Related History	Reports or observations of: • Estimated intake of food less than estimated or measured needs • Limited supply of food in home • Dieting, food faddism • Refusal to eat • Physical activity more than recommended amount • Medications that affect appetite, e.g., stimulants for ADHD
Client History	• Malnutrition • Illness or physical disability • Mental illness, dementia, confusion • Athlete, dancer, gymnast • Vitamin/mineral deficiency

Diagnosis

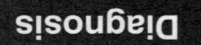

Clinical Domain – Weight

Underweight (NC-3.1)

References

1. Assessment of nutritional status. In: Kleinman R (ed.). *Pediatric Nutrition Handbook*, 5th ed. Elk Grove Village, IL: American Academy of Pediatrics; 2004:407-423.

2. Beck AM, Ovesen LW. At which body mass index and degree of weight loss should hospitalized elderly patients be considered at nutritional risk? *Clin Nutr*. 1998;17:195-198.

3. Blaum CS, Fries BE, Fiatarone MA. Factors associated with low body mass index and weight loss in nursing home residents. *J Gerontol A Biol Sci Med Sci*. 1995;50A:M162-M168.

4. Cook Z, Kirk S, Lawrenson S, Sandford S. Use of BMI in the assessment of undernutrition in older subjects: reflecting on practice. Proceedings of the Nutrition Society. Aug 2005;64:313-317.

5. Position of the American Dietetic Association: Food insecurity and hunger in the United States. *J Am Diet Assoc*. 2006;106:446-458.

6. Position of the American Dietetic Association: Addressing world hunger, malnutrition, and food insecurity. *J Am Diet Assoc*. 2003;103:1046-1057.

7. Position of the American Dietetic Association: Nutrition intervention in the treatment of anorexia nervosa, bulimia nervosa, and eating disorder not otherwise specified (EDNOS). *J Am Diet Assoc*. 2006;106:2073-2082.

8. Ranhoff AH, Gjoen AU, Mowe M. Screening for malnutrition in elderly acute medical patients: the usefulness of MNA-SF. *J Nutr Health Aging*. Jul-Aug 2005;9:221-225.

9. Reynolds MW, Fredman L, Langenberg P, Magaziner J. Weight, weight change, and mortality in a random sample of older community-dwelling women. *J Am Geriatr Soc*. 1999;47:1409-1414.

10. Schneider SM, Al-Jaouni R, Pivot X, Braulio VB, Rampal P, Hebuerne X. Lack of adaptation to severe malnutrition in elderly patients. *Clin Nutr*. 2002;21:499-504.

11. Spear BA. Adolescent growth and development. *J Am Diet Assoc*. 2002 (suppl);102:S23- S29.

12. Sullivan DH, Walls RC. Protein-energy undernutrition and the risk of mortality within six years of hospital discharge. *J Am Coll Nutr*. 1998;17:571-578.

Updated: 2009 Edition

Involuntary Weight Loss (NC-3.2)

Definition

Decrease in body weight that is not planned or desired.

Note: May not be an appropriate nutrition diagnosis when changes in body weight are due to fluid.

Etiology (Cause/Contributing Risk Factors)

Factors gathered during the nutrition assessment process that contribute to the existence or the maintenance of pathophysiological, psychosocial, situational, developmental, cultural, and/or environmental problems:

- Physiological causes increasing nutrient needs due to prolonged catabolic illness, trauma, malabsorption
- Lack of or limited access to food, e.g., economic constraints, restricting food given to elderly and/or children
- Cultural practices that affect ability to access food
- Prolonged hospitalization
- Psychological causes such as depression and disordered eating
- Lack of self-feeding ability

Signs/Symptoms (Defining Characteristics)

A typical cluster of subjective and objective signs and symptoms gathered during the nutrition assessment process that provide evidence that a problem exists; quantify the problem and describe its severity.

Nutrition Assessment Category	Potential Indicators of this Nutrition Diagnosis (one or more must be present)
Biochemical Data, Medical Tests and Procedures	
Anthropometric Measurements	• Weight loss of ≥ 5% within 30 days, ≥ 7.5% in 90 days, or ≥ 10% in 180 days (adults)
Nutrition-Focused Physical Findings	• Fever • Decreased senses, i.e., smell, taste, vision • Increased heart rate • Increased respiratory rate • Loss of subcutaneous fat and muscle stores • Change in way clothes fit • Changes in mental status or function (e.g., depression)

Diagnosis

Clinical Domain – Weight

Involuntary Weight Loss (NC-3.2)

Food/Nutrition-Related History	Reports or observations of: • Normal or usual estimated intake in face of illness • Poor intake, change in eating habits, early satiety, skipped meals • Medications associated with weight loss, such as certain antidepressants
Client History	• Conditions associated with a diagnosis or treatment, e.g., AIDS/HIV, burns, chronic obstructive pulmonary disease, dysphagia, hip/long bone fracture, infection, surgery, trauma, hyperthyroidism (pre- or untreated), some types of cancer or metastatic disease (specify), substance abuse • Cancer chemotherapy

References

1. Collins N. Protein-energy malnutrition and involuntary weight loss: Nutritional and pharmacologic strategies to enhance wound healing. *Expert Opin Pharmacother*. 2003;7:1121-1140.
2. Splett PL, Roth-Yousey LL, Vogelzang JL. Medical nutrition therapy for the prevention and treatment of unintentional weight loss in residential healthcare facilities. *J Am Diet Assoc*. 2003; 103:352-362.
3. Wallace JL, Schwartz RS, LaCroix AZ, Uhlmann RF, Pearlman RA. Involuntary weight loss in older patients: incidence and clinical significance. *J Am Geriatr Soc*. 1995;43:329-337.

Updated: 2009 Edition

Overweight/Obesity (NC-3.3)

Definition
Increased adiposity compared to established reference standards or recommendations, ranging from overweight to morbid obesity.

Etiology (Cause/Contributing Risk Factors)
Factors gathered during the nutrition assessment process that contribute to the existence or the maintenance of pathophysiological, psychosocial, situational, developmental, cultural, and/or environmental problems:

- Decreased energy needs
- Disordered eating pattern
- ✓ Excess energy intake
- ✓ Food- and nutrition-related knowledge deficit
- ✓ Not ready for diet/lifestyle change
- ✓ Physical inactivity
- Increased psychological/life stress

Signs/Symptoms (Defining Characteristics)
A typical cluster of subjective and objective signs and symptoms gathered during the nutrition assessment process that provide evidence that a problem exists; quantify the problem and describe its severity.

Nutrition Assessment Category	Potential Indicators of this Nutrition Diagnosis (one or more must be present)
Biochemical Data, Medical Tests and Procedures	• Measured resting metabolic rate (RMR) less than expected and/or estimated RMR

Anthropometric Measurements	• BMI more than normative standard for age and sex
	  • Overweight 25-29.9
	  • Obesity-grade I 30-34.9
	  • Obesity-grade II 35-39.9
	  • Obesity-grade III 40+
	• Inability to maintain weight or regain of weight
	• Waist circumference more than normative standard for age and sex
	• Increased skinfold thickness
	• Weight for height more than normative standard for age and sex

Nutrition-Focused Physical Findings	• Increased body adiposity

Diagnosis

Clinical Domain – Weight

Overweight/Obesity (NC-3.3)

Food/Nutrition-Related History	Reports or observations of: • Overconsumption of high-fat and/or calorie-density food or beverage • Large portions of food (portion size more than twice than recommended) • Estimated excessive energy intake • Infrequent, low-duration and/or low-intensity physical activity • Large amounts of sedentary activities, e.g., TV watching, reading, computer use in both leisure and work/school • Uncertainty regarding nutrition-related recommendations • Inability to apply nutrition-related recommendations • Unwillingness or disinterest in applying nutrition-related recommendations • Inability to lose a significant amount of excess weight through conventional weight loss intervention • Medications that impact RMR, e.g., midazolam, propranalol, glipizide
Client History	• Conditions associated with a diagnosis or treatment, e.g., hypothyroidism, metabolic syndrome, eating disorder not otherwise specified, depression • Physical disability or limitation • History of familial obesity • History of childhood obesity • History of physical, sexual, or emotional abuse

References

1. Crawford S. Promoting dietary change. *Can J Cardiol*. 1995;11(suppl A):14A-15A.
2. Dickerson RN, Roth-Yousey L. Medication effects on metabolic rate: A systematic review. *J Am Diet Assoc*. 2005;105:835-843.
3. Kumanyika SK, Van Horn L, Bowen D, Perri MG, Rolls BJ, Czajkowski SM, Schron E. Maintenance of dietary behavior change. *Health Psychol*. 2000;19(1 suppl):S42-S56.
4. NHLBI Clinical Guidelines on the Identification, Evaluation, and Treatment of Overweight and Obesity in Adults—Executive Summary. Available at: http://www.nhlbi.nih.gov/guidelines/obesity/ob_tbl2.htm. Accessed January 29, 2007.
5. Position of the American Dietetic Association: Weight management. *J Am Diet Assoc*. 2002;102:1145-1155.
6. Position of the American Dietetic Association: Total diet approach to communicating food and nutrition information. *J Am Diet Assoc*. 2007;107:1224-1232.
7. Position of the American Dietetic Association: The role of dietetics professionals in health promotion and disease prevention. *J Am Diet Assoc*. 2006;106:1875-1884.
8. Position of the American Dietetic Association: Nutrition intervention in the treatment of anorexia nervosa, bulimia nervosa, and eating disorder not otherwise specified (EDNOS). *J Am Diet Assoc*. 2006;106:2073-2082.
9. Shepherd R. Resistance to changes in diet. *Proc Nutr So*c. 2002;61:267-272.
10. U.S. Preventive Services Task Force. Behavioral counseling in primary care to promote a healthy diet. *Am J Prev Med*. 2003;24:93-100.

Updated: 2008 Edition

Involuntary Weight Gain (NC-3.4)

Definition
Weight gain more than that which is desired or planned.

Etiology (Cause/Contributing Risk Factors)
Factors gathered during the nutrition assessment process that contribute to the existence or the maintenance of pathophysiological, psychosocial, situational, developmental, cultural, and/or environmental problems:

- Illness causing unexpected weight gain because of head trauma, immobility, paralysis or related condition
- Chronic use of medications known to cause weight gain, such as use of certain antidepressants, antipsychotics, corticosteroids, certain HIV medications
- Condition leading to excessive fluid weight gains

Signs/Symptoms (Defining Characteristics)
A typical cluster of subjective and objective signs and symptoms gathered during the nutrition assessment process that provide evidence that a problem exists; quantify the problem and describe its severity.

Nutrition Assessment Category	Potential Indicators of this Nutrition Diagnosis (one or more must be present)
Biochemical Data, Medical Tests and Procedures	• Decrease in serum albumin, hyponatremia, elevated fasting serum lipid levels, elevated fasting glucose levels, fluctuating hormone levels
Anthropometric Measurements	• Increased weight, any increase in weight more than planned or desired, such as grams/day or > 10% in 6 months
Nutrition-Focused Physical Findings	• Fat accumulation, excessive subcutaneous fat stores, noticeable change in body fat distribution • Extreme hunger with or without palpitations, tremor, and sweating • Lipodystrophy associated with HIV diagnosis: increase in dorsocervial fat, breast enlargement, increased abdominal girth • Edema • Shortness of breath • Muscle weakness • Fatigue

Diagnosis

Clinical Domain – Weight

Involuntary Weight Gain (NC-3.4)

Food/Nutrition-Related History	Reports or observations of: • Estimated intake inconsistent with estimated or measured energy needs • Changes in recent estimated food intake level • Fluid administration more than requirements • Use of alcohol, narcotics • Medications associated with increased appetite • Physical inactivity or change in physical activity level
Client History	• Conditions associated with a diagnosis or treatment of asthma, psychiatric illnesses, rheumatic conditions, HIV/AIDS, Cushing's syndrome, obesity, Prader-Willi syndrome, hypothyroidism

References

1. Lichtenstein K, Delaney K, Ward D, Palella F. Clinical factors associated with incidence and prevalence of fat atrophy and accumulation (abstract P64). *Antivir Ther*. 2000;5:61-62

2. Heath KV, Hogg RS, Chan KJ, Harris M, Montessori V, O'Shaughnessy MV, Montaner JS. Lipodystrophy-associated morphological, cholesterol and triglyceride abnormalities in a population-based HIV/AIDS treatment database. *AIDS*. 2001;15:231-239.

3. Safri S, Grunfeld C. Fat distribution and metabolic changes in patients with HIV infection. *AIDS*. 1999;13:2493-2505.

4. Sattler F. Body habitus changes related to lipodystrophy. *Clin Infect Dis*. 2003;36:S84-S90.

Updated: 2009 Edition

Food- and Nutrition-Related Knowledge Deficit (NB-1.1)

Definition

Incomplete or inaccurate knowledge about food, nutrition, or nutrition-related information and guidelines, e.g., nutrient requirements, consequences of food behaviors, life stage requirements, nutrition recommendations, diseases and conditions, physiological function, or products.

Etiology (Cause/Contributing Risk Factors)

Factors gathered during the nutrition assessment process that contribute to the existence or the maintenance of pathophysiological, psychosocial, situational, developmental, cultural, and/or environmental problems:

- Harmful beliefs/attitudes about food, nutrition, and nutrition-related topics
- Lack of prior exposure to accurate nutrition-related information
- Lack of understanding of infant/child cues to indicate hunger
- Cultural beliefs that affect ability to learn/apply information
- Impaired cognitive ability, including learning disabilities, neurological or sensory impairment, and/or dementia
- Prior exposure to incorrect information
- Unwilling or disinterested in learning/applying information

Signs/Symptoms (Defining Characteristics)

A typical cluster of subjective and objective signs and symptoms gathered during the nutrition assessment process that provide evidence that a problem exists; quantify the problem and describe its severity.

Nutrition Assessment Category	Potential Indicators of this Nutrition Diagnosis (one or more must be present)
Biochemical Data, Medical Tests and Procedures	
Anthropometric Measurements	
Nutrition-Focused Physical Findings	

Diagnosis

Behavioral-Environmental Domain – Knowledge and Beliefs

Food- and Nutrition-Related Knowledge Deficit (NB-1.1)

Food/Nutrition-Related History	Reports or observations of: • Verbalizes inaccurate or incomplete information • Provides inaccurate or incomplete written response to questionnaire/written tool or is unable to read written tool • No prior knowledge of need for food- and nutrition-related recommendations • Demonstrates inability to apply food- and nutrition-related information, e.g., select food based on nutrition therapy or prepare infant feeding as instructed • Relates concerns about previous attempts to learn information • Verbalizes unwillingness or disinterest in learning information
Client History	• Conditions associated with a diagnosis or treatment, e.g., mental illness • New medical diagnosis or change in existing diagnosis or condition

References

1. Crawford S. Promoting dietary change. *Can J Cardiol*. 1995;11(suppl A):14A-15A.
2. Kumanyika SK, Van Horn L, Bowen D, Perri MG, Rolls BJ, Czajkowski SM, Schron E. Maintenance of dietary behavior change. *Health Psychol*. 2000;19(1 suppl):S42-S56.
3. Position of the American Dietetic Association: Weight management. *J Am Diet Assoc*. 2002;102:1145-1155.
4. Position of the American Dietetic Association: Total diet approach to communicating food and nutrition information. *J Am Diet Assoc* 2007;107:1224-1232.
5. Position of the American Dietetic Association: The role of dietetics professionals in health promotion and disease prevention. *J Am Diet Assoc*. 2006;106:1875-1884.
6. Shepherd R. Resistance to changes in diet. *Proc Nutr Soc*. 2002;61:267-272.
7. U.S. Preventive Services Task Force. Behavioral counseling in primary care to promote a healthy diet. *Am J Prev Med*. 2003;24:93-100.

Harmful Beliefs/Attitudes About Food or Nutrition-Related Topics (NB-1.2)

Use with caution: Be sensitive to patient concerns.

Definition

Beliefs/attitudes or practices about food, nutrition, and nutrition-related topics that are incompatible with sound nutrition principles, nutrition care, or disease/condition (excluding disordered eating patterns and eating disorders).

Etiology (Cause/Contributing Risk Factors)

Factors gathered during the nutrition assessment process that contribute to the existence or the maintenance of pathophysiological, psychosocial, situational, developmental, cultural, and/or environmental problems:

- Disbelief in science-based food and nutrition information
- Lack of prior exposure to accurate nutrition-related information
- Eating behavior serves a purpose other than nourishment (e.g., pica)
- Desire for a cure for a chronic disease through the use of alternative therapy

Signs/Symptoms (Defining Characteristics)

A typical cluster of subjective and objective signs and symptoms gathered during the nutrition assessment process that provide evidence that a problem exists; quantify the problem and describe its severity.

Nutrition Assessment Category	Potential Indicators of this Nutrition Diagnosis (one or more must be present)
Biochemical Data, Medical Tests and Procedures	
Anthropometric Measurements	
Nutrition-Focused Physical Findings	

Diagnosis

Behavioral-Environmental Domain – Knowledge and Beliefs

Harmful Beliefs/Attitudes About Food or Nutrition-Related Topics (NB-1.2)

Food/Nutrition-Related History	Reports or observations of: • Food faddism • Estimated intake that reflects an imbalance of nutrients/food groups • Avoidance of foods/food groups (e.g., sugar, wheat, cooked foods)
Client History	• Conditions associated with a diagnosis or treatment, e.g., obesity, diabetes, cancer, cardiovascular disease, mental illness • Pica • Food fetish

References

1. Chapman GE, Beagan B. Women's perspectives on nutrition, health, and breast cancer. *J Nutr Educ Behav*. 2003;35:135-141.
2. Gonzalez VM, Vitousek KM. Feared food in dieting and non-dieting young women: a preliminary validation of the Food Phobia Survey. *Appetite*. 2004;43:155-173.
3. Jowett SL, Seal CJ, Phillips E, Gregory W, Barton JR, Welfare MR. Dietary beliefs of people with ulcerative colitis and their effect on relapse and nutrient intake. *Clin Nutr*. 2004;23:161-170.
4. Madden H, Chamberlain K. Nutritional health messages in women's magazines: a conflicted space for women readers. *J Health Psychol*. 2004;9:583-597.
5. Peters CL, Shelton J, Sharma P. An investigation of factors that influence the consumption of dietary supplements. *Health Mark Q*. 2003;21:113-135.
6. Position of the American Dietetic Association: Food and nutrition misinformation. *J Am Diet Assoc*. 2006;106:601-607.
7. Povey R, Wellens B, Conner M. Attitudes towards following meat, vegetarian and vegan diets: an examination of the role of ambivalence. *Appetite*. 2001;37:15-26.
8. Putterman E, Linden W. Appearance versus health: does the reason for dieting affect dieting behavior? *J Behav Med*. 2004;27:185-204.
9. Salminen E, Heikkila S, Poussa T, Lagstrom H, Saario R, Salminen S. Female patients tend to alter their diet following the diagnosis of rheumatoid arthritis and breast cancer. *Prev Med*. 2002;34:529-535.

Not Ready for Diet/Lifestyle Change (NB-1.3)

Definition

Lack of perceived value of nutrition-related behavior change compared to costs (consequences or effort required to make changes); conflict with personal value system; antecedent to behavior change.

Etiology (Cause/Contributing Risk Factors)

Factors gathered during the nutrition assessment process that contribute to the existence or the maintenance of pathophysiological, psychosocial, situational, developmental, cultural, and/or environmental problems:

- Harmful beliefs/attitudes about food, nutrition, and nutrition-related topics
- Impaired cognitive ability, including learning disabilities, neurological or sensory impairment, and/or dementia
- Lack of social support for implementing changes
- Denial of need to change
- Perception that time, interpersonal, or financial constraints prevent changes
- Unwilling or disinterested in learning/applying information
- Lack of self-efficacy for making change or demoralization from previous failures at change

Signs/Symptoms (Defining Characteristics)

A typical cluster of subjective and objective signs and symptoms gathered during the nutrition assessment process that provide evidence that a problem exists; quantify the problem and describe its severity.

Nutrition Assessment Category	Potential Indicators of this Nutrition Diagnosis (one or more must be present)
Biochemical Data, Medical Tests and Procedures	
Anthropometric Measurements	
Nutrition-Focused Physical Findings	• Negative body language, e.g., frowning, lack of eye contact, defensive posture, lack of focus, fidgeting (Note: Body language varies by culture.)

Diagnosis

Behavioral-Environmental Domain – Knowledge and Beliefs

Not Ready for Diet/Lifestyle Change (NB-1.3)

Food/Nutrition-Related History	Reports or observations of:
	• Denial of need for food- and nutrition-related changes
	• Inability to understand required changes
	• Failure to keep appointments/schedule follow-up appointments or engage in counseling
	• Previous failures to effectively change target behavior
	• Defensiveness, hostility or resistance to change
	• Lack of efficacy to make change or to overcome barriers to change
Client History	

References

1. Crawford S. Promoting dietary change. *Can J Cardiol*. 1995;11:14A-15A.
2. Greene GW, Rossi SR, Rossi JS, Velicer WF, Fava JS, Prochaska JO. Dietary applications of the Stages of Change Model. *J Am Diet Assoc*. 1999; 99:673-678.
3. Kumanyika SK, Van Horn L, Bowen D, Perri MG, Rolls BJ, Czajkowski SM, Schron E. Maintenance of dietary behavior change. *Health Psychol*. 2000;19:S42-S56.
4. Prochaska JO, Velicer W F. The Transtheoretical Model of behavior change. *Am J Health Promotion*. 1997;12:38–48.
5. Position of the American Dietetic Association: Total diet approach to communicating food and nutrition information. *J Am Diet Assoc*. 2007;107:1224-1232.
6. Position of the American Dietetic Association: The role of dietetics professionals in health promotion and disease prevention. *J Am Diet Assoc*. 2006;106:1875-1884.
7. Resnicow K, Jackson A, Wang T, De A, McCarty F, Dudley W, Baronowski T. A motivational interviewing intervention to increase fruit and vegetable intake through black churches: Results of the Eat for Life trial. *Am J Public Health*. 2001; 91:1686-1693.
8. Shepherd R. Resistance to changes in diet. *Proc Nutr Soc*. 2002;61:267-272.
9. U.S. Preventive Services Task Force. Behavioral counseling in primary care to promote a healthy diet. *Am J Prev Med*. 2003;24:93-100.

Updated: 2008 Edition

Self-Monitoring Deficit (NB-1.4)

Definition

Lack of data recording to track personal progress.

Etiology (Cause/Contributing Risk Factors)

Factors gathered during the nutrition assessment process that contribute to the existence or the maintenance of pathophysiological, psychosocial, situational, developmental, cultural, and/or environmental problems:

- Food- and nutrition-related knowledge deficit concerning self-monitoring
- Lack of social support for implementing changes
- Lack of value for behavior change or competing values
- Perception that lack of resources (e.g., time, financial, or interpersonal) prevent self-monitoring
- Cultural practices that affect the ability to track personal progress
- Impaired cognitive ability, including learning disabilities, neurological or sensory impairment, and/or dementia
- Prior exposure to incompatible information
- Not ready for diet/lifestyle change
- Unwilling or disinterested in tracking progress
- Lack of focus and attention to detail, difficulty with time management and/or organization

Signs/Symptoms (Defining Characteristics)

A typical cluster of subjective and objective signs and symptoms gathered during the nutrition assessment process that provide evidence that a problem exists; quantify the problem and describe its severity.

Nutrition Assessment Category	Potential Indicators of this Nutrition Diagnosis (one or more must be present)
Biochemical Data, Medical Tests and Procedures	• Recorded data inconsistent with biochemical data, e.g., estimated dietary intake is not consistent with biochemical data
Anthropometric Measurements	
Nutrition-Focused Physical Findings	

Diagnosis

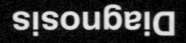

Behavioral-Environmental Domain – Knowledge and Beliefs

Self-Monitoring Deficit (NB-1.4)

Food/Nutrition-Related History	Reports or observations of:
	• Incomplete self-monitoring records, e.g., glucose, food, fluid intake, weight, physical activity, ostomy output records
	• Estimated food intake data inconsistent with weight status or growth pattern data
	• Embarrassment or anger regarding need for self-monitoring
	• Uncertainty of how to complete monitoring records
	• Uncertainty regarding changes that could/should be made in response to data in self-monitoring records
	• No self-management equipment, e.g., no blood glucose monitor, pedometer
Client History	• Diagnoses associated with self-monitoring, e.g., diabetes mellitus, obesity, new ostomy
	• New medical diagnosis or change in existing diagnosis or condition

References

1. American Diabetes Association. Tests of glycemia in diabetes. *Diabetes Care*. 2004;27:S91-S93.
2. Baker RC, Kirschenbaum DS. Weight control during the holidays: highly consistent self-monitoring as a potentially useful coping mechanism. *Health Psychol*. 1998;17:367-370.
3. Berkowitz RI, Wadden TA, Tershakovec AM. Behavior therapy and sibutramine for treatment of adolescent obesity. *JAMA*. 2003;289:1805-1812.
4. Crawford S. Promoting dietary change. *Can J Cardiol*. 1995;11(suppl A):14A-15A.
5. Jeffery R, Drewnowski A, Epstein L, Stunkard A, Wilson G, Wing R. Long-term maintenance of weight loss: current status. *Health Psychol*. 2000;19:5-16.
6. Kumanyika SK, Van Horn L, Bowen D, Perri MG, Rolls BJ, Czajkowski SM, Schron E. Maintenance of dietary behavior change. *Health Psychol*. 2000;19(1 suppl):S42-S56.
7. Lichtman SW, Pisarska K, Berman ER, Pestone M, Dowling H, Offenbacher E, Weisel H, Heshka S, Matthews DE, Heymsfield SB. Discrepancy between self-reported and actual caloric intake and exercise in obese subjects. *N Engl J Med*. 1992;327:1893-1898.
8. Wadden, TA. Characteristics of successful weight loss maintainers. In: Allison DB, Pi-Sunyer FX, eds. *Obesity Treatment: Establishing Goals, Improving Outcomes, and Reviewing the Research Agenda*. New York: Plenum Press; 1995:103-111.

Disordered Eating Pattern (NB-1.5)

Definition

Beliefs, attitudes, thoughts, and behaviors related to food, eating, and weight management, including classic eating disorders as well as less severe, similar conditions that negatively impact health.

Etiology (Cause/Contributing Risk Factors)

Factors gathered during the nutrition assessment process that contribute to the existence or the maintenance of pathophysiological, psychosocial, situational, developmental, cultural, and/or environmental problems:

- Familial, societal, biological/genetic, and/or environmental related obsessive desire to be thin
- Weight regulation/preoccupation significantly influences self-esteem

Signs/Symptoms (Defining Characteristics)

A typical cluster of subjective and objective signs and symptoms gathered during the nutrition assessment process that provide evidence that a problem exists; quantify the problem and describe its severity.

Nutrition Assessment Category	Potential Indicators of this Nutrition Diagnosis (one or more must be present)
Biochemical Data, Medical Tests and Procedures	• Decreased cholesterol, abnormal lipid profiles, hypoglycemia, hypokalemia [anorexia nervosa (AN)] • Hypokalemia and hypochloremic alkalosis [bulimia nervosa (BN)] • Hyponatremia, hypothyroid, elevated BUN (AN) • Urine positive for ketones (AN)
Anthropometric Measurements	• BMI < 17.5, arrested growth and development, failure to gain weight during period of expected growth, weight less than 85% of expected (AN) • BMI > 29 [eating disorder not otherwise specified (EDNOS)] • Significant weight fluctuation (BN)
Nutrition-Focused Physical Findings	• Severely depleted adipose and somatic protein stores (AN) • Lanugo hair formation on face and trunk, brittle listless hair, cyanosis of hands and feet, and dry skin (AN) • Normal or excess adipose and normal somatic protein stores (BN, EDNOS) • Damaged tooth enamel (BN) • Enlarged parotid glands (BN)

Diagnosis

Behavioral-Environmental Domain – Knowledge and Beliefs

Disordered Eating Pattern (NB-1.5)

Nutrition-Focused Physical Findings, cont'd	• Peripheral edema (BN)
	• Skeletal muscle loss (AN)
	• Low body temperature
	• Inability to concentrate (AN)
	• Positive Russell's Sign (BN) callous on back of hand from self-induced vomiting
	• Bradycardia (heart rate < 60 beats/min), hypotension (systolic < 90 mm HG), and orthostatic hypotension (AN)
	• Self-induced vomiting, diarrhea, bloating, constipation, and flatulence (BN); always cold (AN)
	• Muscle weakness, fatigue, dehydration (AN, BN)
	• Denial of hunger (AN)
Food/Nutrition-Related History	Reports or observations of:
	• Avoidance of food or calorie-containing beverages (AN, BN)
	• Avoidance of social events at which food is served
	• Fear of foods or dysfunctional thoughts regarding food or food experiences (AN, BN)
	• Food and weight preoccupation (AN, BN)
	• Knowledgeable about current diet fad (AN, BN, EDNOS)
	• Fasting (AN, BN)
	• Estimated intake of larger quantity of food in a defined time period, a sense of lack of control over eating (BN, EDNOS)
	• Excessive physical activity (AN, BN, EDNOS)
	• Eating much more rapidly than normal, until feeling uncomfortably full, consuming large amounts of food when not feeling physically hungry; eating alone because of embarrassment, feeling very guilty after overeating (EDNOS)
	• Eats in private (AN, BN)
	• Irrational thoughts about food's affect on the body (AN, BN, EDNOS)
	• Pattern of chronic dieting
	• Excessive reliance on nutrition terming and preoccupation with nutrient content of foods
	• Inflexibility with food selection
	• Misuse of laxatives, enemas, diuretics, stimulants, and/or metabolic enhancers (AN,BN)

Disordered Eating Pattern (NB-1.5)

Client History	
	• Diagnosis, e.g., anorexia nervosa, bulimia nervosa, binge eating, eating disorder not otherwise specified, amenorrhea
	• History of mood and anxiety disorders (e.g., depression, obsessive/compulsive disorder [OCD]), personality disorders, substance abuse disorders
	• Family history of ED, depression, OCD, anxiety disorders (AN, BN)
	• Irritability, depression (AN, BN)
	• Anemia
	• Leukopenia
	• Cardiac arrhythmias, bradycardia (AN, BN)

References

1. Anderson GH, Kennedy SH, eds. *The Biology of Feast and Famine*. New York: Academic Press; 1992.

2. American Psychiatric Association. *Diagnostic and statistical manual for mental disorders (fourth edition, text revision)*. APA Press: Washington DC; 2000.

3. American Psychiatric Association. Practice guidelines for the treatment of patients with eating disorders. *Am J Psychiatry*. 2000;157 (suppl):1-39.

4. Cooke RA, Chambers JB. Anorexia nervosa and the heart. *Br J Hosp Med*. 1995;54:313-317.

5. Fisher M. Medical complications of anorexia and bulimia nervosa. *Adol Med Stat of the Art Reviews*. 1992;3:481-502.

6. Gralen SJ, Levin MP, Smolak L, Murnen SK. Dieting and disordered eating during early and middle adolescents: Do the influences remain the same? *Int J Eating Disorder*. 1990;9:501-512.

7. Harris JP, Kriepe RE, Rossback CN. QT prolongation by isoproterenol in anorexia nervosa. *J Adol Health*. 1993;14:390-393.

8. Kaplan AS, Garfunkel PE, eds. *Medical Issues and the Eating Disorders: The Interface*. New York: Brunner/Manzel Publishers; 1993.

9. Keys A, Brozek J, Henschel A, Mickelson O, Taylor HL. *The Biology of Human Starvation*, 2nd vol. Minneapolis, MN: University of Minnesota Press; 1950.

10. Kirkley BG. Bulimia: clinical characteristics, development, and Etiology. *J Am Diet Assoc*. 1986;86:468-475.

11. Kreipe RE, Uphoff M. Treatment and outcome of adolescents with anorexia nervosa. *Adolesc Med*.1992;16:519-540.

12. Kreipe RE, Birndorf DO. Eating disorders in adolescents and young adults. *Medical Clinics of North America*. 2000;84:1027-1049.

13. Mordasini R, Klose G, Greter H. Secondary type II hyperlipoproteinemia in patients with anorexia nervosa. *Metabolism*. 1978;27:71-79.

14. Position of the American Dietetic Association: Nutrition intervention in the treatment of anorexia nervosa, bulimia nervosa, and eating disorder not otherwise specified (EDNOS). *J Am Diet Assoc*. 2006;106:2073-2082.

15. Rock C, Yager J. Nutrition and eating disorders: a primer for clinicians. *Int J Eat Disord*. 1987;6:267-280.

16. Rock, CL. Nutritional and medical assessment and management of eating disorders. *Nutr Clin Care*. 1999;2:332-343.

17. Schebendach J, Reichert-Anderson P. Nutrition in Eating Disorders. In: *Krause's Nutrition and Diet Therapy*. Mahan K, Escott-Stump S (eds). McGraw- Hill: New York, NY; 2000.

18. Silber T. Anorexia nervosa: Morbidity and mortality. Pediar Ann. 1984; 13:851-859.

19. Swenne I. Heart risk associated with weight loss in anorexia nervosa and eating disorders: electrocardiographic changes during the early phase of refeeding. *Acta Paediatr*. 2000;89:447-452.

20. Turner JM, Bulsara MK, McDermott BM, Byrne GC, Prince RL, Forbes DA. Predictors of low bone density in young adolescent females with anorexia nervosa and other dieting disorders. *Int J Eat Disord*. 2001;30:245-251.

Diagnosis

Behavioral-Environmental Domain – Knowledge and Beliefs

Limited Adherence to Nutrition-Related Recommendations (NB-1.6)

Definition
Lack of nutrition-related changes as per intervention agreed on by client or population.

Etiology (Cause/Contributing Risk Factors)
Factors gathered during the nutrition assessment process that contribute to the existence or the maintenance of pathophysiological, psychosocial, situational, developmental, cultural, and/or environmental problems:

- Lack of social support for implementing changes
- Lack of value for behavior change or competing values
- Perception that lack of resources (e.g., time, financial, or interpersonal) prevent changes
- Previous lack of success in making health-related changes
- Food and nutrition-related knowledge deficit concerning how to make nutrition-related changes
- Unwilling or disinterested in applying/learning information

Signs/Symptoms (Defining Characteristics)
A typical cluster of subjective and objective signs and symptoms gathered during the nutrition assessment process that provide evidence that a problem exists; quantify the problem and describe its severity.

Nutrition Assessment Category	Potential Indicators of this Nutrition Diagnosis (one or more must be present)
Biochemical Data, Medical Tests and Procedures	• Expected laboratory outcomes are not achieved
Anthropometric Measurements	• Expected anthropometric outcomes are not achieved
Nutrition-Focused Physical Findings	• Negative body language, e.g., frowning, lack of eye contact, fidgeting (Note: body language varies by culture)

Limited Adherence to Nutrition-Related Recommendations (NB-1.6)

Food/Nutrition-Related History	Reports or observations of:
	• Expected food/nutrition-related outcomes are not achieved
	• Inability to recall agreed on changes
	• Failure to complete any agreed on homework
	• Lack of compliance or inconsistent compliance with plan
	• Failure to keep appointments or schedule follow-up appointments
	• Lack of appreciation of the importance of making recommended nutrition-related changes
	• Uncertainty as to how to consistently apply food/nutrition information
Client History	

References

1. Crawford S. Promoting dietary change. *Can J Cardiol*. 1995;11(suppl A):14A-15A.

2. Kumanyika SK, Van Horn L, Bowen D, Perri MG, Rolls BJ, Czajkowski SM, Schron E. Maintenance of dietary behavior change. *Health Psychol*. 2000;19(1 suppl):S42-S56.

3. Position of the American Dietetic Association: Total diet approach to communicating food and nutrition information. *J Am Diet Assoc*. 2007;107:1224-1232.

4. Shepherd R. Resistance to changes in diet. *Proc Nutr Soc*. 2002;61:267-272.

5. U.S. Preventive Services Task Force. Behavioral counseling in primary care to promote a healthy diet. *Am J Prev Med*. 2003;24:93-100.

Diagnosis

Undesirable Food Choices (NB-1.7)

Definition

Food and/or beverage choices that are inconsistent with Dietary Reference Intakes (DRIs), US Dietary Guidelines, or MyPyramid, or with targets defined in the nutrition prescription or Nutrition Care Process.

Etiology (Cause/Contributing Risk Factors)

Factors gathered during the nutrition assessment process that contribute to the existence or the maintenance of pathophysiological, psychosocial, situational, developmental, cultural, and/or environmental problems:

- Lack of prior exposure to accurate nutrition-related information
- Cultural practices that affect the ability to learn/apply information
- Impaired cognitive ability, including learning disabilities, neurological or sensory impairment, and/or dementia
- High level of fatigue or other side effect of medical, surgical or radiological therapy
- Lack of or limited access to recommended foods
- Perception that lack of resources (e.g., time, financial, or interpersonal) prevent selection of food choices consistent with recommendations
- Food allergies and aversions impeding food choices consistent with guidelines
- Lacks motivation and or readiness to apply or support systems change
- Unwilling or disinterested in learning/applying information
- Psychological causes such as depression and disordered eating

Signs/Symptoms (Defining Characteristics)

A typical cluster of subjective and objective signs and symptoms gathered during the nutrition assessment process that provide evidence that a problem exists; quantify the problem and describe its severity.

Nutrition Assessment Category	Potential Indicators of this Nutrition Diagnosis (one or more must be present)
Biochemical Data, Medical Tests and Procedures	• Elevated lipid panel
Anthropometric Measurements	
Nutrition-Focused Physical Findings	• Findings consistent with vitamin/mineral deficiency or excess

Undesirable Food Choices (NB-1.7)

Food/Nutrition-Related History	Reports or observations of:
	• Estimated intake inconsistent with DRIs, US Dietary Guidelines, MyPyramid, or other methods of measuring diet quality, such as, the Healthy Eating Index (e.g., omission of entire nutrient groups, disproportionate intake [e.g., juice for young children])
	• Inaccurate or incomplete understanding of the guidelines
	• Inability to apply guideline information
	• Inability to select (e.g., access), or unwillingness, or disinterest in selecting, food consistent with the guidelines
Client History	• Conditions associated with a diagnosis or treatment, e.g., mental illness

References

1. Birch LL, Fisher JA. Appetite and eating behavior in children. *Pediatr Clin North Am*.1995;42:931-953.
2. Butte N, Cobb K, Dwyer J, Graney L, Heird W, Richard K. The start healthy feeding guidelines for infants and toddlers. *J Am Diet Assoc*. 2004:104:3:442-454.
3. Position of the American Dietetic Association: Weight management. *J Am Diet Assoc*. 2002;102:1145-1155.
4. Dolecek TA, Stamlee J, Caggiula AW, Tillotson JL, Buzzard IM. Methods of dietary and nutritional assessment and intervention and other methods in the multiple risk factor intervention trial. *Am J Clin Nutr*. 1997;65(suppl):196S-210S.
5. Epstein LH, Gordy CC, Raynor HA, Beddome M, Kilanowski CK, Paluch R. Increasing fruit and vegetable intake and decreasing fat and sugar intake in families at risk for childhood obesity. *Obesity Res*. 2001;9:171-178.
6. Freeland-Graves J, Nitzke S. Total diet approach to communicating food and nutrition information. *J Am Diet Assoc*. 2002;102:100-108.
7. French SA. Pricing effects on food choices. *J Nutr*. 2003;133:S841-S843.
8. Glens K, Basil M, Mariachi E, Goldberg J, Snyder D. Why Americans eat what they do: taste, nutrition, cost, convenience and weight control concerns as influences on food consumption. *J Am Diet Assoc*. 1998;98:1118-1126.
9. Hampl JS, Anderson JV, Mullis R. The role of dietetics professionals in health promotion and disease prevention. *J Am Diet Assoc*. 2002;102:1680-1687.
10. Lin SH, Guthrie J, Frazao E. American children's' diets are not making the grade. *Food Review*. 2001;24: 8-17.
11. Satter E. Feeding dynamics: helping children to eat well. *J Pediatr Health Care*. 1995;9:178-184.
12. Story M, Holt K, Sofka D, eds. *Bright futures in practice: Nutrition*, 2nd Ed. Arlington, VA: National Center for Education in Maternal Child Health; 2002.
13. Pelto GH, Levitt E, Thairu L. Improving feeding practices, current patterns, common constraints and the design of interventions. *Food Nutr Bull*. 2003;24:45-82.

Updated: 2008 Edition

Diagnosis

Physical Inactivity (NB-2.1)

Definition

Low level of activity/sedentary behavior to the extent that it reduces energy expenditure and impacts health.

Etiology (Cause/Contributing Risk Factors)

Factors gathered during the nutrition assessment process that contribute to the existence or the maintenance of pathophysiological, psychosocial, situational, developmental, cultural, and/or environmental problems:

- Harmful beliefs/attitudes about physical activity
- Injury, lifestyle change, condition (e.g., advanced stages of cardiovascular disease, obesity, kidney disease), physical disability or limitation that reduces physical activity or activities of daily living
- Food and nutrition-related knowledge deficit concerning health benefits of physical activity
- Lack of prior exposure to accurate nutrition-related information
- Lack of role models, e.g., for children
- Lack of social support for implementing changes
- Lack of or limited access to safe exercise environment and/or equipment
- Lack of value for behavior change or competing values
- Time constraints
- Financial constraints that may prevent sufficient level of activity (e.g., cost of equipment or shoes or club membership to gain access)

Signs/Symptoms (Defining Characteristics)

A typical cluster of subjective and objective signs and symptoms gathered during the nutrition assessment process that provide evidence that a problem exists; quantify the problem and describe its severity.

Nutrition Assessment Category	Potential Indicators of this Nutrition Diagnosis (one or more must be present)
Biochemical Data, Medical Tests and Procedures	
Anthropometric Measurements	• Obesity—BMI > 30 (adults), BMI >95th percentile (pediatrics > 3 years)
Nutrition-Focused Physical Findings	• Excessive subcutaneous fat and low muscle mass

Physical Inactivity (NB-2.1)

Food/Nutrition-Related History	Reports or observations of: • Infrequent, low duration and/or low intensity physical activity • Large amounts of sedentary activities, e.g., TV watching, reading, computer use in both leisure and work/school • Low level of NEAT (non-exercise activity thermogenesis) expended by physical activities other than planned exercise, e.g., sitting, standing, walking, fidgeting • Low cardiorespiratory fitness and/or low muscle strength • Medications that cause somnolence and decreased cognition
Client History	• Medical diagnoses that may be associated with or result in decreased activity, e.g., arthritis, chronic fatigue syndrome, morbid obesity, knee surgery • Psychological diagnosis, e.g., depression, anxiety disorders

References

1. Position of the American Dietetic Association: Weight management. *J Am Diet Assoc.* 2002;102:1145-1155.
2. Position of the American Dietetic Association: Total diet approach to communicating food and nutrition information. *J Am Diet Assoc.* 2007;107:1224-1232.
3. Position of the American Dietetic Association: The role of dietetics professionals in health promotion and disease prevention. *J Am Diet Assoc.* 2006;106:1875-1884.
4. Levine JA, Lanninghav-Foster LM, McCrady SK, Krizan AC, Olson LR, Kane PH, Jensen MD, Clark MM. Interindividual variation in posture allocation: Possible role in human obesity. *Science.* 2005;307:584-586.

Updated: 2008 Edition

Diagnosis

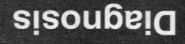

Behavioral-Environmental Domain – Physical Activity and Function

Excessive Physical Activity (NB-2.2)

Definition

Involuntary or voluntary physical activity or movement that interferes with energy needs, growth, or exceeds that which is necessary to achieve optimal health.

Etiology (Cause/Contributing Risk Factors)

Factors gathered during the nutrition assessment process that contribute to the existence or the maintenance of pathophysiological, psychosocial, situational, developmental, cultural, and/or environmental problems:

- Disordered eating
- Irrational beliefs/attitudes about food, nutrition, and fitness
- "Addictive" behaviors/personality

Signs/Symptoms (Defining Characteristics)

A typical cluster of subjective and objective signs and symptoms gathered during the nutrition assessment process that provide evidence that a problem exists; quantify the problem and describe its severity.

Nutrition Assessment Category	Potential Indicators of this Nutrition Diagnosis (one or more must be present)
Biochemical Data, Medical Tests and Procedures	• Elevated liver enzymes, e.g., LDH, AST • Altered micronutrient status, e.g., decreased serum ferritin, zinc, and insulin-like growth factor-binding protein • Increased hematocrit • Possibly elevated cortisol levels
Anthropometric Measurements	• Weight loss, arrested growth and development, failure to gain weight during period of expected growth (related usually to disordered eating)
Nutrition-Focused Physical Findings	• Depleted adipose and somatic protein stores (related usually to disordered eating) • Chronic muscle soreness

Excessive Phyisical Activity (NB-2.2)

Food/Nutrition-Related History	Reports or observations of: • Continued/repeated high levels of exercise exceeding levels necessary to improve health and/or athletic performance • Exercise daily without rest/rehabilitation days • Exercise while injured/sick • Forsaking family, job, social responsibilities to exercise • Overtraining
Client History	• Conditions associated with a diagnosis or treatment, e.g., anorexia nervosa, bulimia nervosa, binge eating, eating disorder not otherwise specified, amenorrhea, stress fractures • Chronic fatigue • Evidence of addictive, obsessive, or compulsive tendencies • Suppressed immune function • Frequent and/or prolonged injuries and/or illnesses

References

1. Aissa-Benhaddad A, Bouix D, Khaled S, Micallef JP, Mercier J, Bringer J, Brun JF. Early hemorheologic aspects of overtraining in elite athletes. *Clin Hemorheol Microcirc*. 1999;20:117-125.

2. American Psychiatric Association. *Diagnostic and Statistical Manual of Mental Disorders*. 4th Ed. Washington, DC: American Psychiatric Association; 1994.

3. Davis C, Brewer H, Ratusny D. Behavioral frequency and psychological commitment: necessary concepts in the study of excessive exercising. *J Behav Med*. 1993;16:611-628.

4. Davis C, Claridge G. The eating disorder as addiction: a psychobiological perspective. *Addict Behav*. 1998;23:463-475.

5. Davis C, Kennedy SH, Ravelski E, Dionne M. The role of physical activity in the development and maintenance of eating disorders. *Psychol Med*. 1994;24:957-967.

6. Klein DA, Bennett AS, Schebendach J, Foltin RW, Devlin MJ, Walsh BT. Exercise "addiction" in anorexia nervosa: model development and pilot data. *CNS Spectr*. 2004;9:531-537.

7. Lakier-Smith L. Overtraining, excessive exercise, and altered immunity: is this a helper-1 vs helper-2 lymphocyte response? *Sports Med*. 2003;33:347-364.

8. Position of the American Dietetic Association: Nutrition intervention in the treatment of anorexia nervosa, bulimia nervosa, and eating disorder not otherwise specified (EDNOS). *J Am Diet Assoc*. 2006;106:2073-2082.

9. Shephard RJ, Shek PN. Acute and chronic over-exertion: do depressed immune responses provide useful markers? *Int J Sports Med*. 1998;19:159-171.

10. Smith LL. Tissue trauma: the underlying cause of overtraining syndrome? *J Strength Cond Res*. 2004;18:185-193.

11. Urhausen A, Kindermann W. Diagnosis of overtraining: what tools do we have. *Sports Med*. 2002;32:95-102.

Updated: 2009 Edition

Diagnosis

Behavioral-Environmental Domain – Physical Activity and Function

Inability or Lack of Desire to Manage Self-Care (NB-2.3)

Definition

Lack of capacity or unwillingness to implement methods to support healthful food- and nutrition-related behavior.

Etiology (Cause/Contributing Risk Factors)

Factors gathered during the nutrition assessment process that contribute to the existence or the maintenance of pathophysiological, psychosocial, situational, developmental, cultural, and/or environmental problems:

- Food- and nutrition-related knowledge deficit concerning self-care
- Lack of social support for implementing changes
- Lack of developmental readiness to perform self-management tasks, e.g., pediatrics
- Lack of value for behavior change or competing values
- Perception that lack of resources (e.g., time, financial, or interpersonal) prevent self-care
- Cultural practices that affect ability to manage self-care
- Impaired cognitive ability, including learning disabilities, neurological or sensory impairment, and/or dementia
- Prior exposure to incompatible information
- Not ready for diet/lifestyle change
- Unwilling or disinterested in learning/applying information
- Lack of or limited access to self-management tools or decision guides

Signs/Symptoms (Defining Characteristics)

A typical cluster of subjective and objective signs and symptoms gathered during the nutrition assessment process that provide evidence that a problem exists; quantify the problem and describe its severity.

Nutrition Assessment Category	Potential Indicators of this Nutrition Diagnosis (one or more must be present)
Biochemical Data, Medical Tests and Procedures	
Anthropometric Measurements	
Nutrition-Focused Physical Findings	

Inability or Lack of Desire to Manage Self-Care (NB-2.3)

Food/Nutrition-Related History	Reports or observations of: • Inability to interpret data or self-management tools • Embarrassment or anger regarding need for self-monitoring • Uncertainty regarding changes could/should be made in response to data in self-monitoring records
Client History	• Diagnoses that are associated with self-management, e.g., diabetes mellitus, obesity, cardiovascular disease, renal or liver disease • Conditions associated with a diagnosis or treatment, e.g., cognitive or emotional impairment • New medical diagnosis or change in existing diagnosis or condition

References

1. Position of the American Dietetic Association: Providing nutrition services for infants, children, and adults with developmental disabilities and special health care needs. *J Am Diet Assoc*. 2004;104:97-107.
2. Crawford S. Promoting dietary change. *Can J Cardiol*. 1995;11(suppl A):14A-15A.
3. Falk LW, Bisogni CA, Sobal J. Diet change processes of participants in an intensive heart program. *J Nutr Educ*. 2000;32:240-250.
4. Glasgow RE, Hampson SE, Strycker LA, Ruggiero L. Personal-model beliefs and social-environmental barriers related to diabetes self-management. *Diabetes Care*. 1997;20:556-561.
5. Keenan DP, AbuSabha R, Sigman-Grant M, Achterberg C, Ruffing J. Factors perceived to influence dietary fat reduction behaviors. *J Nutr Educ*.1999;31:134-144.
6. Kumanyika SK, Van Horn L, Bowen D, Perri MG, Rolls BJ, Czajkowski SM, Schron E. Maintenance of dietary behavior change. *Health Psychol*. 2000;19(1 suppl):S42-S56.
7. Sporny, LA, Contento, Isobel R. Stages of change in dietary fat reduction: Social psychological correlates. *J Nutr Educ*. 1995;27:191.

Diagnosis

Impaired Ability to Prepare Foods/Meals (NB-2.4)

Definition

Cognitive or physical impairment that prevents preparation of foods/fluids.

Etiology (Cause/Contributing Risk Factors)

Factors gathered during the nutrition assessment process that contribute to the existence or the maintenance of pathophysiological, psychosocial, situational, developmental, cultural, and/or environmental problems:

- Impaired cognitive ability, including learning disabilities, neurological or sensory impairment, and/or dementia
- Loss of mental or cognitive ability, e.g., dementia
- Physical disability
- High level of fatigue or other side effect of therapy

Signs/Symptoms (Defining Characteristics)

A typical cluster of subjective and objective signs and symptoms gathered during the nutrition assessment process that provide evidence that a problem exists; quantify the problem and describe its severity.

Nutrition Assessment Category	Potential Indicators of this Nutrition Diagnosis (one or more must be present)
Biochemical Data, Medical Tests and Procedures	
Anthropometric Measurements	
Nutrition-Focused Physical Findings	
Food/Nutrition-Related History	Reports or observations of: • Decreased overall estimated intake • Excessive consumption of convenience foods, pre-prepared meals, and foods prepared away from home resulting in an inability to adhere to nutrition prescription • Uncertainty regarding appropriate foods to prepare based on nutrition prescription • Inability to purchase and transport foods to one's home
Client History	• Conditions associated with a diagnosis or treatment, e.g., cognitive impairment, cerebral palsy, paraplegia, vision problems, rigorous therapy regimen, recent surgery

Impaired Ability to Prepare Foods/Meals (NB-2.4)

References

1. Andren E, Grimby G. Activity limitations in personal, domestic and vocational tasks: a study of adults with inborn and early acquired mobility disorders. *Disabil Rehabil*. 2004;26:262-271.
2. Andren E, Grimby G. Dependence in daily activities and life satisfaction in adult subjects with cerebral palsy or spina bifida: a follow-up study. *Disabil Rehabil*. 2004;26:528-536.
3. Fortin S, Godbout L, Braun CM. Cognitive structure of executive deficits in frontally lesioned head trauma patients performing activities of daily living. *Cortex*. 2003;39:273-291.
4. Godbout L, Doucet C, Fiola M. The scripting of activities of daily living in normal aging: anticipation and shifting deficits with preservation of sequencing. *Brain Cogn*. 2000;43:220-224.
5. Position of the American Dietetic Association: Providing nutrition services for infants, children, and adults with developmental disabilities and special health care needs. *J Am Diet Assoc*. 2004;104:97-107.
6. Position of the American Dietetic Association: Food insecurity and hunger in the United States. *J Am Diet Assoc*. 2006;106:446-458.
7. Position of the American Dietetic Association: Addressing world hunger, malnutrition, and food insecurity. *J Am Diet Assoc*. 2003;103:1046-1057.
8. Sandstrom K, Alinder J, Oberg B. Descriptions of functioning and health and relations to a gross motor classification in adults with cerebral palsy. *Disabil Rehabil*. 2004;26:1023-1031.

Updated: 2009 Edition

Diagnosis

Behavioral-Environmental Domain – Physical Activity and Function

Poor Nutrition Quality of Life (NQOL) (NB-2.5)

Definition
Diminished patient/client perception of quality of life in response to nutrition problems and recommendations.

Etiology (Cause/Contributing Risk Factors)
Factors gathered during the nutrition assessment process that contribute to the existence or the maintenance of pathophysiological, psychosocial, situational, developmental, cultural, and/or environmental problems:

- Food and nutrition knowledge–related deficit
- Not ready for diet/lifestyle change
- Negative impact of current or previous medical nutrition therapy (MNT)
- Food or activity behavior-related difficulty
- Poor self-efficacy
- Altered body image
- Food insecurity
- Lack of social support for implementing changes

Signs/Symptoms (Defining Characteristics)
A typical cluster of subjective and objective signs and symptoms gathered during the nutrition assessment process that provide evidence that a problem exists; quantify the problem and describe its severity.

Nutrition Assessment Category	Potential Indicators of this Nutrition Diagnosis (one or more must be present)
Biochemical Data, Medical Tests and Procedures	
Anthropometric Measurements	
Nutrition-Focused Physical Findings	

Poor Nutrition Quality of Life (NQOL) (NB-2.5)

Food/Nutrition-Related History	Reports or observations of: • Unfavorable NQOL rating • Unfavorable ratings on measure of QOL, such as, SF-36 (multipurpose health survey form with 36 questions) or EORTC QLQ-C30 (quality of life tool developed for patient/clients with cancer) • Food insecurity/unwillingness to use community services that are available • Frustration or dissatisfaction with MNT recommendations • Frustration over lack of control • Inaccurate or incomplete information related to MNT recommendations • Inability to change food- or activity-related behavior • Concerns about previous attempts to learn information • MNT recommendations affecting socialization • Unwillingness or disinterest in learning information
Client History	• New medical diagnosis or change in existing diagnosis or condition • Recent other lifestyle or life changes, e.g., quit smoking, initiated exercise, work change, home relocation • Lack of social and familial support • Ethnic and cultural related issues

References

1. Aaronson NK., Ahmedzai S, Bullinger M. The EORTC core quality of life questionnaire: Interim results of an international field study. In: Osoba D. ed. *Effect of Cancer on Quality of Life*. Boca Raton, FL: CRC Press 1991: 185-203.

2. Barr JT, Schumacher GE. The need for a nutrition-related quality-of-life measure. *J Am Diet Assoc*. 2003;103:177-180.

3. Barr JT, Schumacher GE. Using focus groups to determine what constitutes quality of life in clients receiving medical nutrition therapy: First steps in the development of a nutrition quality-of-life survey. *J Am Diet Assoc*. 2003;103:844-851.

4. NQOL instrument and annotated bibliography. Available at: http://www.bouve.neu.edu (key word search: quality of life). Accessed January 29, 2007.

5. Ware JE. *SF-36 Health Survey: Manual and Interpretation Guide*. Lincoln, RI: Quality Metric Inc; 2003

Updated: 2008 Edition

Diagnosis

Behavioral-Environmental Domain – Physical Activity and Function

Self-Feeding Difficulty (NB-2.6)

Definition
Impaired actions to place food or beverages in mouth.

Etiology (Cause/Contributing Risk Factors)
Factors gathered during the nutrition assessment process that contribute to the existence or the maintenance of pathophysiological, psychosocial, situational, developmental, cultural, and/or environmental problems:

- Physiological difficulty causing inability to physically grasp cups and utensils, support and/or control head and neck, coordinate hand movement to mouth, close lips (or any other suckling issue), bend elbow or wrist, sit with hips square and back straight
- Limited physical strength or range of motion
- Lack of or limited access to foods and/or adaptive eating devices conducive for self-feeding
- Limited vision
- Impaired cognitive ability, including learning disabilities, neurological or sensory impairment, and/or dementia
- Reluctance or avoidance of self-feeding

Signs/Symptoms (Defining Characteristics)
A typical cluster of subjective and objective signs and symptoms gathered during the nutrition assessment process that provide evidence that a problem exists; quantify the problem and describe its severity.

Nutrition Assessment Category	Potential Indicators of this Nutrition Diagnosis (one or more must be present)
Biochemical Data, Medical Tests and Procedures	
Anthropometric Measurements	• Weight loss
Nutrition-Focused Physical Findings	• Dry mucous membranes, hoarse or wet voice, tongue extrusion • Poor lip closure, drooling • Shortness of breath

Self-Feeding Difficulty (NB-2.6)

Food/Nutrition-Related History	Reports or observations of:
	• Being provided with foods that may not be conducive to self-feeding, e.g., peas, broth-type soups
	• Dropping of cups, utensils
	• Emotional distress, anxiety, or frustration surrounding mealtimes
	• Failure to recognize foods
	• Forgets to eat
	• Inappropriate use of food
	• Refusal to eat or chew
	• Dropping of food from utensil (splashing and spilling of food) on repeated attempts to feed
	• Lack of strength or stamina to lift utensils and/or cup
	• Utensil biting
Client History	• Conditions associated with a diagnosis or treatment of, e.g., neurological disorders, Parkinson's, Alzheimer's, Tardive dyskinesia, multiple sclerosis, stroke, paralysis, developmental delay
	• Physical limitations, e.g., fractured arms, traction, contractures
	• Surgery requiring recumbent position
	• Dementia/organic brain syndrome
	• Dysphagia
	• Tremors

References

1. Consultant Dietitians in Healthcare Facilities. *Dining Skills Supplement: Practical Interventions for Caregivers of Eating Disabled Older Adults*. Pensacola, FL: American Dietetic Association; 1992.

2. Morley JE. Anorexia of aging: physiological and pathologic. *Am J Clin Nutr*. 1997; 66:760-773.

3. Position of the American Dietetic Association: Providing nutrition services for infants, children, and adults with developmental disabilities and special health care needs. *J Am Diet Assoc*. 2004;104:97-107.

4. Sandman P, Norberg A, Adolfsson R, Eriksson S, Nystrom L. Prevalence and characteristics of persons with dependency on feeding at institutions. *Scand J Caring Sci*. 1990;4:121-127.

5. Siebens H, Trupe E, Siebens A, Cooke F, Anshen S, Hanauer R, Oster G. Correlates and consequences of feeding dependency. *J Am Geriatr Soc*. 1986;34:192-198.

6. Vellas B, Fitten LJ, eds. *Research and Practice in Alzheimer's Disease*. New York, NY: Springer Publishing Company; 1998.

Updated: 2009 Edition

Diagnosis

Behavioral-Environmental Domain – Food Safety and Access

Intake of Unsafe Food (NB-3.1)

Definition

Intake of food and/or fluids intentionally or unintentionally contaminated with toxins, poisonous products, infectious agents, microbial agents, additives, allergens, and/or agents of bioterrorism.

Etiology (Cause/Contributing Risk Factors)

Factors gathered during the nutrition assessment process that contribute to the existence or the maintenance of pathophysiological, psychosocial, situational, developmental, cultural, and/or environmental problems:

- Food and nutrition-related knowledge deficit concerning potentially unsafe food
- Lack of knowledge about proper food/feeding, (infant and enteral formula, breast milk) storage, and preparation
- Exposure to contaminated water or food, e.g., community outbreak of illness documented by surveillance and/or response agency
- Mental illness, confusion, or altered awareness
- Lack of or limited access to food storage equipment/facilities, e.g., refrigerator
- Lack of or limited access to safe food supply, e.g., inadequate markets with safe, uncontaminated food

Signs/Symptoms (Defining Characteristics)

A typical cluster of subjective and objective signs and symptoms gathered during the nutrition assessment process that provide evidence that a problem exists; quantify the problem and describe its severity.

Nutrition Assessment Category	Potential Indicators of this Nutrition Diagnosis (one or more must be present)
Biochemical Data, Medical Tests and Procedures	• Positive stool culture for infectious causes, such as listeria, salmonella, hepatitis A, E. coli, cyclospora • Toxicology reports for drugs, medicinals, poisons in blood or food samples
Anthropometric Measurements	
Nutrition-Focused Physical Findings	• Evidence of dehydration, e.g., dry mucous membranes, damaged tissues • Diarrhea, cramping, bloating, fever, nausea, vomiting, vision problems, chills, dizziness, headache

Intake of Unsafe Food (NB-3.1)

Food/Nutrition-Related History	Reports or observations of intake of potential unsafe foods: • Mercury content of fish, non-food items (pregnant and lactating women) • Raw eggs, unpasteurized milk products, soft cheeses, undercooked meats (infants, children, immunocompromised persons, pregnant and lactating women, and elderly) • Wild plants, berries, mushrooms • Unsafe food/feeding storage and preparation practices (enteral and infant formula, breast milk)
Client History	• Conditions associated with a diagnosis or treatment, e.g., foodborne illness, such as, bacterial, viral, and parasitic infection, mental illness, dementia • Poisoning by drugs, medicinals, and biological substances • Poisoning from poisonous food stuffs and poisonous plants • Cardiac, neurologic, respiratory changes

References

1. Centers for Disease Control and Prevention. Diagnosis and Management of Foodborne Illnesses: A Primer for Physicians and Other Health Care Professionals. Available at: www.cdc.gov/mmwr/preview/mmwrhtml/rr5304a1.htm. Accessed July 2, 2004.
2. Food Safety and Inspection Service. The Fight BAC Survey Tool and Data Entry Tool. Available at: www.fsis.usda.gov/OA/fses/bac_datatool.htm. Accessed July 2, 2004.
3. Gerald BL, Perkin JE. Food and water safety. *J Am Diet Assoc.* 2003;103:1203-1218.
4. Partnership for Food Safety Education. Four steps. Available at: http://www.fightbac.org/foursteps.cfm?section=4. Accessed July 2, 2004.

Diagnosis

Behavioral-Environmental Domain – Food Safety and Access

Limited Access to Food (NB-3.2)

Definition
Diminished ability to acquire a sufficient quantity and variety of healthful food based upon the U.S. Dietary Guidelines or MyPyramid. Limitation to food because of concerns about weight or aging.

Etiology (Cause/Contributing Risk Factors)
Factors gathered during the nutrition assessment process that contribute to the existence or the maintenance of pathophysiological, psychosocial, situational, developmental, cultural, and/or environmental problems:

- Caregiver intentionally or unintentionally not providing access to food, e.g., unmet needs for food or eating assistance, excess of poor nutritional quality food, abuse/neglect
- Community and geographical constraints for shopping and transportation
- Food and nutrition-related knowledge deficit concerning sufficient quantity or variety of culturally appropriate healthful food
- Lack of financial resources or lack of access to financial resources to purchase a sufficient quantity or variety of culturally appropriate healthful foods
- Lack of food planning, purchasing, and preparation skills
- Limited, absent, or failure to participate in community supplemental food programs, e.g., food pantries, emergency kitchens, or shelters, with a sufficient variety of culturally appropriate healthful foods
- Failure to participate in federal food programs such as WIC, National School Breakfast/Lunch Program, food stamps
- Schools lacking nutrition/wellness policies or application of policies ensuring convenient, appetizing, competitively priced culturally appropriate healthful foods at meals, snacks, and school sponsored activities.
- Physical or psychological limitations that diminish ability to shop, e.g., walking, sight, mental/emotional health

Signs/Symptoms (Defining Characteristics)
A typical cluster of subjective and objective signs and symptoms gathered during the nutrition assessment process that provide evidence that a problem exists; quantify the problem and describe its severity.

Nutrition Assessment Category	Potential Indicators of this Nutrition Diagnosis (one or more must be present)
Biochemical Data, Medical Tests and Procedures	• Indicators of macronutrient or vitamin/mineral status as indicated by biochemical findings

Limited Access to Food (NB-3.2)

Anthropometric Measurements	• Growth failure, based on National Center for Health Statistics (NCHS) growth standards • Underweight, BMI <18.5 (adults)
Nutrition-Focused Physical Findings	• Findings consistent with vitamin/mineral deficiency • Hunger
Food/Nutrition-Related History	Reports or observations of: • Food faddism or harmful beliefs and attitudes of parent or caregiver • Belief that aging can be slowed by dietary limitations and extreme exercise • Estimated inadequate intake of food and/or specific nutrients • Limited supply of food in home • Limited variety of foods
Client History	• Malnutrition, vitamin/mineral deficiency • Illness or physical disability • Conditions associated with a diagnosis or treatment, e.g., mental illness, dementia • Lack of suitable support systems

References

1. Position of the American Dietetic Association: Food insecurity and hunger in the United States. *J Am Diet Assoc*. 2006;106:446-458.
2. Position of the American Dietetic Association: Addressing world hunger, malnutrition, and food insecurity. *J Am Diet Assoc*. 2003;103:1046-1057.

Updated: 2008 Edition

Diagnosis

NCP Step 3. Nutrition Intervention

What is the purpose of a nutrition intervention? The purpose is to resolve or improve the identified nutrition problem by planning and implementing appropriate nutrition interventions that are tailored to the patient/client's* needs.

How does a dietetics practitioner determine a nutrition intervention? The selection of nutrition interventions is driven by the nutrition diagnosis and its etiology. Nutrition intervention strategies are purposefully selected to change nutritional intake, nutrition-related knowledge or behavior, environmental conditions, or access to supportive care and services. Nutrition intervention goals provide the basis for monitoring progress and measuring outcomes.

How are the Nutrition Intervention strategies organized? In four categories:

Food and/or Nutrient Delivery	Nutrition Education	Nutrition Counseling	Coordination of Nutrition Care
An individualized approach for food/nutrient provision, including meals and snacks, enteral and parenteral feeding, and supplements	A formal process to instruct or train a patient/client in a skill or to impart knowledge to help patients/clients voluntarily manage or modify food choices and eating behavior to maintain or improve health	A supportive process, characterized by a collaborative counselor-patient relationship, to set priorities, establish goals and create individualized action plans that acknowledge and foster responsibility for self-care to treat an existing condition and promote health	Consultation with, referral to, or coordination of nutrition care with other health care providers, institutions, or agencies that can assist in treating or managing nutrition-related problems

What does Nutrition Intervention involve? Nutrition intervention entails two distinct and interrelated components—planning and implementing. Planning the nutrition intervention involves: (a) prioritizing nutrition diagnoses, (b) consulting ADA's Evidence-Based Nutrition Practice Guidelines and other practice guides, (c) determining patient-focused expected outcomes for each nutrition diagnosis, (d) conferring with patient/client/caregivers, (e) defining a nutrition intervention plan and strategies, (f) defining time and frequency of care, and (g) identifying resources needed. Implementation is the action phase and involves: (a) communication of the nutrition care plan, (b) carrying out the plan.

Critical thinking during this step…

- Setting goals and prioritizing
- Defining the nutrition prescription or basic plan
- Making interdisciplinary connections
- Initiating behavioral and other nutrition interventions
- Matching nutrition intervention strategies with client needs, nutrition diagnosis, and values
- Choosing from among alternatives to determine a course of action
- Specifying the time and frequency of care

Are dietetics practitioners limited to the Nutrition Intervention terms defined? Nutrition intervention terminology includes commonly used strategies and emphasizes the application of evidence-based strategies matched to appropriate circumstances. Evaluation of the nutrition intervention terminology is ongoing and will guide future modifications. Dietetics practitioners can propose additions or revisions using the Procedure for Nutrition Controlled Vocabulary/Terminology Maintenance/Review available from ADA.

*Patient/client refers to individuals, groups, family members, and/or caregivers.

Detailed information about this step can be found in the American Dietetic Association's International Dietetics and Nutrition Terminology (IDNT) Reference Manual: Standardized Language for the Nutrition Care Process, Second Edition.

Intervention

Nutrition Care Process Step 3.
Nutrition Intervention

Introduction

Nutrition intervention is the third step in the Nutrition Care Process, preceded by nutrition assessment and nutrition diagnosis. Nutrition intervention is defined as purposefully planned actions intended to positively change a nutrition-related behavior, environmental condition, or aspect of health status for an individual (and his/her family or caregivers), target group, or the community at large. A dietetics practitioner works in conjunction with the patient/client(s) and other health care providers, programs, or agencies during the nutrition intervention phase.

While nutrition intervention is one step in the process, it consists of two interrelated components—planning and implementation. Planning involves prioritizing the nutrition diagnoses, conferring with the patient/client and/or others, reviewing practice guides and policies, and setting goals and defining the specific nutrition intervention strategy. Implementation of the nutrition intervention is the action phase that includes carrying out and communicating the plan of care, continuing data collection, and revising the nutrition intervention strategy, as warranted, based on the patient/client response.

When drafting the specific nutrition intervention terms, the Standardized Language Committee strived to include information necessary for medical record documentation, billing, and for research. These terms intentionally distinguish between two distinct nutrition interventions, such as nutrition education and nutrition counseling. However, the patient/client care plan can include more that one nutrition intervention that may be implemented simultaneously during the actual interaction with the patient/client.

The nutrition intervention terminology is organized into four domains—Food and/or Nutrient Delivery, Nutrition Education, Nutrition Counseling, and Coordination of Nutrition Care. Each domain defines classes of nutrition interventions. Reference sheets for each term define the nutrition intervention, list typical details of the nutrition intervention, and illustrate the potential connection to the nutrition diagnoses.

The nature of a single nutrition intervention encounter with a patient/client can be described in many ways. It could include face-to-face contact with the patient/client or an encounter via electronic mail (e-mail) or telephone. The encounter may involve an individual or group and may be described in varying increments of contact time. Throughout the course of nutrition care, the dietetics practitioner and patient/client might engage in several encounters (i.e., interactions, visits, contacts) aimed at helping the patient/client implement the nutrition intervention(s). Nutrition interventions in the Food and/or Nutrient Delivery class and Coordination of Nutrition Care class may occur without direct patient/client contact (e.g., change in enteral formula).

At all levels of practice, dietetics practitioners are competent to provide many types of nutrition interventions. However, dietetics practitioners' roles and responsibilities vary with experience, education, training, practice setting, employer expectations, and local standards of care. Responsible dietetics practitioners ensure that they are competent to practice by participating in continuing education activities and obtaining necessary education, training, and credentials related to their area of practice. The Scope of Dietetics Practice and Framework documents (available at www.eatright.org in the Practice section) provide guidance to the dietetics practitioner in identifying activities within and outside the Scope of Practice. The ADA Code of Ethics, Dietetic Practice Groups, and specialty groups also have documents that help identify appropriate dietetics practitioner roles and responsibilities.

Individualized nutrition interventions, based on a patient/client's needs identified through nutrition assessment and nutrition diagnosis, are the product of this step of the Nutrition Care Process. Using a standardized terminology for describing the nutrition interventions extends the ability of the dietetics practitioner to document, communicate, and research the impact of nutrition care on health and disease.

What is New in this Edition Related to Nutrition Intervention?

There are no changes to the Nutrition Intervention standardized language in this edition; however, a reference sheet for defining and describing a Nutrition Prescription is included with the nutrition intervention reference sheets.

Nutrition Intervention Components

Planning and implementation are the two components of nutrition intervention. These components are interrelated, and the dietetics practitioner will make decisions about the nutrition intervention when both planning and implementation are feasible.

Planning the Nutrition Intervention

As a dietetics practitioner plans the nutrition intervention, he/she prioritizes the nutrition diagnoses, based on the severity of the problem, safety, patient/client need, likelihood that the nutrition intervention will impact the problem, and the patient/client perception of importance.

To determine which nutrition diagnosis can be positively impacted, a dietetics practitioner needs to examine the relationship between each aspect of the nutrition diagnosis and the nutrition intervention. It has been previously established that the nutrition diagnosis states the problem, etiology, and the signs and symptoms based on data from the nutrition assessment.

Relationships

Nutrition Assessment	Nutrition Diagnosis	Nutrition Intervention	Nutrition Monitoring & Evaluation

Problem	**Etiology**	**Signs & Symptoms**

The nutrition intervention is directed, whenever possible, at the etiology or cause of the problem identified in the PES (i.e., problem, etiology, and signs/symptoms) statements. In some cases, it is not possible to direct the nutrition intervention at the etiology if the etiology cannot be changed by a dietetics practitioner. For example, if Excessive Energy Intake (NI-1.5) is caused by depression, the nutrition intervention is aimed at reducing the impact of the signs and symptoms of the problem, e.g., weight gain due to energy intake more than estimated needs.

Note: Whenever possible, dietetics practitioners direct the nutrition intervention at the etiology of the problem. In some cases, practitioners may need to direct the nutrition intervention at the signs and symptoms if the etiology can not be changed by the dietetics practitioner.

Intervention

Edition: 2009

Relationships

| Nutrition Assessment | Nutrition Diagnosis | Nutrition Intervention | Nutrition Monitoring & Evaluation |

| Problem | Etiology | Signs & Symptoms |

Follow-up monitoring of the signs and symptoms is used to determine the impact of the nutrition intervention on the etiology of the problem.

Relationships

| Nutrition Assessment | Nutrition Diagnosis | Nutrition Intervention | Nutrition Monitoring & Evaluation |

| Problem | Etiology | Signs & Symptoms |

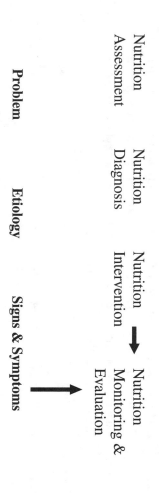

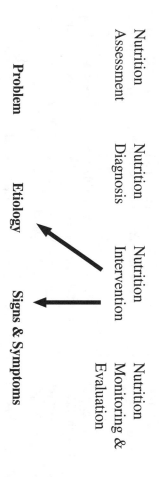

During the planning phase to choose the most appropriate nutrition intervention, the dietetics practitioner uses evidence-based guidelines, institutional policies and procedures, care maps, and other resources for recommended nutrition interventions to reach medical nutrition therapy goals, desired behavior changes, and/or expected outcomes. ADA's Evidence-Based Nutrition Practice Guidelines provide evidence-based recommendations for nutrition interventions. Dietetics practitioners should carefully examine resources to determine if the recommendations are evidence-based.

Nutrition Prescription

An essential part of planning the nutrition intervention is detailing the Nutrition Prescription. The nutrition prescription concisely states the patient/client's individualized recommended dietary intake of energy and/or selected foods or nutrients based on current reference standards and dietary guidelines and the patient/client's health condition and nutrition diagnosis. It is determined using the assessment data, the nutrition diagnosis statement (PES), current evidence, policies and procedures, and patient/client values and preferences. The nutrition prescription either drives the nutrition intervention selection or is the context within which the nutrition intervention should be implemented. With the nutrition prescription defined, the dietetics practitioner identifies the specific nutrition intervention strategies and establishes the patient/client-focused goals to be accomplished. A reference sheet defining a nutrition prescription and its components is included with the nutrition intervention reference sheets.

The **nutrition prescription** concisely states the patient/client's individualized recommended dietary intake of energy and/or selected foods or nutrients based on current reference standards and dietary guidelines and the patient/client's health condition and nutrition diagnosis. A **nutrition prescription reference sheet** is included following this introduction to Step 3.

Intervention

Goal Setting

This is the time to establish clear patient/client goals that are measurable, achievable, and time-defined. It is most desirable to set goals jointly with the patient/client; however, this is not always possible, such as in the case of patients/clients receiving enteral or parenteral nutrition. In goal setting, the individual(s) responsible for the associated actions to achieve the goals is/are clearly identified.

These steps are essential because it is impossible to assess the impact of the nutrition intervention without quantifying or qualifying the goals so they can be measured. If the goals are not achievable, even the most appropriate nutrition intervention could be judged as unsuccessful. Additionally, the time for achieving the individual goals should be delineated into short-term (next visit) and long-term goals (over the course of the nutrition intervention).

The parties responsible for establishing the goals and the associated actions—such as joint development with patient/client and/or family or solely provider-directed (e.g., patient/client unable to participate in interaction and family/other not available)—need to be documented.

Planning Summary:

- Prioritize the nutrition diagnoses, based on problem severity, safety, patient/client need, likelihood that the nutrition intervention will impact the problem, and patient/client perception of importance
- Consult ADA's Evidence-Based Nutrition Practice Guidelines and other practice guides/policies
- Confer with patient/client and other caregivers, or refer to policies throughout planning step
- Detail the nutrition prescription and identify the specific nutrition intervention strategies
- Determine patient/client-focused goals/expected outcomes
- Define time and frequency of care

Implementing the Nutrition Intervention

Implementation is the action portion of the nutrition intervention in which dietetics practitioners carry out and communicate the plan of care to all relevant parties, continue the data collection that was initiated with the nutrition assessment, and revise the nutrition intervention based on the patient/client response.

Once a dietetics practitioner has verified that the nutrition intervention is occurring, the data collected will also provide evidence of the response(s) and potentially lead to revision of the nutrition intervention.

Implementation Summary:

- Action phase
  - Communicate the plan of care
  - Carry out the plan
  - Continue data collection
- Other aspects
  - Individualize nutrition intervention
  - Collaborate with other colleagues
  - Follow-up and verify that nutrition intervention is occurring
  - Adjust intervention strategies, if needed, as response occurs

344

Intervention

Nutrition Intervention Terms

The Standardized Language Committee identified four domains of nutrition interventions—Food and/or Nutrient Delivery, Nutrition Education, Nutrition Counseling, and Coordination of Care—and defined classes within them. These domains and classes are intended to be used by all dietetics practitioners in all nutrition intervention settings (e.g., community, public health, home care, long-term care, private practice, and pediatric and adult acute care). Currently, the nutrition intervention terms are being tested for usability and validity in clinical settings. The specific nutrition intervention domains and classes are:

Food and/or Nutrient Delivery (ND) refers to an individualized approach for food/ nutrient provision.

Meal and Snacks (ND-1)—meals are regular eating events that include a variety of foods consisting of grains and/or starches, meat and/or meat alternatives, fruits and vegetables, and milk or milk products. A snack is defined as food served between regular meals.

Enteral and Parenteral Nutrition (ND-2)—nutrition provided through the gastrointestinal tract via tube, catheter, or stoma that delivers nutrients distal to the oral cavity (enteral) or the administration of nutrients intravenously (centrally or peripherally) (parenteral).

Supplements (ND-3)—foods or nutrients that are not intended as a sole item or a meal or diet, but that are intended to provide additional nutrients.

Medical Food Supplement (ND-3.1)—commercial or prepared foods or beverages intended to supplement the nutrient intake in energy, protein, carbohydrate, fiber, and/or fat, which may also contribute to vitamin and mineral intake.

Vitamin and Mineral Supplement (ND-3.2)—a product that is intended to supplement vitamin or mineral intake.

Bioactive Substance Supplement (ND-3.3)—a product that is intended to supplement bioactive substances (e.g., plant stanol and sterol esters, psyllium).

Feeding Assistance (ND-4)—accommodation or assistance in eating designed to restore the patient/client's ability to eat independently, support adequate nutrient intake, and reduce the incidence of unplanned weight loss and dehydration.

Feeding Environment (ND-5)—adjustment of the physical environment, temperature, convenience, and attractiveness of the location where food is served that impacts food consumption.

Nutrition-Related Medication Management (ND-6)—modification of a drug or herbal to optimize patient/client nutritional or health status.

Nutrition Education (E) is a formal process to instruct or train a patient/client in a skill or to impart knowledge to help patients/clients voluntarily manage or modify food choices and eating behavior to maintain or improve health.

Initial/Brief Nutrition Education (E-1)—instruction or training intended to build or reinforce basic nutrition-related knowledge, or to provide essential nutrition-related information until patient/ client returns.

Comprehensive Nutrition Education (E-2)—instruction or training intended to lead to in-depth nutrition-related knowledge and/or skills in given topics.

Nutrition Counseling (C) is a supportive process, characterized by a collaborative counselor-patient/client relationship, to set priorities, establish goals, and create individualized action plans that acknowledge and foster responsibility for self-care to treat an existing condition and promote health.

Theoretical basis/approach (C-1)—the theories or models used to design and implement an intervention. Theories and theoretical models consist of principles, constructs and variables, which offer systematic explanations of the human behavior change process. Behavior change theories and models provide a research-based rational for designing and tailoring nutrition interventions

Intervention

to achieve the desired effect. A theoretical framework for curriculum and treatment protocols, it guides determination of: (a) what information patients/clients need at different points in the behavior change process, (b) what tools and strategies may be best applied to facilitate behavior change, and (c) outcome measures to assess effectiveness in interventions or components of interventions.

Strategies (C-2)—An evidence-based method or plan of action designed to achieve a particular goal. Application of behavior change theories in nutrition practice has provided practitioners with a collection of evidence-based strategies to promote behavior change. Some strategies target change in motivation and intention to change, and others target behavior change. Dietetics practitioners selectively apply strategies based upon patient/client goals and objectives, and their personal counseling philosophy and skill.

Dietetics practitioners engaging in nutrition counseling are asked to indicate for each encounter both the theoretical basis or approach they are using (may be multiple) and the strategy or strategies they are using within a particular encounter.

Coordination of Nutrition Care (RC) is consultation with, referral to, or coordination of nutrition care with other health care providers, institutions, or agencies that can assist in treating or managing nutrition-related problems.

Coordination of Other Care During Nutrition Care (RC-1)—facilitating services or interventions with other professionals, institutions, or agencies on behalf of the patient/client prior to discharge from nutrition care.

Discharge and Transfer of Nutrition Care to New Setting or Provider (RC-2)—discharge planning and transfer of nutrition care from one level or location of care to another.

Nutrition Education vs. Nutrition Counseling

As mentioned earlier, it is intentional to separate nutrition education from nutrition counseling even though a dietetics practitioner may use both of these nutrition interventions during a single encounter.

More than one type of intervention, e.g. nutrition education and nutrition counseling, may be applied within a single encounter or in sequential encounters. The appropriate nutrition intervention domain(s) and class(es) are selected based on the nutrition assessment, diagnosis and patient/client needs and interests, and reported on the care plan. For example, the dietetics professional could refer the client to a nutrition education class to address knowledge barriers, and spend individual counseling time exploring ambivalence to change (motivational interviewing) and food/nutrition access issues. Group classes are frequently designed to impart knowledge and are therefore nutrition education. These may include didactic classes, supermarket tours, and/or cooking demonstrations. Nutrition counseling may address a variety of etiologies such as beliefs and attitudes, behavior, and access to healthful food. Nutrition counseling is process characterized as an interpersonal helping relationship, which begins by exploring the way the patient/client thinks and feels as well as his or her current dietary habits, for the purpose of facilitating dietary change.

During the nutrition encounter, the following attitudinal, knowledge, and environmental barriers to change (etiologies) may be identified: lack of motivation, lack of knowledge and/or lack of financial resources. When knowledge related etiologies are addressed via knowledge transfer within a counseling session, nutrition education is the intervention applied. The dietetics practitioner would then use different intervention techniques to address barriers identified. These may include:

• Nutrition counseling (C-1 or C-2) using the motivational interviewing strategy to address lack of motivation, and development of an action plan to facilitate a patient/client link with community/government food/nutrition resources.

• Nutrition education (E-1 or E-2) in a group or individual setting to address knowledge deficits related to disease/condition, interpreting lab results, self-management parameters, selection of healthful foods/meals and food preparation and cooking.

Intervention

Nutrition counseling and education interventions are separated to highlight the differences between them and to show the true nature of the interaction(s) between dietetics practitioner and patient/client. This will assist a practitioner in thinking about providing distinct education and counseling approaches, while moving seamlessly between these two activities.

Uses of Nutrition Interventions Based on Practice Setting

The typical uses of nutrition interventions may vary by practice setting, but they are not limited based upon the practice setting.

- Food and/or Nutrient Delivery nutrition interventions will commonly be used by dietetics practitioners in institutional settings (e.g., hospitals, long-term care) and home care.

- Nutrition Education interventions—Initial/Brief Education (E-1) will be utilized more often in institutionalized settings and Comprehensive Education (E-2) will be utilized more often in outpatient/noninstitutionalized settings (e.g., outpatient offices, private practice, community).

- Nutrition Counseling will likely be used more by dietetics practitioners in outpatient/noninstitutionalized settings (e.g., outpatient offices, private practice, community) due to the nature of the nutrition intervention and the practice setting.

- Coordination of Nutrition Care interventions will be used by dietetics practitioners in a variety of practice settings.

It is important to reiterate that these are typical uses of specific nutrition interventions. Dietetics practitioners in any practice setting can use the complete array of nutrition interventions as appropriate and necessary.

Nutrition Intervention Reference Sheets

A reference sheet for each nutrition intervention has been developed that includes the nutrition intervention label and its definition, descriptive details of the nutrition intervention, and the nutrition diagnoses with which the nutrition intervention might typically be used. Additional considerations pertinent to the nutrition intervention are also included. A partial example of a nutrition intervention reference sheet follows here:

Example

Feeding Assistance (ND-4)

Defined as accommodation or assistance in eating designed to restore the patient/client's ability to eat independently, support adequate nutrient intake, and reduce the incidence of unplanned weight loss and dehydration.

Details of Nutrition Intervention: A typical nutrition intervention might be further described with the following details:

- Recommends, implements, or orders adaptive equipment, feeding position, feeding cues, meal set-up, or mouth care to facilitate eating
- Recommends, designs, or implements a restorative dining program
- Recommends, designs, or implements a feeding assistance training program
- Recommends, designs, or implements menu selections that foster, promote, and maintain independent eating

Encounter Details

A single nutrition intervention encounter (i.e., interactions, visits, contacts, sessions) includes time spent reviewing the medical record or patient/client information, time spent interacting with other health care professionals involved in patient/client care, and direct (i.e., face-to-face) or indirect (e.g., electronic, phone) contact with the patient/client and his/her family or caregiver. With the expanded use of electronic communication has come the growth of nutrition interventions and are available following this chapter.

These reference sheets are designed to assist dietetics practitioners with consistent and correct utilization of the nutrition interventions and are available following this chapter.

Intervention

interventions via methods like e-mail and webinars (seminars on the Internet), along with phone and teleconference encounters.

Encounters may involve an individual or group where:

- An individual is one person with his/her family or caregiver
- A group is intended to meet more than one individual's needs

A typical method to indicate contact time in ambulatory care is in increments of 15 minutes (one unit = 15 minutes). Naturally, throughout a course of nutrition care, the dietetics practitioner and patient/client might engage in several encounters.

Roles and Responsibilities

Dietetics practice is such that practitioners differ in their need, desire, opportunity, experience, or credentials to perform various nutrition interventions. Generalist dietetics practitioners may maintain competence in a wide variety of nutrition interventions, while specialty dietetics practitioners may develop in-depth expertise with a few nutrition interventions. Some of the nutrition interventions described in the reference sheets (e.g., nutrition counseling, enteral and parenteral nutrition, or nutrition-related medication management) may require specialty or advanced education and/or training.

Practice roles and responsibilities may vary according to employer expectations or institutional tradition. Regulations, in certain practice settings and/or licensure laws, may be interpreted as restricting intervention to that authorized by order of a physician or others. Protocols may be used to allow interventions to be implemented or modified. Clinical privileges allow dietetics practitioners to autonomously intervene according to a specified scope of practice. Obtaining clinical privileges or being granted authority to make independent changes to a patient/client's nutrition prescription or nutrition intervention may be needed. In some situations, such as private practice or community settings, a dietetics practitioner may have complete autonomy. Further, depending on the setting, the dietetics practitioner may assume various levels of autonomy for different nutrition interventions. Examples are provided below:

- *Implements the specified nutrition intervention; recommends initiating, modifying, or discontinuing a nutrition intervention as appropriate.* On completion of a nutrition assessment, the dietetics practitioner may recommend (verbally or by writing) refinements, modifications, or alternative nutrition interventions that require affirmation before they can be implemented.

  Example: The dietetics practitioner assesses a patient/client on a general diet and notices elevated serum cholesterol and triglyceride levels. The dietetics practitioner recommends a modification of the nutrition prescription to the physician or nurse practitioner, and modifies the nutrition prescription upon affirmation of the recommendation.

- *Implements, within the parameters of an approved protocol or algorithm, the initiation, modification, or discontinuance of a nutrition intervention.* On completion of a nutrition assessment, the dietetics practitioner modifies the original nutrition intervention within preapproved parameters.

  Example: The dietetics practitioner assesses a patient/client with a general nutrition prescription and notices elevated serum cholesterol, triglyceride, and blood glucose levels. According to an approved treatment algorithm, the dietetics practitioner can implement a "heart healthy" nutrition prescription for any patient/client with a serum cholesterol level more than 200 mg/dL. The dietetics practitioner changes the nutrition prescription to "heart healthy," initiates patient/client nutrition education, and documents the change and other details of the nutrition intervention in the medical record. Because the algorithm does not specify the nutrition intervention for hyperglycemia, the dietetics practitioner must provide (verbally or in writing) recommendations for an additional carbohydrate restriction or management in the nutrition prescription, then await affirmation before implementation.

- *Independently orders the initiation, modification, or discontinuance of a nutrition intervention based on a scope of practice.* Authority may be specified in an approved clinical privileging document or inherent in the setting. On completion of the nutrition assessment, the dietetics practitioner is able to initiate, modify, or discontinue a nutrition intervention based on independent clinical judgment.

Intervention

Example: The dietetics practitioner assesses a patient/client with a general nutrition prescription, and notices elevated serum cholesterol, triglyceride levels, and blood glucose levels. In this setting, a dietetics practitioner has the autonomy to order, change, and implement nutrition prescriptions designed to manage disorders of lipid, carbohydrate, protein, and energy metabolism. The dietetics practitioner changes the nutrition prescription to "heart healthy" with consistent carbohydrate intake and initiates patient/client nutrition education and other details of the nutrition intervention as appropriate.

The table provides examples of the common level of autonomy in a few practice settings:

Setting	Common Triggers	Common Levels of Autonomy
Inpatient	Physician or advanced practice nurse **orders** a diet or **requests** a consultation or the patient is **identified** at risk by screening criteria.	• Implements the specified nutrition intervention; recommends initiating, modifying, or discontinuing a nutrition intervention. • Implements, within the parameters of an approved protocol or algorithm, initiation, modification, or discontinuance of a nutrition intervention. • Independently orders initiation, modification, or discontinuance of a nutrition intervention based on a scope of practice. Authority is usually specified in an approved clinical privileging document.
Outpatient	Physician or advanced practice nurse **refers** the patient/client or the patient/client is **self-referred**.	• Implements the specified nutrition intervention; recommends initiating, modifying, or discontinuing a nutrition intervention. • Implements, within the parameters of an approved protocol or algorithm, initiation, modification, or discontinuance of a nutrition intervention. • Independently orders initiation, modification, or discontinuance of a nutrition intervention based on a scope of practice. Authority may be specified in an approved clinical privileging document or inherent in practice setting.
Private Practice	Physician or advanced practice nurse **refers** the patient/client or the patient/client is **self-referred**.	• Independently orders initiation, modification, or discontinuance of a nutrition intervention based on scope of practice.
Community	Client is **self-referred** or is identified at risk by screening criteria.	• Independently orders initiation, modification, or discontinuance of a nutrition intervention based on scope of practice.

Summary

Using defined nutrition intervention terminology will assist the profession in communicating within the profession and also among a variety of other health care providers. It will also be instrumental in documenting and researching the impact the profession has on specific diagnoses and/or etiologies in all patient/client populations. The nutrition intervention reference sheets are a tool that dietetics practitioners can use to select strategies and implement this aspect of the Nutrition Care Process. Finally, evaluation of the nutrition intervention terminology is planned and will guide possible future modifications.

As mentioned earlier, the Scope of Dietetics Practice and Framework documents provide guidance to the dietetics practitioner in identifying activities within and outside the Scope of Dietetics Practice. All Scope of Dietetics Practice documents are available on the ADA website, www.eatright.org, in the Nutrition Care Process section. Dietetic Practice Groups and specialty organizations have documents that help identify appropriate practitioner roles and responsibilities and dietetics practitioners should refer to these reports for guidance.

349

Intervention

References

1. Davis AM, Baker SS, Leary RA. Advancing clinical privileges for support practitioners: the dietitian as a model. *Nutr Clin Pract*. 1995;10:98-103.

2. Hager M. Hospital therapeutic diet orders and the Centers for Medicare & Medicaid Services: Steering through regulations to provide quality nutrition care and avoid survey citations. *J Am Diet Assoc*. 2006;106:198-204.

3. Kieselhorst KJ, Skates J, Pritchett E. American Dietetic Association: Standards of practice in nutrition care and updated standards of professional performance. *J Am Diet Assoc*. 2005;105:641-645.

4. Kulkarni K, Boucher J, Daly A, Shwide-Slavin C, Silvers B, Maillet JO, Pritchett E. American Dietetic Association: Standards of practice and standards of professional performance for registered dietitians (generalist, specialty, and advanced) in diabetes care. *J Am Diet Assoc*. 2005;105:819-824.

5. Lacey K, Pritchett E. Nutrition care process and model: ADA adopts road map to quality care and outcomes management. *J Am Diet Assoc*. 2003;103:1061-1072.

6. Mahan L, Escott-Stump S. *Krause's Food, Nutrition, & Diet Therapy*. 11th ed. Philadelphia, PA: Saunders; 2000.

7. Miller R, Rollnick S. *Motivational Interviewing: Preparing People for Change*, 2nd ed. New York, NY: Guilford Press; 2002.

8. Moreland K, Gotfried M, Vaughn L. Development and implementation of the clinical privileges for dietitian nutrition order writing program at a long-term acute-care hospital. *J Am Diet Assoc*. 2002;102:72-74.

9. Myers EF, Barnhill G, Bryk J. Clinical privileges: missing piece of the puzzle for clinical standards that elevate responsibilities and salaries for registered dietitians. *J Am Diet Assoc*. 2002;102:123-132.

10. O'Sullivan Maillet J, Skates J, Pritchett E. American Dietetic Association: Scope of dietetics practice framework. *J Am Diet Assoc*. 2005;105:634-640.

11. Silver H, Wellman N. Nutrition diagnosing and order writing: value for practitioners, quality for clients. *J Am Diet Assoc*. 2003;103:1470-1472.

Intervention

Nutrition Intervention Terminology

Problem _____

Etiology _____

Signs/Symptoms _____

Nutrition Prescription

The patient's/client's individualized recommended dietary intake of energy and/or selected foods or nutrients based on current reference standards and dietary guidelines and the patient's/client's health condition and nutrition diagnosis _(specify)_.

Intervention #1 _____

Goal(s) _____

Intervention #2 _____

Goal(s) _____

Intervention #3 _____

Goal(s) _____

FOOD AND/OR NUTRIENT DELIVERY ND

Meal and Snacks (1)
Regular eating event (meal); food served between regular meals (snack).

- ☐ General/healthful diet — ND-1.1
- ☐ Modify distribution, type, or amount of food and nutrients within meals or at a specified time — ND-1.2
- ☐ Specific foods/beverages or groups — ND-1.3
- ☐ Other — ND-1.4
  (specify)

Enteral and Parenteral Nutrition (2)
Nutrition provided through the GI tract via tube, catheter, or stoma (enteral) or intravenously (centrally or peripherally) (parenteral).

- ☐ Initiate EN or PN — ND-2.1
- ☐ Modify rate, concentration, composition or schedule — ND-2.2
- ☐ Discontinue EN or PN — ND-2.3
- ☐ Insert enteral feeding tube — ND-2.4
- ☐ Site care — ND-2.5
- ☐ Other — ND-2.6
  (specify)

Supplements (3)

Medical Food Supplements (3.1)
Commercial or prepared foods or beverages that supplement energy, protein, carbohydrate, fiber, fat intake.

- Type
  - ☐ Commercial beverage — ND-3.1.1
  - ☐ Commercial food — ND-3.1.2
  - ☐ Modified beverage — ND-3.1.3
  - ☐ Modified food — ND-3.1.4
  - ☐ Purpose — ND-3.1.5
  (specify)

Vitamin and Mineral Supplements (3.2)
Supplemental vitamins or minerals.

- ☐ Multivitamin/mineral — ND-3.2.1
- ☐ Multi-trace elements — ND-3.2.2
- ☐ Vitamin — ND-3.2.3
  - ☐ A (1)
  - ☐ C (2)
  - ☐ D (3)
  - ☐ E (4)
  - ☐ K (5)
  - ☐ Thiamin (6)
  - ☐ Riboflavin (7)
  - ☐ Niacin (8)
  - ☐ Folate (9)
  - ☐ B6 (10)
  - ☐ B12 (11)
  - ☐ Other _(specify)_ (12)
- ☐ Mineral — ND-3.2.4
  - ☐ Calcium (1)
  - ☐ Chloride (2)
  - ☐ Iron (3)
  - ☐ Magnesium (4)
  - ☐ Potassium (5)
  - ☐ Phosphorus (6)
  - ☐ Sodium (7)
  - ☐ Zinc (8)
  - ☐ Other _(specify)_ (9)

Bioactive Substance Supplement (3.3)
Supplemental bioactive substances.

- ☐ Initiate — ND-3.3.1
- ☐ Dose change — ND-3.3.2
- ☐ Form change — ND-3.3.3
- ☐ Route change — ND-3.3.4
- ☐ Administration schedule — ND-3.3.5
- ☐ Discontinue — ND-3.3.6
  (specify)

Feeding Assistance (4)
Accommodation or assistance in eating.

- ☐ Adaptive equipment — ND-4.1
- ☐ Feeding position — ND-4.2
- ☐ Meal set-up — ND-4.3
- ☐ Mouth care — ND-4.4
- ☐ Other — ND-4.5
  (specify)

Feeding Environment (5)
Adjustment of the factors where food is served that impact food consumption.

- ☐ Lighting — ND-5.1
- ☐ Odors — ND-5.2
- ☐ Distractions — ND-5.3
- ☐ Table height — ND-5.4
- ☐ Table service/set up — ND-5.5
- ☐ Room temperature — ND-5.6
- ☐ Other — ND-5.7
  (specify)

Nutrition-Related Medication Management (6)
Modification of a drug or herbal to optimize patient/client nutritional or health status.

- ☐ Initiate — ND-6.1
- ☐ Dose change — ND-6.2
- ☐ Form change — ND-6.3
- ☐ Route change — ND-6.4
- ☐ Administration schedule — ND-6.5
- ☐ Discontinue — ND-6.6
  (specify)

NUTRITION EDUCATION E

Initial/Brief Nutrition Education (1)
Build or reinforce basic or essential nutrition-related knowledge.

- ☐ Purpose of the nutrition education — E-1.1
- ☐ Priority modifications — E-1.2
- ☐ Survival information — E-1.3
- ☐ Other — E-1.4
  (specify)

Comprehensive Nutrition Education (2)
Instruction or training leading to in-depth nutrition-related knowledge or skills.

- ☐ Purpose of the nutrition education — E-2.1
- ☐ Recommended modifications — E-2.2

Comprehensive Nutrition Education (2), cont'd
- ☐ Advanced or related topics — E-2.3
- ☐ Result interpretation — E-2.4
- ☐ Skill development — E-2.5
- ☐ Other — E-2.6
  (specify)

NUTRITION COUNSELING C

Theoretical Basis/Approach (1)
The theories or models used to design and implement an intervention.

- ☐ Cognitive-Behavioral Theory — C-1.1
- ☐ Health Belief Model — C-1.2
- ☐ Social Learning Theory — C-1.3
- ☐ Transtheoretical Model/ Stages of Change — C-1.4
- ☐ Other — C-1.5

Strategies (2)
Selectively applied evidence-based methods or plans of action designed to achieve a particular goal.

- ☐ Motivational interviewing — C-2.1
- ☐ Goal setting — C-2.2
- ☐ Self-monitoring — C-2.3
- ☐ Problem solving — C-2.4
- ☐ Social support — C-2.5
- ☐ Stress management — C-2.6
- ☐ Stimulus control — C-2.7
- ☐ Cognitive restructuring — C-2.8
- ☐ Relapse prevention — C-2.9
- ☐ Rewards/contingency management — C-2.10
- ☐ Other — C-2.11
  (specify)

COORDINATION OF NUTRITION CARE RC

Coordination of Other Care During Nutrition Care (1)
Facilitating services with other professionals, institutions, or agencies during nutrition care.

- ☐ Team meeting — RC-1.1
- ☐ Referral to RD with different expertise — RC-1.2
- ☐ Collaboration/referral to other providers — RC-1.3
- ☐ Referral to community agencies/ programs _(specify)_ — RC-1.4

Discharge and Transfer of Nutrition Care to New Setting or Provider (2)
Discharge planning and transfer of nutrition care from one level or location of care to another.

- ☐ Collaboration/referral to other providers — RC-2.1
- ☐ Referral to community agencies/ programs _(specify)_ — RC-2.2

Intervention

Nutrition Intervention Terms and Definitions

Nutrition Intervention Term	Term Number	Definition	Reference Sheet Page Numbers
DOMAIN: FOOD AND/OR NUTRIENT DELIVERY	ND	Individualized approach for food/nutrient provision.	
Meals and Snacks	ND-1	Meals are defined as regular eating events that include a variety of foods consisting of grains and/or starches, meat and/or meat alternatives, fruits and vegetables, and milk or milk products. A snack is defined as food served between regular meals.	360-361
Enteral and Parenteral Nutrition	ND-2	Enteral nutrition is defined as nutrition provided through the gastrointestinal (GI) tract via tube, catheter, or stoma that delivers nutrients distal to the oral cavity. Parenteral nutrition is defined as the administration of nutrients intravenously, centrally (delivered into a large-diameter vein, usually the superior vena cava adjacent to the right atrium) or peripherally (delivered into a peripheral vein, usually of the hand or forearm).	362-363
Supplements	ND-3	Foods or nutrients that are not intended as a sole item or a meal or diet, but that are intended to provide additional nutrients.	
Medical Food Supplements	ND-3.1	Commercial or prepared foods or beverages intended to supplement energy, protein, carbohydrate, fiber, and/or fat intake that may also contribute to vitamin and mineral intake.	364-365
Vitamin and Mineral Supplements	ND-3.2	A product that is intended to supplement vitamin or mineral intake.	366-367
Bioactive Substance Supplement	ND-3.3	A product that is intended to supplement bioactive substances (e.g., plant stanol and sterol esters, psyllium).	368
Feeding Assistance	ND-4	Accommodation or assistance in eating designed to restore the patient's/client's ability to eat independently, support adequate nutrient intake, and reduce the incidence of unplanned weight loss and dehydration.	369-370
Feeding Environment	ND-5	Adjustment of the physical environment, temperature, convenience, and attractiveness of the location where food is served that impacts food consumption.	371-372
Nutrition-Related Medication Management	ND-6	Modification of a drug or herbal to optimize patient/client nutritional or health status.	373-374

Nutrition Intervention Terms and Definitions

Nutrition Intervention Term	Term Number	Definition	Reference Sheet Page Numbers
DOMAIN: NUTRITION EDUCATION	E	Formal process to instruct or train a patient/client in a skill or to impart knowledge to help patients/clients voluntarily manage or modify food choices and eating behavior to maintain or improve health.	
Initial/Brief Nutrition Education	E-1	Instruction or training intended to build or reinforce basic nutrition-related knowledge, or to provide essential nutrition-related information until patient/client returns.	375-376
Comprehensive Nutrition Education	E-2	Instruction or training intended to lead to in-depth nutrition-related knowledge and/or skills in given topics.	377-378
DOMAIN: NUTRITION COUNSELING	C	A supportive process, characterized by a collaborative counselor-patient/client relationship, to set priorities, establish goals, and create individualized action plans that acknowledge and foster responsibility for self-care to treat an existing condition and promote health.	
Theoretical basis/approach	C-1	The theories or models used to design and implement an intervention. Theories and theoretical models consist of principles, constructs and variables, which offer systematic explanations of the human behavior change process. Behavior change theories and models provide a research-based rational for designing and tailoring nutrition interventions to achieve the desired effect. A theoretical framework for curriculum and treatment protocols, it guides determination of: 1) what information patients/clients need at different points in the behavior change process, 2) what tools and strategies may be best applied to facilitate behavior change, and 3) outcome measures to assess effectiveness in interventions or components of interventions.	379-391
Strategies	C-2	An evidence-based method or plan of action designed to achieve a particular goal. Application of behavior change theories in nutrition practice has provided practitioners with a collection of evidence-based strategies to promote behavior change. Some strategies target change in motivation and intention to change, and others target behavior change. Dietetics practitioners selectively apply strategies based upon patient/client goals and objectives, and their personal counseling philosophy and skill.	392-399

Nutrition Intervention Terms and Definitions

Nutrition Intervention Term	Term Number	Definition	Reference Sheet Page Numbers
DOMAIN: COORDINATION OF NUTRITION CARE	RC	Consultation with, referral to, or coordination of nutrition care with other providers, institutions, or agencies that can assist in treating or managing nutrition-related problems.	
Coordination of Other Care During Nutrition Care	RC-1	Facilitating services or interventions with other professionals, institutions, or agencies on behalf of the patient/client prior to discharge from nutrition care.	400-402
Discharge and Transfer of Nutrition Care to New Setting or Provider	RC-2	Discharge planning and transfer of nutrition care from one level or location of care to another.	403-404

Nutrition Prescription

Definition

The patient's/client's individualized recommended dietary intake of energy and/or selected foods or nutrients based on current reference standards and dietary guidelines and the patient's/client's health condition and nutrition diagnosis

Purpose

To communicate the nutrition professional's diet/nutrition recommendation based upon a thorough nutrition assessment

Indicators

- Recommend regular diet
- Recommend modified diet
  - Recommended energy/nutrient modification
    - Calorie modification (specify, e.g., calories/day, calories/kg/day)
    - Recommended carbohydrate modification
      - Diabetic diet (specify, e.g., distribution)
      - Amount (specify, e.g., grams/day, grams/kg/min, percent of calories)
      - Other (specify, e.g., no concentrated sweets)
    - Recommended protein level (specify, e.g., grams/day, grams/kg/day, percent of calories)
    - Recommended fat level (specify, e.g., grams/day, grams/kg/day, percent of calories)
      - Fat restricted diet (specify, e.g., grams/day)
      - Therapeutic lifestyle change diet
      - Recommended saturated fat level (specify, e.g., grams/day, percent of calories)
      - Recommended unsaturated fat level (specify, e.g., grams/day, percent of calories)
      - Recommended cholesterol intake (specify, e.g., mg/day)
    - Recommended vitamin intake
      - Vitamin A (µg/day)
      - Vitamin C (mg/day)
      - Vitamin D (µg/day)
      - Vitamin E (mg/day)
      - Vitamin K (µg/day)
      - Thiamin (mg/day)
      - Riboflavin (mg/day)
      - Niacin (mg/day)
      - Vitamin B6 (mg/day)
      - Folate (µg/day)
      - Vitamin B12 (µg/day)
      - Multivitamin

Nutrition Intervention

Nutrition Prescription

- Recommended mineral intake
  - Calcium (mg/day)
  - Iron (mg/day)
  - Magnesium (mg/day)
  - Phosphorus (mg/day)
  - Zinc (mg/day)
  - Potassium (g/day)

  - Sodium (mg/day)
  - Chloride (mg/day)
  - Multimineral
  - Multi-trace element

  - Recommended fluid level (specify, e.g., mL/day, mL/kg/day, mL/calories expended, mL/m^2/day, mL output)
  - Recommended fiber level (specify, e.g., type, grams/day, grams/1000 kcals/day)
  - Recommended level of bioactive substances (specify, e.g., substance, amount)
- Recommended enteral nutrition order (specify, e.g., formula, rate/schedule)
  - Tube feeding modulars (specify, e.g., carbohydrate, protein, fat, fiber)
- Recommended parenteral nutrition order (specify, e.g., solution, rate, access)
- Recommend liquid diet
  - Clear liquid
  - Full liquid
- Recommended texture modification (specify, e.g., mechanical soft, puree)
- Recommended liquid consistency modification (specify, e.g., thin, nectar, honey, pudding)
- Recommended food intake
  - Grain group intake (specify, e.g., servings, exchanges, amounts)
  - Fruit and vegetable intake (specify, e.g., servings, exchanges, amounts)
  - Meat, poultry, fish, eggs, beans, nut intake (specify, e.g., servings, exchanges, amounts)
  - Milk and milk product intake (specify, e.g., servings, exchanges, amounts)
  - Fat foods (specify, e.g., type, servings, exchanges, amounts)

Note: The nutrition prescription can be used as a comparative standard for nutrition assessment and nutrition monitoring and evaluation.

Nutrition Prescription

References

The following are some suggested references; other references may be appropriate.

1. American Diabetes Association. Standards of Medical Care in Diabetes–2006. *Diabetes Care*. 2006;29:S4-S42.

2. American Dietetic Association Evidence-Analysis Library, 2007. Available at: http://www.ada.portalxm.com/eal/. Accessed on December 2, 2007.

3. American Dietetic Association. Nutrition Care Manual. 2004. Available at: www.nutritioncaremanual.org.

4. American Heart Association Nutrition Committee: Lichtenstein, A, Appel, L, Brands M, Carnethon M, Daniels S, Franch HA, Franklin B, Kris-Etherton P, Harris WS, Howard B, Karanja N, Lefevre M, Rudel L, Sacks F, Van Horn L, Winston M, Wylie-Rosett J. Diet and lifestyle recommendations revision 2006: a scientific statement from the American Heart Association Nutrition Committee. *Circulation*, 2006, 114(1) 82-96.

5. American Society for Parenteral and Enteral Nutrition Board of Directors and The Clinical Guidelines Task Force. Guidelines for the use of parenteral and enteral nutrition in adult and pediatric patients: Specific guidelines for disease - adults. *J Parenter Enteral Nutr*. 2002;26(Suppl):S61-S96.

6. American Society for Parenteral and Enteral Nutrition Board of Directors and The Clinical Guidelines Task Force. Guidelines for the use of parenteral and enteral nutrition in adult and pediatric patients: Life cycle and metabolic conditions. *J Parenter Enteral Nutr*. 2002; 26(Suppl):S45-S60.

7. American Society for Parenteral and Enteral Nutrition Board of Directors and The Clinical Guidelines Task Force. Guidelines for the use of parenteral and enteral nutrition in adult and pediatric patients: Specific guidelines for disease - pediatrics. *J Parenter Enteral Nutr*. 2002;26(Suppl):S111-S138.

8. Appel LJ, Moore TJ, Obarzanek E, Vollmer WM, Svetkey LP, Sacks FM, Bray GA, Vogt TM, Cutler JA, Windhauser MM, Lin P, Karanja N, Simons-Morton D, McCullough M, Swain J, Steele P, Evans MA, Miller ER, Harsha DW. A clinical trial of the effects of dietary patterns on blood pressure. *N Eng J Med*. 1997;336:1117-1124.

9. Bantle JP, Wylie-Rosett J, Albright AL, Apovian CM, Clark NG, Franz MJ, Hoogwerf BJ, Lichtenstein AH, Mayer-Davis E, Mooradian AD, Wheeler ML. Nutrition recommendations and interventions for diabetes-2006: a position statement of the American Diabetes Association. *Diabetes Care*, 2006, 29(9):2140-2157.

10. Committee on Nutrient Relationships in Seafood – National Academies. *Seafood choices: Balancing Benefits and Risks*. National Academies Press. 2006.

11. Compher C. Frankenfield D, Keim N, Roth-Yousey L. Best practice methods to apply to measurement of resting metabolic rate in adults: A systematic review. *J Am Diet Assoc*. 2006;106:881-903.

12. Frankenfield D, Roth-Yousey L, Compher C. Comparison of predictive equations for resting metabolic rate in healthy nonobese adults: A systematic review. *J Am Diet Assoc*. 2005;105:775-789.

13. Gartner LM, Greer FR, American Academy of Pediatrics Committee on Nutrition. Prevention of rickets and vitamin D deficiency: new guidelines for vitamin D Intake. *Pediatrics*.2003:111:908-10.

14. Institute of Medicine, Food and Nutrition Board. *Dietary Reference Intakes for Energy, Carbohydrate, Fiber, Fat, Fatty Acids, Cholesterol, Protein and Amino Acids*. Food and Nutrition Board. National Academy of Sciences. Washington, DC: National Academy Press; 2002. Available at: www.iom.edu/Object.File/Master/21/372/DRI%20Tables%20after%20electrolytes%20plus%20micro-macroEAR_2.pdf

15. National Academy of Sciences, Institute of Medicine. *Dietary Reference Intakes for Calcium, Phosphorus, Magnesium, Vitamin D, and Fluoride*. Washington, DC: National Academy Press; 1997.

16. National Academy of Sciences, Institute of Medicine. *Dietary Reference Intakes: Thiamin, riboflavin, niacin, vitamin B6, folate, vitamin B12, pantothenic acid, biotin, and choline*. National Academy Press. Washington, DC, 1998.

17. National Academy of Sciences, Institute of Medicine. *Dietary Reference Intakes for Vitamin A, Vitamin K, Arsenic, Boron, Chromium, Copper, Iodine, Iron, Manganese, Molybdenum, Nickel, Silicon, Vanadium, and Zinc*. National Academy Press, Washington, DC, 2001.

18. National Academy of Sciences, Institute of Medicine. *Dietary Reference Intakes: Vitamin C, Vitamin E, Selenium, and Carotenoids*. National Academy Press, Washington, DC, 2000.

19. National Academy of Sciences, Institute of Medicine. *Dietary Reference Intakes for Water, Potassium, Sodium, Chloride, and Sulfate*. Washington DC: National Academy Press; 2004.

20. US Department of Health and Human Services. National Institutes of Health. National Heart, Lung and Blood Institute. Third Report of the Expert Panel on Detection, Evaluation, and Treatment of High Blood Cholesterol in Adults (Adult Treatment Panel III), 2001

21. US Departments of Agriculture and Health and Human Services. Dietary Guidelines for Americans 2005. Available at: www.healthierus.gov/dietaryguidelines.

22. USDA Nutrient Data Laboratory, National Nutrient Database for Standard Reference. Available at: http://www.nal.usda.gov/fnic/foodcomp/search/. Accessed on December 1, 2007.

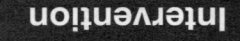

Food and/or Nutrient Delivery Domain

Meals and Snacks (ND-1)

Definition

Meals are defined as regular eating events that include a variety of foods consisting of grains and/or starches, meat and/or meat alternatives, fruits and vegetables, and milk or milk products. A snack is defined as food served between regular meals.

Details of Intervention

A typical intervention might be further described with the following details:

- Recommend, implement, or order an appropriate distribution of type or quantity of food and nutrients within meals or at specified times
- Identify specific food/beverage(s) or groups for meals and snacks

Typically used with the following

Nutrition Diagnostic Terminology Used in PES Statements	Common Examples (not intended to be inclusive)
Nutrition Diagnoses	• Increased energy expenditure (NI-1.2) • Excessive fat intake (NI-5.6.2) • Excessive carbohydrate intake (NI-5.8.2) • Inconsistent carbohydrate intake (NI-5.8.4)
Etiology	• Lack of access to healthful food choices, e.g., food provided by caregiver • Physiologic causes, e.g., increased energy needs due to increased activity level or metabolic change, malabsorption • Psychological causes, e.g., disordered eating • Difficulty chewing, swallowing, extreme weakness

Meals and Snacks (ND-1)

Signs and Symptoms	Biochemical Data, Medical Tests and Procedures
	• Serum cholesterol level > 200 mg/dL
	• Hemoglobin A1C > 6%
	Physical Assessment
	• Weight change
	• Dental caries
	• Diarrhea in response to carbohydrate feeding
	Food/Nutrition History
	• Cultural or religious practices that do not support modified food/nutrition intake
	• Changes in physical activity
	• Intake of inappropriate foods
	Client History
	• Conditions associated with diagnosis or treatment, e.g., surgery, trauma, sepsis, diabetes mellitus, inborn errors of metabolism, digestive enzyme deficiency, obesity
	• Chronic use of medications that increase or decrease nutrient requirements or impair nutrient metabolism

Other considerations (e.g., patient/client negotiation, patient/client needs and desires, and readiness to change)

- Compliance skills and abilities
- Economic concerns with purchasing special food items
- Willingness/ability to change behavior to comply with diet
- Availability/access to a qualified practitioner for follow-up and monitoring

References

1. Lacey K, Pritchett E. Nutrition Care Process and Model: ADA adopts road map to quality care and outcomes management. *J Am Diet Assoc*. 2003;103:1061-1071.

Food and/or Nutrient Delivery Domain

Enteral and Parenteral Nutrition (ND-2)

Definition

Enteral nutrition is defined as nutrition provided through the gastrointestinal (GI) tract via tube, catheter, or stoma that delivers nutrients distal to the oral cavity. Parenteral nutrition is defined as the administration of nutrients intravenously, centrally (delivered into a large-diameter vein, usually the superior vena cava adjacent to the right atrium) or peripherally (delivered into a peripheral vein, usually of the hand or forearm).

Details of Intervention

A typical intervention might be further described with the following details:

- Recommend, implement, or order changes in the rate, composition, schedule, and/or duration of feeding
- Recommend, implement, or order the initiation, route, and discontinuation of enteral nutrition
- Insert the feeding tube, provide tube site care; administer feedings
- Change dressings and provide line care
- Review changes in the intervention with the patient/client(s) and/or caregivers

Typically used with the following

Nutrition Diagnostic Terminology Used in PES Statements	Common Examples (not intended to be inclusive)
Nutrition Diagnoses	- Swallowing difficulties (NC-1.1) - Altered GI function (NC-1.4) - Inadequate oral food/beverage intake (NI-2.1) - Inadequate intake from enteral/parenteral nutrition infusion (NI-2.3) - Excessive intake from parenteral nutrition infusion (NI-2.4)
Etiology	- Altered gastrointestinal tract function, inability to absorb nutrients - Inability to chew/swallow

Enteral and Parenteral Nutrition (ND-2)

Signs and Symptoms	Physical Assessment
	• Weight loss > 10% in 6 months, > 5% in 1 month
	• Obvious muscle wasting
	• Skin turgor (tenting, edema)
	• Growth failure
	• Insufficient maternal weight gain
	• BMI < 18.5
	Food/Nutrition History
	• Intake < 75% of requirements (insufficient intake)
	• Existing or expected inadequate intake for 7-14 days
	Client History
	• Malabsorption, maldigestion
	• Emesis
	• Diffuse peritonitis, intestinal obstruction, paralytic ileus, intractable diarrhea or emesis, gastrointestinal ischemia, or perforated viscus, short-bowel syndrome

Other considerations (e.g., patient/client negotiation, patient/client needs and desires, and readiness to change)

- End-of-life issues, ethical considerations, patient/client rights and family/caregiver issues
- Other nutrient intake (oral, parenteral, or enteral nutrition)
- Enteral formulary composition and product availability
- Availability/access to a qualified practitioner for follow-up and monitoring
- Economic constraints that limit availability of food/enteral/parenteral products

References

1. A.S.P.E.N. Board of Directors and Standards Committee. Definition of terms, style, and conventions used in A.S.P.E.N. guidelines and standards. *Nutr Clin Pract*. 2005;20:281-285.

2. A.S.P.E.N. Board of Directors and the Clinical Guidelines Task Force. Guidelines for the use of parenteral and enteral nutrition in adult and pediatric patients. *J Parenter Enteral Nutr*. 2002;26:1SA-138SA.

3. McClave SA, Lowen CC, Kleber MJ, Nicholson JF, Jimmerson SC, McConnell JW, Jung LY. Are patients fed appropriately according to their caloric requirements? *J Parenter Enteral Nutr*. 1998;22:375-381.

4. Mirtallo J, Canada T, Johnson D, Kumpf V, Petersen C, Sacks G, Seres D, Guenter P. Task force for the revision of safe practices for parenteral nutrition. *J Parenter Enteral Nutr*. 2004;28:S39-S70.

Intervention

Food and/or Nutrient Delivery Domain

Medical Food Supplements (ND-3.1)

Definition

Commercial or prepared foods or beverages intended to supplement energy, protein, carbohydrate, fiber, and/or fat intake that may also contribute to vitamin and mineral intake.

Details of Intervention

A typical intervention might be further described with the following details:

- Recommend, implement, or order changes in an individualized feeding plan including the initiation, composition, type, frequency, timing, and discontinuation of oral supplements
- Describe the purpose of the supplement (e.g., to supplement energy, protein, carbohydrate, fiber, and/or fat intake)

Typically used with the following

Nutrition Diagnostic Terminology Used in PES Statements	Common Examples (not intended to be inclusive)
Nutrition Diagnoses	• Inadequate oral food/beverage intake (NI-2.1) • Inadequate fluid intake (NI-3.1) • Increased nutrient needs (NI-5.1)
Etiology	• Neurologic deficit (stroke) • Difficulty chewing or swallowing • Food allergies or intolerance • Altered GI function • Partial GI obstruction

Medical Food Supplements (ND-3.1)

Signs and Symptoms	Physical Examination Findings
	• Weight loss > 10% in 6 months or > 5% in 1 month
	• Obvious muscle wasting
	• Poor skin turgor (tenting or edema)
	Food/Nutrition History
	• Insufficient usual food/beverage intake
	Client History
	• Diagnosis consistent with elevated nutrient needs
	• Potential for repletion of nutritional status
	• Ability to feed self
	• Choking on foods, oral/facial trauma
	• Insufficient vitamin-mineral intake

Other considerations (e.g., patient/client negotiation, patient/client needs and desires, and readiness to change)

• Appetite sufficient to take medical food supplements

• System constraints that prevent meeting the client's preferences for specific flavors, textures, foods and the timing of feedings

• Availability of feeding assistance

• Economic concerns and product/food availability

References

1. Milne AC, Avenell A, Potter J. Meta-analysis: Protein and energy supplementation in older people. *Ann Intern Med*. 2006;144:37-48.

Intervention

Vitamin and Mineral Supplements (ND-3.2)

Definition

A product that is intended to supplement vitamin or mineral intake.

Details of Intervention

A typical intervention might be further described with the following details:

- Recommend, implement, or order initiation, change in administration schedule and dose/form/route, or discontinuation of a vitamin and/or mineral supplement

Typically used with the following

Nutrition Diagnostic Terminology Used in PES Statements	Common Examples (not intended to be inclusive)
Nutrition Diagnoses	• Inadequate vitamin intake (NI-5.9.1) • Excessive vitamin intake (NI-5.9.2) • Inadequate mineral intake (NI-5.10.1) • Excessive mineral intake (NI-5.10.2) • Food–medication interaction (NC-2.3) • Food- and nutrition-related knowledge deficit (NB-1.1) • Undesirable food choices (NB-1.7)
Etiology	• Poor intake of nutrient dense foods that contain vitamins and minerals • Excessive use of vitamin and mineral supplements • Medical diagnosis consistent with altered vitamin and mineral requirements • Malabsorption of vitamins and minerals
Signs and Symptoms	Physical Examination Findings • Cutaneous abnormalities consistent with vitamin and mineral deficiency or excess Food/Nutrition History • Nutrient intake analysis reveals vitamin and mineral intake more or less than recommended • Laboratory or radiologic indexes of vitamin-mineral depletion

Vitamin and Mineral Supplements (ND-3.2)

Other considerations (e.g., patient/client negotiation, patient/client needs and desires, and readiness to change)

- Emerging scientific evidence to support the use of vitamin and mineral supplements in specific populations
- Availability of a qualified practitioner with additional education/training in the use of vitamin and mineral supplements in practice
- Economic considerations and product availability

References

1. Federal Food, Drug and Cosmetic Act. US Code, Title 21, Chapter 9, Subchapter II, Section 321 (ff). 2000 Edition. Available at: http://frwebgate.access.gpo.gov/cgi-bin/getdoc.cgi?dbname=browse_usc&docid=Cite:+21USC321. Accessed April 26, 2005.
2. Position of the American Dietetic Association: Fortification and nutritional supplements. *J Am Diet Assoc*. 2005;105:1300-1311.

Food and/or Nutrient Delivery Domain

Bioactive Substance Supplement (ND-3.3)

Definition

A product that is intended to supplement bioactive substances (e.g., plant stanol and sterol esters, psyllium).

Details of Intervention

A typical intervention might be further described with the following details:

- Recommend, implement, or order initiation, change in administration schedule or dose/form/route, or discontinuation of a bioactive substances (e.g., soluble fiber, soy protein, fish oils, plant sterol and stanol esters)

Typically used with the following

Nutrition Diagnostic Terminology Used in PES Statements	Common Examples (not intended to be inclusive)
Nutrition Diagnoses	• Inadequate bioactive substance intake (NI-4.1) • Excessive bioactive substance intake (NI-4.2) • Excessive alcohol intake (NI-4.3) • Food–medication interaction (NC-2.3) • Food- and nutrition-related knowledge deficit (NB-1.1) • Undesirable food choices (NB-1.7)
Etiology	• Poor intake of bioactive substance–containing foods • Excessive use of bioactive substance supplements
Signs and Symptoms	Food/Nutrition History • Nutrient intake analysis reveals bioactive substance intake more or less than recommended Client History • Medical diagnosis associated with increased bioactive substance need

Other considerations (e.g., patient/client negotiation, patient/client needs and desires, and readiness to change)

- Emerging scientific evidence to support the use of bioactive supplements in specific populations
- Availability of a qualified practitioner with additional education/training in the use of bioactive supplements in practice

References

1. Position of the American Dietetic Association: Functional foods. *J Am Diet Assoc*. 2004;104:814-826.

Feeding Assistance (ND-4)

Definition

Accommodation or assistance in eating designed to restore the patient /client's ability to eat independently, support adequate nutrient intake, and reduce the incidence of unplanned weight loss and dehydration.

Details of Intervention

A typical intervention might be further described with the following details:

- Recommend, implement, or order adaptive equipment, feeding position, feeding cues, meal set-up, or mouth care to facilitate eating
- Recommend, design, or implement a restorative dining program
- Recommend, design, or implement a feeding assistance training program
- Recommend, design, or implement menu selections that foster, promote, and maintain independent eating

Typically used with the following

Nutrition Diagnostic Terminology Used in PES Statements	Common Examples (not intended to be inclusive)
Nutrition Diagnoses	• Inadequate energy intake (NI-1.4) • Inadequate oral/food beverage intake (NI-2.1) • Involuntary weight loss (NC-3.2)
Etiology	• Physical disability • Poor food/nutrient intake • Decreased memory/concentration problems
Signs and Symptoms	Physical Examination Findings • Dropping the utensils or food • Weight loss Client History • Cerebral palsy, stroke, dementia • Refusal to use prescribed adaptive eating devices, or follow prescribed positioning techniques

Food and/or Nutrient Delivery Domain

Feeding Assistance (ND-4)

Other considerations (e.g., patient/client negotiation, patient/client needs and desires, and readiness to change)

- Acceptance of feeding assistance/feeding devices
- Poor environment to foster adequate intake
- Lack of individual to provide assistance at meal time
- Lack of training in methods of feeding assistance
- Lack of available physical therapy, occupational therapy, or speech therapy evaluations
- Ability to understand the reasoning behind the recommendations and then want to make personal changes

References

1. Consultant Dietitians in Health Care Facilities. *Eating Matters: A Training Manual for Feeding Assistants*. Chicago, IL: Consultant Dietitians in Health Care Facilities, American Dietetic Association; 2003.

2. Niedert K, Dorner B, eds. *Nutrition Care of the Older Adult*, 2nd edition. Chicago, IL: Consultant Dietitians in Health Care Facilities, American Dietetic Association; 2004.

3. Position of the American Dietetic Association: Liberalization of the diet prescription improves quality of life for older adults in long-term care. *J Am Diet Assoc*. 2005;105:1955-1965.

4. Position of the American Dietetic Association: Providing nutrition services for infants, children, and adults with developmental disabilities and special health care needs. *J Am Diet Assoc*. 2004;104:97-107.

5. Robinson GE, Leif B, eds. *Nutrition Management and Restorative Dining for Older Adults: Practical Interventions for Caregivers*. Chicago, IL: Consultant Dietitians in Health Care Facilities, American Dietetic Association; 2001.

6. Russell C, ed. *Dining Skills: Practical Interventions for the Caregivers of Older Adults with Eating Problems*. Chicago, IL: Consultant Dietitians in Health Care Facilities, American Dietetic Association; 2001.

7. Simmons SF, Osterweil D, and Schnelle JF. Improving food intake in nursing home residents with feeding assistance: A staffing analysis. *J Gerontol A Biol Sci Med Sci*. 2001;56:M790-M794.

8. Simmons SF, Schnelle JF. Individualized feeding assistance care for nursing home residents: Staffing requirements to implement two interventions. *J Gerontol A Biol Sci Med Sci*. 2004;59:M966-M973.

Feeding Environment (ND-5)

Definition
Adjustment of the physical environment, temperature, convenience, and attractiveness of the location where food is served that impacts food consumption.

Details of Intervention
A typical intervention might be further described with the following details:

- Recommend, implement, or order changes in table service/colors/set up/height, room temperature and lighting, meal schedule, menu choice, appetite enhancers, proper positioning, and minimize distractions and odors
- Recommend, implement, or order seating arrangements considering groupings that inspire social interactions

Typically used with the following

Nutrition Diagnostic Terminology Used in PES Statements	Common Examples (not intended to be inclusive)
Nutrition Diagnoses	• Inadequate oral food/beverage intake (NI-2.1) • Disordered eating pattern (NB-1.5) • Self-feeding difficulty (NB-2.6)
Etiology	• Dementia • Inability to stick to task/easily distracted by others
Signs and Symptoms	Food/Nutrition History • Changes in appetite attributed to mealtime surroundings • Easily distracted from eating • Food sanitation and safety issues • Available foods not of the patient's choosing • Decline in patient/client ability to eat independently Client History • Pacing, wandering, changes in affect

Other considerations (e.g., patient/client negotiation, patient/client needs and desires, and readiness to change)

- Resources available to improve/modify the feeding environment

Food and/or Nutrient Delivery Domain

Feeding Environment (ND-5)

References

1. Niedert K, Dorner B, eds. *Nutrition Care of the Older Adult*, 2nd edition. Chicago, IL: Consultant Dietitians in Health Care Facilities, American Dietetic Association; 2004.

2. Position of the American Dietetic Association: Liberalization of the diet prescription improves quality of life for older adults in long-term care. *J Am Diet Assoc*. 2005;105:1955-1965.

3. Position of the American Dietetic Association: Providing nutrition services for infants, children, and adults with developmental disabilities and special health care needs. *J Am Diet Assoc*. 2004;104:97-107.

4. Robinson GE, Leif B, eds. *Nutrition Management and Restorative Dining for Older Adults: Practical Interventions for Caregivers*. Chicago, IL: Consultant Dietitians in Health Care Facilities, American Dietetic Association; 2001.

5. Russell C, ed. *Dining Skills: Practical Interventions for the Caregivers of Older Adults with Eating Problems*. Consultant Dietitians in Health Care Facilities. Chicago, IL: American Dietetic Association; 2001.

Nutrition-Related Medication Management (ND-6)

Definition
Modification of a drug or herbal to optimize patient/client nutritional or health status.

Details of Intervention
A typical intervention might be further described with the following details:

- Recommend, implement, order initiation, changes in dose/form/route, change in administration schedule, or discontinuance of medications or herbals including insulin, appetite stimulants, digestive enzymes, or probiotics

Typically used with the following

Nutrition Diagnostic Terminology Used in PES Statements	Common Examples (not intended to be inclusive)
Nutrition Diagnoses	- Altered GI function (NC-1.4) - Impaired nutrient utilization (NC-2.1) - Food–medication interaction (NC-2.3)
Etiology	- Appetite insufficient resulting in adequate nutrient intake - Frequent hypo- or hyperglycemia - Pancreatic insufficiency - Malabsorption of fat, protein, lactose, or other carbohydrates - Polypharmacy and medication abuse - Drug toxicity
Signs and Symptoms	Physical Examination Findings - Thin, wasted appearance Food/Nutrition History - Sufficient oral intake - Report of herbal use Client History - Diabetes with poorly controlled blood sugar

Food and/or Nutrient Delivery Domain

Nutrition-Related Medication Management (ND-6)

Other considerations (e.g., patient/client negotiation, patient/client needs and desires, and readiness to change)

- Availability/access to a clinical pharmacist
- Availability of a qualified practitioner with appropriate pharmacology training and/or education

References

1. Position of the American Dietetic Association: Integration of medical nutrition therapy and pharmacotherapy. *J Am Diet Assoc*. 2003;103:1363-1370.
2. Kris-Etherton P, Pearson T. Over-the-counter statin medications: Emerging opportunities for RDs. *J Am Diet Assoc*. 2000;100:1126-1130.
3. Moyers B. Medications as adjunct therapy for weight loss: Approved and off-label agents in use. *J Am Diet Assoc*. 2005;105:948-959.

Initial/Brief Nutrition Education (E-1)

Definition
Instruction or training intended to build or reinforce basic nutrition-related knowledge, or to provide essential nutrition-related information until patient/client returns.

Details of Intervention
A typical intervention might be further described with the following details:

- Discuss the purpose of the nutrition education intervention
- Communicate relationship between nutrition and specific disease/health issue
- Begin instruction of nutrition issue of most concern to patient/client's health and well-being
- Provide basic nutrition-related educational information until client is able to return for comprehensive education

Typically used with the following

Nutrition Diagnostic Terminology Used in PES Statements	Common Examples (not intended to be inclusive)
Nutrition Diagnoses	• Food–medication interaction (NC-2.3) • Food- and nutrition-related knowledge deficit (NB-1.1) • Harmful beliefs/attitudes about food- or nutrition-related topics (NB-1.2) • Self-monitoring deficit (NB-1.4) • Other: Any diagnoses related to inadequate, excessive, inappropriate, or inconsistent intake
Etiology	• Capacity for learning • Knowledge deficit related to newly diagnosed medical condition • Interest and/or motivation • Medical or surgical procedure requiring modified diet • Unable to distinguish legitimate from false information
Signs and Symptoms	Food/Nutrition History • Unable to explain purpose of the nutrition prescription or rationale for nutrition prescription in relationship to disease/health • Expresses need for additional information or clarification of education or additional time to learn information • Unable to select appropriate foods or supplements • Unable to choose appropriate timing, volume, or preparation/handling of foods

Nutrition Education Domain

Initial/Brief Nutrition Education (E-1)

Other considerations (e.g., patient/client negotiation, patient/client needs and desires, and readiness to change)

- Met with several providers in one day and is unable or unwilling to receive more nutrition education at this time
- Profile reflects complicated situation warranting additional education/instruction
- Being discharged from the hospital
- Caregiver unavailable at time of nutrition education
- Baseline knowledge
- Learning style
- Other education and learning needs, e.g., new medication or other treatment administration

References

1. Position of the American Dietetic Association: Total diet approach to communicating food and nutrition information. *J Am Diet Assoc* 2007;107:1224-1232.
2. Holli BB, Calabrese RJ, O'Sullivan-Maillet J. *Communication and education skills for dietetics professionals.* 4th ed. New York, NY: Lipincott Williams and Wilkins; 2003.
3. Sahyoun NR, Pratt CA, Anderson A. Evaluation of nutrition education interventions for older adults: A proposed framework. *J Am Diet Assoc.* 2004;104:58-69.
4. Contento I. The effectiveness of nutrition education and implications for nutrition education policy, programs, and research: a review of research. *J Nutr Ed.* 1995;27: 279-283.
5. Medeiros LC, Butkus SN, Chipman H, Cox RH, Jones L, Little D. A logic model framework for community nutrition education. *J Nutr Educ Behav.* 2002;37: 197-202.

Comprehensive Nutrition Education (E-2)

Definition

Instruction or training intended to lead to in-depth nutrition-related knowledge and/or skills in given topics.

Details of Intervention

A typical intervention might be further described with the following details:

- Provide information related to purpose of the nutrition prescription
- Initiate thorough instruction of relationship between nutrition and disease/health
- Explain detailed or multiple nutrition prescription modifications recommended given patient/client situation
- Introduce more advanced nutrition topics related to patient/condition (e.g., saturated and trans fatty acid intake vs. total fat intake, menu planning, food purchasing)
- Support skill development (e.g., glucometer use, home tube feeding and feeding pump training, cooking skills/preparation)
- Commence training on interpreting medical or other results to modify nutrition prescription (e.g., distribution of carbohydrates throughout the day based on blood glucose monitoring results)

Typically used with the following

Nutrition Diagnostic Terminology Used in PES Statements	Common Examples (not intended to be inclusive)
Nutrition Diagnoses	• Food–medication interaction (NC-2.3) • Food- and nutrition-related knowledge deficit (NB-1.1) • Harmful beliefs/attitudes about food- or nutrition-related topics (NB-1.2) • Self-monitoring deficit (NB-1.4) • Other: Any diagnoses related to inadequate or excessive, inappropriate, or inconsistent intake
Etiology	• Deficient understanding of relevant nutrition-related topics • Exposure to incorrect food and nutrition information • Lack of skill in self management techniques
Signs and Symptoms	Food/Nutrition History • Expresses desire for knowledge/information • Food and nutrient intake assessment indicates food choice incompatible with recommendations

Nutrition Education Domain

Comprehensive Nutrition Education (E-2)

Other considerations (e.g., patient/client negotiation, patient/client needs and desires, and readiness to change)

- Profile reflects complicated situation warranting additional education/instruction
- Increased capacity and willingness to learn information
- Quality of life may be enhanced with in-depth nutrition education and understanding
- Baseline knowledge
- Lifestyle factors
- Education approaches that enhance knowledge/skill transfer

References

1. Position of the American Dietetic Association: Total diet approach to communicating food and nutrition information. *J Am Diet Assoc*. 2007;107:1224-1232.
2. Carmona RH. Improving health literacy: Preventing obesity with education. *J Am Diet Assoc*. 2005;105:S9-S10.
3. Contento I. The effectiveness of nutrition education and implications for nutrition education policy, programs, and research: a review of research. *J Nutr Educ*. 1995;27: 279-283.
4. Holli BB, Calabrese RJ, O'Sullivan-Maillet J. *Communication and education skills for dietetics professionals*. 4th ed. New York, NY: Lipincott Williams and Wilkins; 2003.
5. Holmes AL, Sanderson B, Maisiak R, Brown R, Bittner V. Dietitian services are associated with improved patient outcomes and the MEDFICTS dietary assessment questionnaire is a suitable outcome measure in cardiac rehabilitation. *J Am Diet Assoc*. 2005;105:1533-1540.
6. Medeiros LC, Butkus SN, Chipman H, Cox RH, Jones L, Little D. A logic model framework for community nutrition education. *J Nutr Educ Behav*. 2005;37:197-202.
7. Sahyoun NR, Pratt CA, Anderson A. Evaluation of nutrition education interventions for older adults: A proposed framework. *J Am Diet Assoc*. 2004;104:58-69.

Theoretical Basis/Approach (C-1)

Definition

The theories or models used to design and implement an intervention. Theories and theoretical models consist of principles, constructs and variables, which offer systematic explanations of the human behavior change process. Behavior change theories and models provide a research-based rationale for designing and tailoring nutrition interventions to achieve the desired effect. A theoretical framework for curriculum and treatment protocols, it guides determination of: 1) what information patients/clients need at different points in the behavior change process, 2) what tools and strategies may be best applied to facilitate behavior change, and 3) outcome measures to assess effectiveness in interventions or components of interventions.

Application Guidance

One or more of the following theories or theoretical models may influence a practitioner's counseling style or approach. Practitioners are asked to identify those theories (C-1) that most influence the intervention being documented. An intervention might also incorporate tools and strategies derived from a variety of behavior change theories and models. The practitioner is also asked to indicate which strategies (C-2) they used in a particular intervention session.

Details of Intervention

A typical intervention might be further described with the following details:

The following theories and models have proven valuable in providing a theoretical framework for evidence-based individual and interpersonal level nutrition interventions. Other theories may be useful for community level interventions (e.g., Community Organization, Diffusion of Innovations, Communication Theory).

- Cognitive-Behavioral Theory
- Health Belief Model
- Social Learning Theory
- Transtheoretical Model/Stages of Change

Additional information regarding each of the above theories and models can be found within this reference sheet.

Nutrition Counseling Domain

Theoretical Basis/Approach (C-1)

Typically used with the following

Nutrition Diagnostic Terminology Used in PES Statements	Common Examples (not intended to be inclusive)
Nutrition Diagnoses	• Overweight/obesity (NC-3.3) • Harmful beliefs/attitudes about food or nutrition-related topics (NB-1.2) • Not ready for diet/lifestyle change (NB-1.3) • Self-monitoring deficit (NB-1.4) • Disordered eating pattern (NB-1.5) • Limited adherence to nutrition-related recommendations (NB-1.6) • Undesirable food choices (NB-1.7) • Physical inactivity (NB-2.1) • Excessive exercise (NB-2.2) • Inability or lack of desire to manage self care (NB 2.3) • Poor nutrition quality of life (NB-2.5) • Other: Any diagnoses related to inadequate, excessive, inappropriate, or inconsistent intake
Etiology	• New medical diagnosis • Harmful beliefs/attitudes about food, nutrition, and nutrition-related topics • Lack of value for behavior change, competing values • Cultural/religious practices that interfere with implementation of the nutrition prescription • Lack of efficacy to make changes or to overcome barriers to change • Lack of focus/attention to detail, difficulty with time management and/or organization • Perception that time, interpersonal, or financial constraints prevent change • Prior exposure to incorrect or incompatible information • Not ready for diet/lifestyle change • Lack of caretaker or social support for implementing changes • High level of fatigue or other side effect of medical condition

Theoretical Basis/Approach (C-1)

Signs and Symptoms (Defining Characteristics)	Food/Nutrition History
	• Frustration with MNT recommendations
	• Previous failures to effectively change target behavior
	• Defensiveness, hostility, or resistance to change
	• Sense of lack of control of eating
	• Inability to apply food- and nutrition-related information/guidelines
	• Inability to change food- and nutrition-related behavior
	• Absent or incomplete self-monitoring records
	• Inability to problem-solve/self manage
	• Irrational thoughts about self and effects of food intake
	• Unrealistic expectations
	• Inflexibility with food selection
	• Evidence of excessive, inadequate, inappropriate, or inconsistent intake related to needs

Other considerations (e.g., patient/client negotiation, patient/client needs and desires, and readiness to change)

- Lifestyle factors
- Language barrier
- Educational level
- Culture
- Socioeconomic status

References

1. Glanz K. Current theoretical bases for nutrition intervention and their uses. In Coulston AM, Rock CL, Monsen E. *Nutrition in the Prevention and Treatment of Disease*. San Diego, CA: Academy Press; 2001:83-93.

2. U.S. Department of Health and Human Services, National Institutes of Health, National Cancer Institute. Theory at a Glance: A Guide for Health Promotion Practice, Spring 2005. Available at: http://www.cancer.gov/PDF/481f5d53-63df-41bc-bfaf-5aa48ee1da4d/TAAG3.pdf, Accessed on January 22, 2007.

3. Powers MA, Carstensen K, Colon K, Rickheim P, Bergenstal RM. Diabetes BASICS: education, innovation, revolution. *Diabetes Spectrum*. 2006;19:90-98.

4. Glanz K, Rimer BK, Lewis FM. *Health Behavior and Health Education: Theory Research and Practice,* 3rd ed. San Francisco, CA:Jossey-Bass Publishers; 2002.

Intervention

Nutrition Counseling Domain

Theoretical Basis/Approach (C-1)
Cognitive-Behavioral Theory

Description

Cognitive-behavioral theory (CBT) is based on the assumption that all behavior is learned and is directly related to internal factors (e.g., thoughts and thinking patterns) and external factors (e.g., environmental stimulus and reinforcement) that are related to the problem behaviors. Application involves use of both cognitive and behavioral change strategies to effect behavior change.

Implication for Counseling Interventions

CBT, derived from an educational model, is based upon the assumption that most emotional and behavioral reactions are learned and can be unlearned. The goal of CBT is to facilitate client identification of cognitions and behaviors that lead to inappropriate eating or exercise habits and replace these with more rational thoughts and actions.

The process is:
- Goal directed
- Process oriented
- Facilitated through a variety of problem solving tools

Behavioral and cognitive techniques to modify eating and exercise habits are taught for continuous application by the patient/client. Practitioners implement Cognitive-Behavioral Theory by partnering with clients to study their current environment to:
- Identify determinants or antecedents to behavior that contribute to inappropriate eating/exercise
- Identify resultant inappropriate behavior (e.g., overeating, vomiting)
- Analyze consequences of this behavior (cognitions, positive and negative reinforcers and punishments, e.g., decreased anxiety, feeling over full, losing or gaining weight)
- Make specific goals to modify the environment/cognitions to reduce target behaviors

Cognitive and behavioral strategies used to promote change in diet and physical activity may include:

- Goal setting
- Self-monitoring
- Problem solving
- Social support
- Stress management
- Stimulus control
- Cognitive restructuring
- Relapse prevention
- Rewards/contingency management

Theoretical Basis/Approach (C-1)
Cognitive-Behavioral Theory

References

1. Fabricatore AN. Behavior therapy and cognitive-behavioral therapy of obesity: Is there a difference? *J Am Diet Assoc*. 2007:107:92-99.

2. Brownell KD, Cohen LR. Adherence to Dietary Regimens 2: Components of effective interventions. *Behav Med*. 1995;20:155–163.

3. Kiy AM. Cognitive-behavioral and psychoeducational counseling and therapy. In: Helm KK, Klawitter B. *Nutrition Therapy: Advanced Counseling Skills*. Lake Dallas, TX: Helms Seminars; 1995:135-154.

4. Foster GD. Clinical implications for the treatment of obesity. *Obesity*. 2006;14:182S-185S.

5. Berkel LA, Poston WS 2d, Reeves RS, Foreyt JP. Behavioral interventions for obesity. *J Am Diet Assoc*. 2005;105:S35-S43.

Nutrition Counseling Domain

Theoretical Basis/Approach (C-1)
Health Belief Model

Description

The Health Belief Model is a psychological model, which focuses on an individual's attitudes and beliefs to attempt to explain and predict health behaviors. The HBM is based on the assumption that an individual will be motivated to take health-related action if that person 1) feels that a negative health condition (e.g., diabetes) can be avoided or managed, 2) has a positive expectation that by taking a recommended action, he/she will avoid negative health consequences (e.g., good blood glucose control will preserve eye sight), and believes he/she can successfully perform a recommended health action (e.g., I can use carbohydrate counting and control my diet).

Implication for Counseling Interventions

The Health Belief Model is particularly helpful to practitioners planning interventions targeted to individuals with clinical nutrition-related risk factors, such as diabetes, high blood cholesterol and/or hypertension. The six major constructs of the model have been found to be important in impacting an individual's motivation to take health-related action. The following table provides definitions and application guidance for the key constructs of the theory. Motivational interviewing strategies may be appropriate to address perceived susceptibility, severity, benefits and barriers. Behavioral strategies are most appropriate once the patient/client begins to take action to modify his/her diet.

These six constructs are useful components in designing behavior change programs. It is important for the practitioner to understand the patient's perception of the health threat and potential benefits of treatment. According to the HBM, an asymptomatic diabetic may not be compliant with his/her treatment regiment if he/she does not:

- believe he or she has diabetes (susceptibility)
- believe diabetes will seriously impact his/her life (perceived seriousness)
- believe following the diabetic diet will decrease the negative effects of diabetes (perceived benefits)
- believe the effort to follow the diet is worth the benefit to be gained (perceived barriers)
- have stimulus to initiate action (cue to action)
- have confidence in their ability to achieve success (self-efficacy)

Theoretical Basis/Approach (C-1)

Health Belief Model

Construct	Definition	Strategies
Perceived susceptibility	Client's belief or opinion of the personal threat a health condition represents for them; client opinion regarding whether they have the condition (e.g., diabetes or hypertension) or their chance of getting the disease or condition	• Educate on disease/condition risk factors • Tailor information to the client • Ask client if they think they are at risk or have the disease/condition • Guided discussions • Motivational interviewing (express empathy, open-ended questions, reflective listening, affirming, summarizing, and eliciting self-motivation statements)
Perceived severity	Client's belief about the impact a particular health threat will have on them and their lifestyle	• Educate on consequences of the disease/condition; show graphs, statistics • Elicit client response • Discuss potential impact on client's lifestyle • Motivational interviewing
Perceived benefits and barriers	Client's belief regarding benefits they will derive from taking nutrition-related action; perceived benefits versus barriers--client's perception of whether benefits will outweigh the sacrifices and efforts involved in behavior change	• Clearly define benefits of nutrition therapy • Role models, testimonials • Explore ambivalence and barriers • Imagine the future • Explore successes • Summarize and affirm the positive
Cues to action	Internal or external triggers that motivate or stimulate action	• How-to education • Incentive programs • Link current symptoms to disease/condition • Discuss media information • Reminder phone calls/mailings • Social support
Self-efficacy	Client confidence in their ability to successfully accomplish the necessary action	• Skill training/demonstration • Introduce alternatives and choices • Behavior contracting; small, incremental goals • Coaching, verbal reinforcement

Nutrition Counseling Domain

Theoretical Basis/approach (C-1)
Health Belief Model

References

1. Glanz K. Current theoretical bases for nutrition intervention and their uses. In Coulston AM, Rock CL, Monsen E. *Nutrition in the Prevention and Treatment of Disease*. San Diego, Ca: Academy Press; 2001:83-93.

2. U.S. Department of Health and Human Services, National Institutes of Health, National Cancer Institute. Theory at a Glance: A Guide for Health Promotion Practice, Spring 2005. Available at: http://www.cancer.gov/PDF/481f5d53-63df-41bc-bfaf-5aa48ee1da4d/TAAG3.pdf, Accessed on January 22, 2007.

3. Powers MA, Carstensen K, Colon K, Rickheim P, Bergenstal RM. Diabetes BASICS: education, innovation, revolution. *Diabetes Spectrum*. 2006;19:90-98.

Theoretical Basis/Approach (C-1)
Social Learning Theory

Description
Social learning theory, also known as Social Cognitive Theory, provides a framework for understanding, predicting, and changing behavior. The theory identifies a dynamic, reciprocal relationship between environment, the person, and behavior. The person can be both an agent for change and a responder to change. It emphasizes the importance of observing and modeling behaviors, attitudes and emotional reactions of others. Determinants of behavior include goals, outcome expectations and self-efficacy. Reinforcements increase or decrease the likelihood that the behavior will be repeated (1).

Implication for Counseling Interventions
Social Learning Theory is rich in concepts applicable to nutrition counseling. The following table provides definitions and application guidance for the key concepts of the theory.

Concept	Definition	Strategies
Reciprocal Determinism	A person's ability to change a behavior is influenced by characteristics within the person (e.g., beliefs), the environment, and the behavior itself (e.g., difficulty doing the behavior). All three interact to influence if the behavior change will happen.	• Consider multiple behavior change strategies targeting motivation, action, the individual and the environment: • Motivational interviewing • Social support • Stimulus control • Demonstration • Skill development training/coaching
Behavioral Capability	The knowledge and skills that are needed for a person to change behavior	• Comprehensive education • Demonstration • Skill development training/coaching
Expectations	For a person to do a behavior, they must believe that the behavior will result in outcomes important to them	• Motivational interviewing • Model positive outcomes of diet/exercise

Nutrition Counseling Domain

Theoretical Basis/Approach (C-1)

Social Learning Theory

Self-Efficacy	Confidence in ability to take action and persist in action	• Break task down to component parts • Demonstration/modeling • Skill development training/coaching • Reinforcement • Small, incremental goals/behavioral contracting
Observational Learning	When a person learns how to do a behavior by watching credible others do the same behavior	• Demonstrations • Role modeling • Group problem-solving sessions
Reinforcement	Response to a behavior that will either increase or decrease the likelihood that the behavior will be repeated	• Affirm accomplishments • Encourage self reward/self-reinforcement • Incentives for process components of change (e.g., keeping a food diary)

References

1. Glanz K. Current theoretical bases for nutrition intervention and their uses. In Coulston AM, Rock CL, Monsen E. *Nutrition in the Prevention and Treatment of Disease*. San Diego, Ca: Academy Press; 2001:83-93.

2. U.S. Department of Health and Human Services, National Institutes of Health, National Cancer Institute. Theory at a Glance: A Guide for Health Promotion Practice, Spring 2005. Available at: http://www.cancer.gov/PDF/481f5d53-63df-41bc-bfaf-5aa48ee1da4d/TAAG3.pdf. Accessed on January 22, 2007.

3. Bandura A. *Social Foundations of Thought and Action: A Social Cognitive Theory*. Englewood Cliffs, NJ: Prentice-Hall; 1986.

4. Bandura A. *Self-Efficacy: The Exercise of Control*. New York, NY: W.H. Freeman; 1997.

5. Glanz K, Rimer BK, Lewis FM. *Health Behavior and Health Education: Theory Research and Practice*, 3rd ed. San Francisco, Ca:Jossey-Bass Publishers, 2002.

Theoretical Basis/Approach (C-1)
Transtheoretical Model/Stages of Change

Definition

A theoretical model of intentional health behavior change that describes a sequence of cognitive (attitudes and intentions) and behavioral steps people take in successful behavior change. The model, developed by Prochaska and DiClemente, is composed of a core concept known as Stages of Change, a series of independent variables, the Processes of Change, and outcome measures including decision balance and self-efficacy. The model has been used to guide development of effective interventions for a variety of health behaviors.

Implication for Counseling Interventions

One of the defining characteristics of this model is that it describes behavior change not as a discrete event (e.g., today I am going to stop overeating), but as something that occurs in stages, over time. The five stages reflect an individual's attitudes, intentions and behavior related to change of a specific behavior and include the following:

- Precontemplation – no recognition of need for change; no intention to take action within the next 6 months
- Contemplation – recognition of need to change; intends to take action within the next 6 months
- Preparation – intends to take action in the next 30 days and has taken some behavioral steps in that direction
- Action – has made changes in target behavior for less than 6 months
- Maintenance – has changed target behavior for more than 6 months

Determination of a patient/client stage of change is relatively simple, involving a few questions regarding intentions and current diet. One of the appealing aspects of the theory is that the Process of Change construct describes cognitive and behavioral activities or strategies, which may be applied at various stages to move a person forward through the stages of change. This movement is not always linear, and patients can cycle in and out of various stages. The model has been used to effectively tailor interventions to the needs of clients at various stages. Knowing a patient/client's stage of change can help a practitioner determine:

- Whether intervention now is appropriate
- The type and content of intervention to use (motivational versus action oriented)
- Appropriate and timely questions about past efforts, pros and cons of change, obstacles, challenges and potential strategies
- The amount of time to spend with the patient

The following table provides guidance for applying stages and processes of change to the adoption of healthful diets.

Nutrition Counseling Domain

Theoretical Basis/Approach (C-1)
Transtheoretical Model/Stages of Change

Table 3

General guidelines for applying stages and processes of change ot adoption of heathful diets

State of readiness	Key strategies for moving to next stage	Treatment do's at this stage	Treatment don'ts at this stage
Precontemplation	Increased information and awareness, emotional acceptance	• Provide personalized information. • Allow client to express emotions about his or her disease or about the need to make dietary changes.	• Do not assume client has knowledge or expect that providing information will automatically lead to behavior change. • Do not ignore client's emotional adjustment to the need for dietary change, which could override ability to process relevant information.
Contemplation	Increased confidence in one's ability to adopt recommended behaviors	• Discuss and resolve barriers to dietary change. • Encourage support networks. • Give positive feedback about a client's abilities. • Help to clarify ambivalence about adopting behavior and emphasize expected benefits.	• Do not ignore the potential impact of family menbers, and others, or client's ability to comply. • Do not be alarmed or critical of a client's ambivalence.
Preparation	Resolution of abivalence, firm commitment, and specific action plan	• Encourage client to set specific, achievable goals (e.g., use 1% milk instead of whole milk). • Reinforce small changes that client may have already achieved.	• Do not recommend general behavior changes (e.g., "Eat less fat"). • Do not refer to small changes as "not good enough."
Action	Behavioral skill training and social support	• Refer to education program for self-management skills. • Provide self-help materials.	• Do not refer clients to information-only classes.
Maintenance	Problem-solving skills and social and environmental support	• Encourage client to anticipate and plan for potential difficulties (e.g., maintaining dietary changes on vacation). • Collect information about local resources (e.g., support groups, shopping guides). • Encourage client to "recycle" if he or she has a lapse or relapse. • Recommend more challenging dietary changes if client is motivated.	• Do not assume that intial action means permanent change. • Do not be discouraged or judgmental about a lapse or relapse.

Source: Kristal AR, Glanz K, Curry S, Patterson RE. How can stages of change be best used in dietary interventions? *J Am Diet Assoc.*1999;99:683.

Theoretical Basis/Approach (C-1)
Transtheoretical Model/Stages of Change

Prochaska recommends the following strategies, which target motivation, be used in the early stages of change: consciousness raising, dramatic relief (e.g., emotional arousal via role playing or personal testimonials), environmental reevaluation (e.g., empathy training and family interactions), social liberation (e.g., advocacy, empowerment) and self-reevaluation (e.g., value clarification, healthy role models and imagery). These strategies are very consistent with motivational interviewing techniques. In the later stages of change, behavioral strategies are most appropriate.

References

1   Kristal AR, Glanz K, Curry S, Patterson RE. How can stages of change be best used in dietary interventions? *J Am Diet Assoc*. 1999;99:679-684.

2. Nothwehr F, Snetselaar L, Yang J, Wu H. Stage of change for healthful eating and use of behavioral strategies. *J Am Diet Assoc*. 2006;106:1035-1041.

3. Green GW, Rossi SR, Rossi JS, Velicer WF, Fava JL, Prochaska JO. Dietary applications of the stages of change model. *J Am Diet Assoc*. 1999;99:673-678.

4. Glanz K. Current theoretical bases for nutrition intervention and their uses. In Coulston AM, Rock CL, Monsen E. *Nutrition in the Prevention and Treatment of Disease*. San Diego, CA: Academy Press; 2001:83-93.

5. Prochaska JO, Norcross JC, DiClemente V. *Changing for Good: A Revolutionary Six-Stage Program for Overcoming Bad Habits and Moving Your Life Positively Forward*. New York, NY: Avon Books Inc; 1994

Strategies (C-2)

Definition

An evidence-based method or plan of action designed to achieve a particular goal. Application of behavior change theories in nutrition practice has provided practitioners with a collection of evidence-based strategies to promote behavior change. Some strategies target change in motivation and intention to change, and others target behavior change. Practitioners selectively apply strategies based upon patient/client goals and objectives, and their personal counseling philosophy and skill.

Application Guidance

An intervention typically incorporates tools and strategies derived from a variety of behavior change theories and models. The practitioner is asked to indicate which strategies (C-2) he/she used in a particular intervention session along with the theories (C-1), which most influence the intervention being documented.

Details of Intervention

A typical intervention might be further described with the following details:

The following strategies have proven valuable in providing effecting nutrition-related behavior change.

- Motivational interviewing
- Goal setting
- Self-monitoring
- Problem solving
- Social support
- Stress management
- Stimulus control
- Cognitive restructuring
- Relapse prevention
- Rewards/contingency management

Additional information regarding each of the above strategies can be found within this reference sheet.

Strategies (C-2)

Typically used with the following

Nutrition Diagnostic Terminology Used in PES Statements	Common Examples (not intended to be inclusive)
Nutrition Diagnoses	• Overweight/obesity (NC-3.3) • Harmful beliefs/attitudes about food or nutrition-related topics (NB-1.2) • Not ready for diet/lifestyle change (NB-1.3) • Self-monitoring deficit (NB-1.4) • Disordered eating pattern (NB-1.5) • Limited adherence to nutrition-related recommendations (NB-1.6) • Undesirable food choices (NB-1.7) • Physical inactivity (NB-2.1) • Excessive exercise (NB-2.2) • Inability or lack of desire to manage self care (NB 2.3) • Poor nutrition quality of life (NB-2.5) • Other: Any diagnoses related to inadequate, excessive, inappropriate, or inconsistent intake
Etiology	• New medical diagnosis • Harmful beliefs/attitudes about food, nutrition, and nutrition-related topics • Lack of value for behavior change, competing values • Cultural/religious practices that interfere with implementation of the nutrition prescription • Lack of efficacy to make changes or to overcome barriers to change • Lack of focus/attention to detail, difficulty with time management and/or organization • Perception that time, interpersonal, or financial constraints prevent change • Prior exposure to incorrect or incompatible information • Not ready for diet/lifestyle change • Lack of caretaker or social support for implementing changes • High level of fatigue or other side effect of medical condition

Nutrition Counseling Domain

Strategies (C-2)

Signs and Symptoms *(Defining Characteristics)*	Food/Nutrition History
	• Frustration with MNT recommendations
	• Previous failures to effectively change target behavior
	• Defensiveness, hostility, or resistance to change
	• Sense of lack of control of eating
	• Inability to apply food- and nutrition-related information/guidelines
	• Inability to change food- and nutrition-related behavior
	• Absent or incomplete self-monitoring records
	• Inability to problem-solve/self manage
	• Irrational thoughts about self and effects of food intake
	• Unrealistic expectations
	• Inflexibility with food selection
	• Evidence of excessive, inadequate, inappropriate, or inconsistent intake related to needs

Other considerations (e.g., patient/client negotiation, patient/client needs and desires, and readiness to change)

- Lifestyle factors
- Language barrier
- Educational level
- Culture
- Socioeconomic status

References

1. Glanz K. Current theoretical bases for nutrition intervention and their uses. In Coulston AM, Rock CL, Monsen E. *Nutrition in the Prevention and Treatment of Disease*. San Diego, CA: Academy Press; 2001:83-93.
2. U.S. Department of Health and Human Services, National Institutes of Health, National Cancer Institute. Theory at a Glance: A Guide for Health Promotion Practice, Spring 2005. Available at: http://www.cancer.gov/PDF/481f5d53-63df-41bc-bfaf-5aa48ee1da4d/TAAG3.pdf, Accessed on January 22, 2007.
3. Powers MA, Carstensen K, Colon K, Rickheim P, Bergenstal RM. Diabetes BASICS: education, innovation, revolution. *Diabetes Spectrum*. 2006;19:90-98.
4. Glanz K, Rimer BK, Lewis FM. *Health Behavior and Health Education: Theory Research and Practice*, 3rd ed. San Francisco, CA: Jossey-Bass Publishers, 2002.

Strategies (C-2)

Strategy descriptions and application guidance

Strategy	Description	Implementation Tips
Motivational interviewing	A directive, client-centered counseling style for eliciting behavior change by helping clients to explore and resolve ambivalence (1). The approach involves selective response to client speech in a way that helps the client resolve ambivalence and move toward change. The four guiding principles that underlie this counseling approach include: • Express empathy • Develop discrepancy • Roll with resistance • Support self-efficacy. The following specific practitioner behaviors are characteristic of the MI style (2): • Expressing acceptance and affirmation • Eliciting and selectively reinforcing the client's own self motivational statements, expressions of problem recognition, concern, desire, intention to change, and ability to change • Monitoring the client's degree of readiness to change, and ensuring that jumping ahead of the client does not generate resistance • Affirming the client's freedom of choice and self-direction The source of motivation is presumed to reside within the client and the counselor encourages the client to explore ambivalence, motivation and possibilities to change, so it is the client who chooses what to change, determines the change plan and strategy. MI is an evidence-based counseling strategy which builds on Carl Roger's client-centered counseling model, Prochaska and DiClemente's transtheoretical model of change, Milton Rokeach's human values theory and Daryl Bern's theory of self-perception.	Tone of counseling: • Partnership • Nonjudgmental • Empathetic/supportive/encouraging • Nonconfrontational • Quiet and eliciting The client does most of the talking and the counselor guides the client to explore and resolve ambivalence by: • Asking open ended questions • Listening reflectively • Summarizing • Affirming • Eliciting self-motivational statements • Shared agenda setting/decision making • Allowing clients to interpret information • Rolling with resistance, rather than confronting • Building discrepancy • Eliciting "change talk" • Negotiating a change plan Motivational interviewing is best applied in situations when a patient is not ready, is unwilling or ambivalent about changing their diet or lifestyle. MI integrates well with the readiness to change model to move individuals from the early stages to the action stage of change. MI is a major paradigm change from the problem solving oriented counseling frequently employed by practitioners. MI is not a set of techniques that can be learned quickly, but a style or approach to counseling.

Nutrition Counseling Domain

Strategies (C-2)

Goal setting	A collaborative activity between the client and the practitioner in which the client decides from all potential activity recommendations what changes he/she will expend effort to implement.	• Appropriate for patients ready to make dietary changes • Coach on goal setting skills • Document and track progress toward short-term and long-term goals • Probe client about pros and cons of proposed goals • Assist client in gaining the knowledge and skills necessary to succeed • Encourage strategies to build confidence (discuss realistic steps and start with easily achievable goals) • Aid clients in building a supportive environment • Celebrate successes
Self-monitoring	A technique that involves keeping a detailed record of behaviors that influence diet and/or weight and may include: • What, when, how much eaten • Activities during eating • Emotions and cognitions related to meals/snacks • Frequency, duration and intensity of exercise • Target nutrient content of foods consumed (i.e., calories, fat, fiber) • Event, thoughts about event, emotional response, behavioral response • Negative self-talk, replacement thoughts • Blood glucose, blood pressure Self-monitoring is associated with improved treatment outcomes.	• Provide rationale and instructions for self-monitoring • Review and identify patterns • Assist with problem solving and goal setting • Celebrate successes • The amount of feedback required typically diminishes as patient/client skill improves
Problem solving	Techniques that are taught to assist clients in identifying barriers to achieving goals, identifying and implementing solutions and evaluating the effectiveness of the solutions (2).	Work collaboratively with client to: • Define the problem • Brainstorm solutions • Weigh pros/cons of potential solutions • Select/implement strategy • Evaluate outcomes • Adjust strategy

Strategies (C-2)

Social support	Increased availability of social support for dietary behavior change. Social support may be generated among an individual's family, church, school, co-workers, health club or community.	A dietetics practitioner may assist a client by: • Establishing a collaborative relationship • Identifying family/community support • Assisting clients in developing assertiveness skills. • Utilize modeling, skill training, respondent and operant conditioning • Conducting education in a group • Encourage family involvement
Stress management	Reaction to stress can cause some clients to loss their appetite and others to overeat. Dietetics practitioners are particularly interested in management of stressful situations, which result in inappropriate eating behaviors.	Two approaches may be used to manage stress, one focuses on changing the environment, and the other focuses on modifying the client's response to stress. Environmental-focused strategies may include: • Guidance on planning ahead • Use of time-management skills • Developing a support system • Building skills to prepare quick and healthful meals • Guidance on eating on the run Emotion-focused strategies may include: • Use of positive self-talk • Building assertiveness in expressing eating desires • Setting realistic goals • Learning to deal appropriately with emotion-driven eating cravings • Relaxation exercises

Nutrition Counseling Domain

Strategies (C-2)

Stimulus control	Identifying and modifying social or environmental cues or triggers to act, which encourage undesirable behaviors relevant to diet and exercise. In accordance with operant conditioning principles, attention is given to reinforcement and rewards.	Review of self-monitoring records with clients may help to identify triggers for undesirable eating Assist client in identifying ways to modify the environment to eliminate triggers. This may include things such as: • Keeping food out of sight • Removing high sugar/high fat snacks from the house • Bringing lunch to work • Establishing a rule – no eating in the car • Help client establish criteria for rewards for desirable behavior • Ensure reward (reinforcement) received only if criteria met
Cognitive restructuring	Techniques used to increase client awareness of their perceptions of themselves and their beliefs related to diet, weight and weight loss expectations.	Self-monitoring and techniques such as the ABC Technique of Irrational Beliefs may help clients to become more aware of thoughts that interfere in their ability to meet behavioral goals Help clients replace dysfunctional thoughts with more rationale ones: • Challenge shoulds, oughts, musts • Decatastrophize expected outcomes • Confront faulty self-perceptions • Decenter by envisioning other perspectives Coach clients on replacing negative self-talk with more positive, empowering and affirming statements
Relapse prevention	Techniques used to help clients prepare to address high-risk situations for relapse with appropriate strategies and thinking. Incorporates both cognitive and behavioral strategies to enhance long-term behavior change outcomes.	Assist clients: • Assess if external circumstances are contributing to lapse e.g., loss of job or support system • Identify high-risk situations for slips • Analyze reactions to slips • Acquire knowledge and skills necessary to address high-risk situations • Gain confidence in their ability to succeed in high-risk situations

Strategies (C-2)

Rewards/contingency management	A **systematic** process by which behaviors can be changed through the use of rewards for specific actions. Rewards may be derived from the client or the provider.	• Provide rewards for desired behaviors e.g., attendance, diet progress, consistent self-monitoring • Rewards can be monetary, prizes, parking space, gift certificates • Assist clients in determining rewards for achievement • Ensure rewards are not received if progress is not made

References

1. Miller WR, Rollnick S. *Motivational Interviewing: Preparing People for Change*. 2nd ed., New York: Guilford Press; 2002

2. Miller WR, Rollnick. S Motivational Interviewing: resources for clinicians, researchers and trainers. Available at: http://www.motivationalinterview.org/clinical/. Accessed January 12, 2007

3. Berg-Smith SM, Stevens VJ, Brown KM, Van Horn L, Gernhofer N, Peters E, Greenberg R, Snetselaar L, Ahrens L, Smith K for the Dietary Intervention Study in Children (DISC) Research Group. A brief motivational intervention to improve dietary adherence in adolescents. *Health Educ Res*. 1999; 14:399-410.

4. Snetselaar L. Counseling for change. In: Mahan LK, Escott-Stump S, eds. *Krause's Food, Nutrition, & Diet Therapy*. 10th ed. Philadelphia: Saunders; 2000.

5. Brug J, Spikmans F, Aartsen C, Breedbveld B, Bes R, Fereira I. Training dietitians in basic motivational interviewing skills results in changes in their counseling style and in lower saturated fat intakes in their patients. *J Nutr Ed Behav*. 2007;39:8-12.

6. DiLillo V, Siegfried NJ, West DS. Incorporating motivational interviewing into behavioral obesity training. *Cogn Behav Prac*. 2003;10:120-130

7. National Heart, Lung, and Blood Institute, National Institute of Diabetes and Digestive and Kidney Diseases. *Clinical Guidelines on the Identification, Evaluation, and Treatment of Overweight and Obesity in Adults: The Evidence Report*. Washington, DC: U.S. Government Printing Office. 1998. Guidelines available at http://www.nhlbi.nih.gov/guidelines/obesity/ob_gdlns.htm.

8. Estabrooks P, Nelson C, Xu S, King D, Bayliss E, Gaglio B, Nutting P, Glasgow R. the frequency and behavioral outcomes of goal choices in the self-management of diabetes. *Diabetes Educ*. 2005;31(3):391-400.

9. Boutelle KN, Kirschenbaum DS. Further support for consistent self-monitoring as a vital component of successful weight control. *Obes Res*. 1998;52:219-224.

10. Foster GD. Clinical implications for the treatment of obesity. *Obesity*. 2006;14:182S-185S.

11. Brownell KD, Cohen LR. Adherence to Dietary Regimens 2: components of effective interventions. *Behav Med*. 1995; 20: 155–163.

12. D'Zurilla TJ, Goldfried MR. Problem solving and behavior modification. *J Abnorm Psychol*. 1971;78:107-126.

13. Barrere M, Toobert D, Angell K, Glasgow R, Mackinnon D. Social support and social-ecological resources as mediators of lifestyle intervention effects for type 2 diabetes. *J Health Psychol*. 2006;11:483-495.

14. Berkel LA, Poston WS 2d, Reeves RS, Foreyt JP. Behavioral Interventions for Obesity. *J Am Diet Assoc*. 2005;105: S35-S43.

15. Snetselaar L. *Nutritional Counseling for Lifestyle Change*. New York:Taylor & Francis Group; 2007: 117-119.

16. Snetselaar LG. *Nutrition Counseling Skills for Medical Nutrition Therapy*. 2nd ed. Gaithersburg, MD: Aspen Press; 2007

17. Fabricatore AN. Behavior therapy and cognitive-behavioral therapy of obesity: Is there a difference? *J Am Diet Assoc*. 2007:107:92-99.

18. Kiy AM. Cognitive-behavioral and psychoeducational counseling and therapy. In: Helm KK, Klawitter B. *Nutrition Therapy: Advanced Counseling Skills*. Lake Dallas, TX: Helms Seminars: 1995:135-154.

19. Irvin JE, Bowers CA, Dunn ME, Wang MC. Efficacy of relapse prevention: A meta-analytic review. *J Consult Clin Psychol*. 1999;67:563-570.

20. Prochaska JO, Norcross JC, DiClemente V. *Changing for Good: A Revolutionary Six-Stage Program for Overcoming Bad Habits and Moving Your Life Positively Forward*. New York, NY: Avon Books Inc; 1994.

Intervention

Coordination of Other Care During Nutrition Care (RC-1)

Definition
Facilitating services or interventions with other professionals, institutions, or agencies on behalf of the patient/client prior to discharge from nutrition care.

Details of Intervention
A typical intervention might be further described with the following details:

- Holding a team meeting to develop a comprehensive plan of care
- A formal referral for care by other dietetics practitioners who provide different expertise
- Collaboration with or referral to others such as the physician, dentist, physical therapist, social worker, occupational therapist, speech therapist, nurse, pharmacist, or other specialist dietitian
- Referral to an appropriate agency/program (e.g., home delivered meals, WIC, food pantry, soup kitchen, food stamps, housing assistance, shelters, rehabilitation, physical and mental disability programs, education training, and employment programs)

Typically used with the following

Nutrition Diagnostic Terminology Used in PES Statements	Common Examples (not intended to be inclusive)
Nutrition Diagnoses	- Inadequate oral food and beverage intake (NI 2.1) - Involuntary weight loss (NC-3.2) - Excessive alcohol intake (NI-4.3) - Inappropriate intake of food fats (NI-5.6.3) - Overweight/obesity (NC-3.3) - Physical inactivity (NB-2.1) - Food–medication interaction (NC-2.3) - Self-feeding difficulty (NB-2.6) - Limited access to food (NB-3.2)

Coordination of Other Care During Nutrition Care (RC-1)

Etiology	Physical Examination Findings • Physical disability with impaired feeding ability, other impairments related to activities of daily living • Growth and development issues Food/Nutrition History • Inadequate intake • Nutrient drug interactions Psychological/Social History • Transportation issues • Food acceptance issues • Developmental issues • Economic considerations impacting food/nutrient intake
Signs and Symptoms	Physical Examination Findings • Weight loss • Unacceptable growth rates compared to standard growth charts Food/Nutrition History • More than 10% weight loss in 6 months • Hyperglycemia and weight loss • Poor wound healing • Client History • Inability to procure food • Anorexia nervosa • Lack of access to food sources • Lack of food preparation skills

Coordination of Nutrition Care Domain

Coordination of Other Care During Nutrition Care (RC-1)

Other considerations (e.g., patient/client negotiation, patient/client needs and desires, and readiness to change)

- Availability of services related to patient/client need (specialty dietitians, clinical pharmacists, speech pathologists, nurse practitioners, etc.)
- Anticipated duration of health care encounter/hospital or long-term care discharge
- Resources available for care
- Medicare/Medicaid/insurance guidelines and restrictions
- Food assistance program (e.g., food stamp program) guidelines and regulations

References

1. Position of the American Dietetic Association. Nutrition, aging, and the continuum of care. *J Am Diet Assoc*. 2000;100:580-595.
2. McLaughlin C, Tarasuk V, Kreiger N. An examination of at-home food preparation activity among low-income, food insecure women. *J Am Diet Assoc*. 2003;103:1506-1512.
3. Greger JL, Maly A, Jensen N, Kuhn J, Monson K, Stocks A. Food pantries can provide nutritionally adequate food packets but need help to become effective referral units for public assistance programs. *J Am Diet Assoc*. 2002;102:1125-1128.
4. Olson CM, Holben DH. Position of the American Dietetic Association: Domestic food and nutrition security. *J Am Diet Assoc*. 2002;102:1840-1847.
5. Millen BE, Ohls JC, Ponza M, McCool AC. The elderly nutrition program: An effective national framework for preventive nutrition interventions. *J Am Diet Assoc*. 2002;102:234-240.

Discharge and Transfer of Nutrition Care to a New Setting or Provider (RC-2)

Definition

Discharge planning and transfer of nutrition care from one level or location of care to another.

Details of Intervention

A typical intervention might be further described with the following details:

- Change in the nutrition prescription with consideration for changes in patient/client schedule, activity level, and food/nutrient availability in the new setting
- Collaboration with or referral to others such as the physician, dentist, physical therapist, social worker, occupational therapist, speech therapist, nurse, pharmacist, or other specialist dietitian
- Referral to an appropriate agency/program (e.g., home delivered meals, WIC, food pantry, soup kitchen, food stamps, housing assistance, shelters, rehabilitation, physical and mental disability programs, education, training and employment programs)

Typically used with the following

Nutrition Diagnostic Terminology Used in PES Statements	Common Examples (not intended to be inclusive)
Nutrition Diagnoses	• Inadequate oral food/beverage intake (NI-2.1)
	• Imbalance of nutrients (NI-5.5)
	• Inappropriate intake of fats (NI-5.6.3)
	• Food–medication interaction (NC-2.3)
	• Underweight (NC-3.1)
	• Overweight/obesity (NC-3.3)
	• Impaired ability to prepare foods/meals (NB-2.4)
	• Self-feeding difficulty (NB-2.6)
Etiology	Food/Nutrition History
	• Long-term insufficient intake mandating home enteral or parenteral nutrition
	• Growth and development considerations requiring intervention in a new setting

Edition: 2009

Intervention

Coordination of Nutrition Care Domain

Discharge and Transfer of Nutrition Care to a New Setting or Provider (RC-2)

Signs and Symptoms	Biochemical Data, Medical Tests and Procedures
	• Abnormal lab values
	Anthropometric Measurements
	• Inappropriate weight status
	• Continuing weight gain or loss
	Food/Nutrition History
	• Inappropriate dietary practices
	• Harmful beliefs and attitudes
	Client History
	• Treatment failure
	• Readmission

Other considerations (e.g., patient/client negotiation, patient/client needs and desires, and readiness to change)

- Availability of discharge planning services, options for care
- Preferences for the level and location of care
- Resources available for care
- Medicare/Medicaid/insurance guidelines and restrictions
- Health literacy
- Ability to implement treatment at home
- Food assistance program (e.g., food stamp program) guidelines and regulations

References

1. Baker EB, Wellman NS. Nutrition concerns for discharge planning for older adults: A need for multidisciplinary collaboration. *J Am Diet Assoc*. 2005;105:603-607.
2. Position of the American Dietetic Association. Nutrition, aging, and the continuum of care. *J Am Diet Assoc*. 2000;100:580-595.

SNAPshot

NCP Step 4. Nutrition Monitoring and Evaluation

What is the purpose of Nutrition Monitoring and Evaluation? The purpose is to determine the amount of progress made and whether goals/expected outcomes are being met. Nutrition monitoring and evaluation identifies patient/client* outcomes relevant to the nutrition diagnosis and intervention plans and goals. Nutrition care outcomes—the desired results of nutrition care—are defined in this step. The change in specific nutrition care indicators, through assessment and reassessment, can be measured and compared to the patient/client's previous status, nutrition intervention goals, or reference standards. The aim is to promote more uniformity within the dietetics profession in assessing the effectiveness of nutrition intervention.

How does a dietetics practitioner determine what to measure for Nutrition Monitoring and Evaluation? Practitioners select nutrition care indicators that will reflect a change as a result of nutrition care. In addition, dietetics practitioners will consider factors such as the nutrition diagnosis and its etiology and signs or symptoms, the nutrition intervention, medical diagnosis, health care outcome goals, quality management goals for nutrition, practice setting, patient/client population, and disease state and/or severity.

How are outcomes used in Nutrition Monitoring and Evaluation organized? In four categories**:

Food/Nutrition-Related History Outcomes	Biochemical Data, Medical Tests, and Procedure Outcomes	Anthropometric Measurement Outcomes	Nutrition-Focused Physical Finding Outcomes
Food and nutrient intake, medication/herbal supplement intake, knowledge, beliefs, food and supplies availability, physical activity, nutrition quality of life	*Lab data (e.g., electrolytes, glucose) and tests (e.g., gastric emptying time, resting indices/percentile ranks, and metabolic rate)*	*Height, weight, body mass index (BMI), growth pattern weight history*	*Physical appearance, muscle and fat wasting, swallow function, appetite, and affect*

What does Nutrition Monitoring and Evaluation involve? Practitioners do three things as part of nutrition monitoring and evaluation—monitor, measure, and evaluate the changes in nutrition care indicators—to determine patient/client progress. Practitioners monitor by providing evidence that the nutrition intervention is or is not changing the patient/client's behavior or status. They measure outcomes by collecting data on the appropriate nutrition outcome indicator(s). Finally, dietetics practitioners compare the current findings with previous status, nutrition intervention goals, and/or reference standards (i.e., criteria) and evaluate the overall impact of the nutrition intervention on the patient/client's health outcomes. The use of standardized indicators and criteria increases the validity and reliability outcome data are collected. All these procedures facilitate electronic charting, coding, and outcomes measurement.

Critical thinking during this step…

- Selecting appropriate indicators/measures
- Using appropriate reference standards for comparison
- Defining where patient/client is in terms of expected outcomes
- Explaining a variance from expected outcomes
- Determining factors that help or hinder progress
- Deciding between discharge and continuation of nutrition care

Are dietetics practitioners limited to the Nutrition Monitoring and Evaluation outcomes terms? A cascade of outcomes of nutrition care have been identified; each outcome has several possible indicators that can be measured depending on the patient/client population, practice setting, and disease state/severity. Dietetics practitioners can propose additions or revisions using the Procedure for Nutrition Controlled Vocabulary/Terminology Maintenance/Review available from ADA.

Detailed information about this step can be found in the American Dietetic Association's International Dietetics and Nutrition Terminology (IDNT) Reference Manual: Standardized Language for the Nutrition Care Process, Second Edition.

*Patient/client refers to individuals, groups, family members, and/or caregivers.

**While the domains, classes, and terms for nutrition assessment and nutrition monitoring and evaluation are combined, there are no nutrition care outcomes associated with the domain entitled Client History. Items from this domain are used for nutrition assessment only and do not change as a result of nutrition intervention.

Monitoring & Evaluation

Edition: 2009

Nutrition Care Process Step 4.
Nutrition Monitoring and Evaluation

Introduction

Since 2003, the ADA has been working to describe and research the initial three steps in the Nutrition Care Process (NCP), Nutrition Assessment, Nutrition Diagnosis, and Nutrition Intervention. These three steps, along with the fourth, Nutrition Monitoring and Evaluation, are described to enhance the ability to communicate within and outside of the profession and improve the consistency and quality of individualized patient/client care and the measurement of patient/client outcomes.

The fourth step is a critical component of the Nutrition Care Process (NCP) because it identifies important measures of change or patient/client outcomes relevant to the nutrition diagnosis and nutrition intervention and describes how best to measure and evaluate these outcomes. The aim is to promote more uniformity within the profession in evaluating the efficacy of nutrition intervention.

In defining a nutrition monitoring and evaluation taxonomy, it was clear that there is substantial overlap between nutrition assessment and nutrition monitoring and evaluation. Many data points may be the same or related; however, the data purpose and use are distinct in these two steps. The items included in the monitoring and evaluation terms are those thought to be useful in evaluating the outcomes of nutrition interventions.

> **Special Note:** The terms patient/client are used in association with the NCP; however, the process is also intended for use with groups. In addition, family members or caregivers are an essential asset to the patient/client and dietetics practitioner in the NCP. Therefore, groups and families and caregivers of patients/clients are implied each time a reference is made to patient/client.

While the Nutrition Care Process steps are not necessarily linear, simply stated, a dietetics practitioner using the process completes a nutrition assessment, identifies and labels the patient/client nutrition diagnosis, and targets the nutrition intervention at the etiology of the nutrition diagnosis. Nutrition monitoring and evaluation determines whether the patient/client is achieving the nutrition intervention goals or desired outcomes (1).

Nutrition care outcomes, those that dietetics practitioners are striving to measure, result directly from the Nutrition Care Process and represent the practitioner's contribution to care. Many dietetics practitioners have been involved in tracking physician-centric or institution-centric health care outcomes, such as length of stay or reduction in health risk profile, but efforts to measure the nutrition-specific contributions to patient/client care have been sporadic and uncoordinated. This section of the publication will focus on describing and defining nutrition care outcomes. Nutrition care outcomes contribute to favorable health care outcomes; however, describing and defining the profession's impact on health care outcomes is beyond the scope of this publication.

The following figure illustrates how nutrition care outcomes are categorized and are linked together in a logical cascade that flows to other health care outcomes that are of concern to other health care providers, health systems, payors, and patients/clients.

Edition: 2009

Cascade of Nutrition Care and Health Care Outcomes

	Nutrition Care Outcomes*				Health Care Outcomes		
Appropriate Nutrition Intervention	Food/Nutrition-Related History	Anthropometric Measurements	Biochemical Data, Medical Tests and Procedures	Nutrition-Focused Physical Findings	Health and Disease Outcomes	Cost Outcomes	Patient Outcomes
	Improved nutrient intake, knowledge, behavior, access, and ability and nutrition quality of life.	Normalization of anthropometric measures.	Normalization of biochemical data, tests, and procedures.	Normalization of physical findings.	↓ Risk. Improvement of disease or condition. Prevention of adverse event.	↓ Diagnostic and treatment costs. ↓ Hospital and outpatient visits.	↓ Disability. ↑ Quality of life.

While the domains, classes, and terms for nutrition assessment and nutrition monitoring and evaluation are combined, there is no Client History Domain in nutrition monitoring and evaluation because there are no nutrition care outcomes associated with Client History. Items in the Client history domain are used for nutrition assessment only and do not change as a result of nutrition intervention.

The ADA has developed a language and methodology to aid in standardizing the dietetics practitioner's approach to nutrition monitoring and evaluation of the Nutrition Care Process. The combined nutrition assessment and nutrition monitoring and evaluation reference sheets, within the nutrition assessment chapter, are based on scientific literature and describe how dietetics practitioners measure nutrition care indicators and evaluate them.

Dietetics practitioners are encouraged to pool or aggregate data from the nutrition monitoring and evaluation step to create an outcomes management system. Like nutrition screening, the outcomes management system is not a part of the Nutrition Care Process. The primary purpose of an outcomes management system is to evaluate the efficacy and efficiency of the entire process.

What Is New in This Edition Related to Nutrition Monitoring and Evaluation?

This edition describes the revision of the nutrition monitoring and evaluation domains, terms, and indicators and maintains the description of monitoring and evaluating outcomes. However, the nutrition monitoring and evaluation reference sheets have been combined with the nutrition assessment terms and moved to the nutrition assessment section. Further, there is also discussion of the comparative standards for evaluating nutrient intake and weight, and information clarifying how to address monitoring and evaluation findings that may be consistent with inadequate intake.

- **Consolidation of the nutrition assessment and nutrition monitoring and evaluation domains, terms, and reference sheets.** Nutrition assessment and nutrition monitoring data have substantial overlap in identification and approach. In both steps, a data element is compared to either the nutrition prescription/goal or a reference standard. While dietetics practitioners use assessment data for identification of whether a nutrition problem or diagnosis exists, the same types of data are collected during assessment and reassessment for the purposes of monitoring and evaluation. Therefore, the domains, terms and reference sheets are combined and described in this chapter.

- **Revision of some specific nutrition monitoring and evaluation terms and nutrition care indicators.** Some of the individual reference sheet terms and/or indicators were changed. All of the changes were made in an attempt to help dietetics practitioners best identify and document what specific markers (indicators) are needed to monitor and evaluate patient/client improvements.

  - At the end of this chapter is a chart detailing where specific Nutrition Monitoring and Evaluation terms can now be found in the combined nutrition assessment and monitoring and evaluation reference sheets.

  - An example of a change now that the nutrition assessment and monitoring and evaluation terms are combined: The Glucose Profile was changed to the Glucose/Endocrine Profile. This term and its definition were expanded to include indicators used for nutrition assessment for identification of endocrine disorders, such as thyroid stimulating hormone, while maintaining indicators for both nutrition assessment and monitoring and evaluation, such as fasting glucose and HgbA1c.

- The reference sheets distinguish between nutrition assessment indicators and nutrition monitoring and evaluation indicators by placing *** after indicators used only for nutrition assessment. In the case of the Glucose/Endocrine Profile, thyroid stimulating hormone*** is a nutrition assessment–only indicator. In contrast to glucose, which is used for both nutrition assessment and nutrition monitoring and evaluation, thyroid stimulating hormone does not change as a result of nutrition intervention.

Note: On the combined nutrition assessment and monitoring and evaluation reference sheets, indicators used only for nutrition assessment (those that do not change as a result of nutrition intervention) have *** after the indicator. In some reference sheets, there are NO indicators with *** because all of the indicators are used for nutrition assessment and monitoring and evaluation.

- **Elimination of intervention-oriented reference sheets in the Behavior class.** Identification of nutrition assessment terms entailed careful examination of etiologies and nutrition diagnoses. This focus on etiologies leads to the decision to eliminate several intervention-oriented behavior reference sheets in favor of realigning monitoring and evaluation indicators with reference sheets related to the root cause of the behavior. For example, the reference sheet "Ability to Prepare Food/Meals" was eliminated, but the concept was added to the "Food and Nutrition Knowledge" reference sheet, because lack of adequate knowledge may be the root cause of an inability to prepare food/snacks. This concept was also included on an expanded "Adherence" reference sheet, because the patient/client may know what to do, but has not exerted the energy needed to do it. Lack of finances, food storage or preparation facilities may be the barrier to preparing food/meals and these concepts are reflected on the "Safe Food/Meal Availability" reference sheet. Finally, the concept was included on the "Nutrition-Related Activities of Daily Living" reference sheet, since cognitive or physical limitations may be the main reason the patient/client is not able to prepare food/meals.

Below is a list of the behavior monitoring and evaluation reference sheets that were eliminated, followed by the titles of reference sheets that now reflect these concepts:

Reference Sheets Eliminated	Reference Sheets That Address Concept
• Ability to Plan Meals/Snacks	• Food and Nutrition Knowledge • Adherence • Nutrition-Related Activities of Daily Living
• Ability to Select Healthful Food/Meals • Ability to Prepare Food/Meals	• Food and Nutrition Knowledge • Adherence • Safe Food/Meal Availability • Nutrition-Related Activities of Daily Living
• Portion Control	• Food and Nutrition Knowledge • Adherence
• Goal Setting • Self-Care Management • Self-Monitoring	• Food and Nutrition Knowledge • Adherence
• Stimulus Control	• Food and Nutrition Knowledge • Adherence • Eating Environment

Monitoring & Evaluation

A **Map** detailing where specific nutrition monitoring and evaluation terms are relocated within the new combined nutrition assessment and nutrition monitoring and evaluation terms list can be found immediately following this introduction.

Edition: 2009

- **Additions to the Behavior class.** The following new reference sheets were added to the Behavior class: Avoidance Behavior, Bingeing and Purging Behavior, and Mealtime Behavior, to provide standardized language to support nutrition assessment and nutrition monitoring and evaluation of these important behaviors.

- **Development of comparative standards reference sheets.** During nutrition assessment and monitoring and evaluation, practitioners determine a patient/client's recommended nutrient intake and often use this information to compare and interpret a patient/client's estimated intake of one or more nutrients. Therefore, comparative standard reference sheets are included with this edition of the reference manual, and a comparative standard reference sheet for recommended body weight/body mass index is also provided following the combined nutrition assessment and monitoring and evaluation reference sheets.

- **Addition of interpretive information for the Dietary Reference Intakes (DRIs).** The DRIs are one reference standard that dietetics professionals can use for comparison of estimated intake. Since the DRIs are for healthy individuals in a particular life stage and gender group, they may not be applicable standards for all clinical scenarios. Specific guidance on how to use the DRIs appropriately is included in this manual on pages 35-37 in the nutrition assessment chapter.

Clarification for Inadequate Intake

The combined nutrition assessment and nutrition monitoring and evaluation reference sheets list the indicators and measures as well as the criteria for comparison, either the nutrition prescription/goal or a reference standard. For example, one may compare total calories per day to the nutrition prescription (e.g., total calories for weight gain as determined by the dietetics professional based upon previous encounters with patient/client) or a reference standard (e.g., DRI calculation for energy).

- Because it is very difficult to measure a patient/client's intake even when enteral and/or parenteral nutrition is provided as the sole source of nutrition, it is recommended that additional data for assessment of nutritional status be considered. Indeed, these measures are estimated intakes.

- As such, the Standardized Language Committee created a clarification statement that should be given professional consideration, in particular when comparing estimated intake to the DRIs, prior to identifying and labeling a patient/client with "Inadequate Intake" (e.g., inadequate vitamin intake, inadequate protein intake). The note is part of the definition for the ten nutrition assessment and monitoring and evaluation reference sheets related to nutrient intake and the eleven nutrition diagnoses with "Inadequate" in the label. An additional nutrition assessment and monitoring and evaluation reference sheet regarding bioactive substance intake contains a special notation described below.

  Note: Whenever possible, nutrient intake data should be considered in combination with clinical, biochemical, anthropometric information, medical diagnosis, clinical status, and/or other factors as well as diet to provide a valid assessment of nutritional status based on a totality of the evidence. (Dietary Reference Intakes. Applications in Dietary Assessment. Institute of Medicine. Washington, D.C.: National Academy Press; 2000.)

The notation from the Institute of Medicine (IOM) advises combining intake data with clinical, biochemical, and other supporting information to complete a valid assessment of nutritional status. While it is acknowledged that inadequate intake is not synonymous with nutritional status, there may be an implied expectation that an inadequate intake over a period of time will lead to a change in nutritional status. The difficulty encountered is in the ability to accurately predict the consequences of intake due to a myriad of factors, such as scientific uncertainty about "nutrient requirements," individual differences, and inaccurate intake assessments.

- Bioactive substances do not have established DRIs. They are not considered essential nutrients because inadequate intakes do not result in biochemical or clinical symptoms of deficiency. However, naturally occurring food components with potential risk or benefit to health are reviewed by the Food and Nutrition Board of the Institute of Medicine and, if sufficient data exist, reference intakes are established. Further, the nutrition assessment and monitoring and evaluation reference sheets note that the criteria for evaluation of intake must be the patient/client goal or nutrition prescription because there are no established minimum requirements or Tolerable Upper Intake Levels. The patient/client goal or nutrition prescription would be based upon an individual goal or research, for example, the ADA Disorders of Lipid Metabolism Evidence-Based Guideline. This guideline considers the evidence supporting intake of plant stanol/sterol esters in the presence of lipid disorders. It is available on the ADA Evidence Analysis Library (EAL).

  Note: Bioactive Substances are not included as part of the Dietary Reference Intakes, and therefore there are no established minimum requirements or Tolerable Upper Intake Levels. However, RDs can assess whether estimated intakes are adequate or excessive using the patient/client goal or nutrition prescription for comparison.

Further information regarding use of the word "inadequate" in the Nutrition Care Process can be found in the chapters on nutrition assessment and nutrition diagnosis and on the ADA website, www.eatright.org, in the Nutrition Care Process section.

Nutrition Care Process and Nutrition Monitoring and Evaluation

Nutrition monitoring and evaluation determines whether the patient/client is meeting the nutrition intervention goals or desired outcomes (1). To reach this point in the process, a nutrition reassessment is needed to identify whether a nutrition-related problem exists.

If a nutrition diagnosis/problem does exist, the dietetics practitioner labels the problem and creates a PES (Problem, Etiology, Signs/Symptoms) statement.

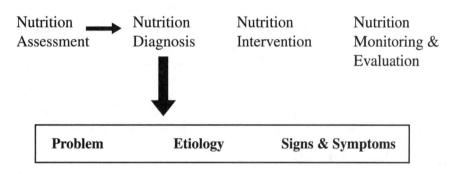

The nutrition intervention is almost always aimed at the etiology (E) of the nutrition diagnosis/problem identified in the PES statement. Less frequently, the nutrition intervention is directed at the signs and symptoms (S) to minimize their impact.

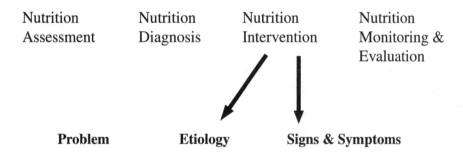

Nutrition monitoring and evaluation determines whether the patient/client is achieving the nutrition intervention goals or desired outcomes.

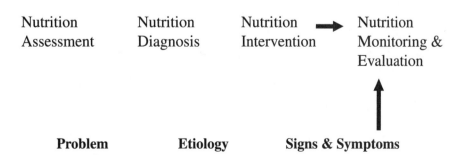

Edition: 2009

Monitoring & Evaluation

Nutrition monitoring and evaluation answers the question, "Is the nutrition intervention strategy working to resolve the nutrition diagnosis, its etiology, and/or signs and symptoms?" This step clearly defines the outcomes specific to nutrition care. For instance, a patient newly diagnosed with hyperlipidemia may have goals related to nutrition knowledge and fat, fiber, and energy intake along with biochemical measures of total cholesterol and LDL cholesterol. The dietetics practitioner may develop an action plan to periodically monitor, evaluates and document nutrition knowledge, intake of fat and/or saturated fat, and/or lab values.

As will be described in greater detail throughout in this chapter, nutrition monitoring and evaluation assesses the patient/client's progress by comparing very specific markers or nutrition care indicators against recognized, science-based standards or baseline. Some of the terminology essential to this step is defined here. Its application to patient/client nutrition care will be covered thoroughly.

Nutrition Monitoring and Evaluation Definitions

Nutrition monitoring—preplanned review and measurement of selected nutrition care indicators of patient/client's status relevant to the defined needs, nutrition diagnosis, nutrition intervention, and outcomes.

Nutrition evaluation—the systematic comparison of current findings with the previous status, nutrition intervention goals, effectiveness of overall nutrition care, or a reference standard.

Nutrition care outcomes—the results of nutrition care that are directly related to the nutrition diagnosis and the goals of the intervention plan.

Nutrition care indicators—markers that can be measured and evaluated to determine the effectiveness of the nutrition care.

Nutrition Care Outcomes

Nutrition care should result in important changes that lead to improved behaviors and/or nutritional status. In outpatient and community settings, this might include improvement in the patient/client's understanding of the food and nutrient needs and their ability and motivation to meet those needs. In hospital settings, this might include an improvement in biochemical parameters or a basic understanding of the nutrition prescription. In long-term care facilities, this might include an improvement in a patient/client's ability to feed himself or herself independently and a reduction in need for supplemental enteral nutrition support.

Nutrition care outcomes are often intermediate outcomes to other broader health care outcomes (e.g., occurrence, duration or severity of acute and chronic disease, infections, wound healing, health care cost, and patient functional ability).

Nutrition care outcomes are distinguished by several characteristics. They:

- Represent results that the practitioner/nutrition care impacted independently
- Can be linked to nutrition intervention goals
- Are measurable with tools and resources available to the practitioner
- Occur in a reasonable time period
- Can be attributed to the nutrition care
- Are logical and biologically or psychologically plausible stepping stones to other health care outcomes (e.g., health and disease, cost, and patient/client outcomes)

Nutrition Care Outcome Categories

Nutrition care outcomes are distinct from health care outcomes because they represent the dietetics practitioner's specific contribution to care. They are categorized into four of the five domains included in nutrition assessment. There is no Client History Domain in nutrition monitoring and evaluation because there are no nutrition care outcomes associated with client history. Items in the Client History Domain are used for nutrition assessment only and do not change as a result of nutrition intervention.

Nutrition Care Outcome Domains

Food/Nutrition-Related History consists of food and nutrient intake, medication and herbal supplement intake, knowledge/beliefs/attitudes, behavior, factors affecting access to food and food/nutrition-related supplies, physical activity and nutrition quality of life.

> **Food and nutrient intake** includes factors such as composition and adequacy of food and nutrient intake, meal and snack patterns, and current and previous diets and/or food modifications, and eating environment.

> **Medication and herbal supplement intake** includes prescription and over-the-counter medications, including herbal preparations and complementary medicine products used.

> **Knowledge/beliefs/attitudes** includes understanding of nutrition-related concepts and conviction of the truth and feelings/emotions toward some nutrition-related statement or phenomenon, along with readiness to change nutrition-related behaviors.

> **Behavior** includes patient/client activities and actions that influence achievement of nutrition-related goals.

> **Factors affecting access to food and food/nutrition-related supplies** includes factors that affect intake and availability of a sufficient quantity of safe, healthful food as well as food/nutrition-related supplies.

> **Physical activity and function** includes physical activity as well as cognitive and physical ability to engage in specific tasks, e.g., breastfeeding and self-feeding.

> **Nutrition-related patient/client-centered measures** consists of patient/client's perception of his/her nutrition intervention and its impact on life.

> **Note:** Whenever possible, nutrient intake data should be considered in combination with clinical, biochemical, anthropometric information, medical diagnosis, clinical status, and/or other factors as well as diet to provide a valid assessment of nutritional status based on a totality of the evidence. (*Dietary Reference Intakes. Applications in Dietary Assessment.* Institute of Medicine. Washington, D.C.: National Academy Press; 2000.)

Anthropometric Measurements include height, weight, body mass index (BMI), growth pattern indices/percentile ranks, and weight history.

Biochemical Data, Medical Tests, and Procedures include laboratory data, (e.g., electrolytes, glucose, and lipid panel) and tests (e.g., gastric emptying time, resting metabolic rate).

Nutrition-Focused Physical Findings include findings from an evaluation of body systems, muscle and subcutaneous fat wasting, oral health, suck/swallow/breathe ability, appetite, and affect.

Edition: 2009

Nutrition Monitoring and Evaluation Components: Monitor, Measure, and Evaluate

In the fourth step of the Nutrition Care Process, dietetics practitioners do the following three things—monitor progress, measure outcomes, and evaluate the outcomes against criteria to determine changes in specific indicators of nutrition care outcomes.

Monitor

Nutrition intervention typically involves activities completed with the patient/client (e.g., self-monitoring record review, education) and actions taken by the patient/client as a result of the intervention (e.g., adjusting insulin dosage based upon self-monitoring, label reading and interpretation, self-feeding with an adapted feeding device). At each encounter, the dietetics practitioner monitors some or all of the nutrition care indicators to determine whether nutrition goals have been achieved or if further intervention is necessary.

In many cases, nutrition monitoring and evaluation will begin with a determination of the patient/client's understanding of the nutrition intervention. Progress may be impacted if the patient/client did not implement the nutrition intervention or did not comprehend how to implement the nutrition intervention.

Measure

Patient/client records, counseling sessions, and classes offer an abundance of potential nutrition care outcomes. The appropriate nutrition care indicators are determined by the nutrition diagnosis and its etiology and signs or symptoms. In addition, the nutrition intervention, medical diagnosis and health care outcome goals, and quality management goals for nutrition may influence the nutrition care indicators chosen. Other factors, such as practice setting, patient/client population, and disease state and/or severity, may also affect the choice of indicator. As noted earlier, nutrition care outcomes and health care outcomes are different and distinct. Only nutrition care outcomes are discussed here.

Sometimes the measurement or data collection will occur during the initial encounter, and other times it will occur at a later date during subsequent encounters. For example, you can measure knowledge change immediately but you may only be able to measure a nutrition-related physical sign and symptom such as laboratory indicator at a subsequent encounter.

Use of standardized indicators and measures will increase the likelihood that valid and reliable measures of change will be collected and facilitate electronic charting, coding, and outcomes measurement.

Evaluate

Comparing the nutrition care indicators against standards shown to produce the desired effect (e.g., < 30% of calories from fat/day) will aid in more consistent and comparable nutrition care changes and outcomes across patient populations, practitioners, and practice settings. The criteria used for comparison may be national, institutional, and/or regulatory standards when available. For data related to the intake of specific nutrients, comparative standards are available in this resource for guiding accurate documentation of a patient/client's recommended nutrient intake and for comparison of the patient/client estimated intake of one or more nutrients.

Fortunately, the monitoring and evaluation step is flexible. Dietetics practitioners select the most appropriate reference standard or goal based upon the patient/client condition and patient care setting. Not all patients/clients may be able to achieve the goals established by a national standard—for example, < 2,300 mg sodium per day from the Dietary Guidelines for Americans (2). Mitigating circumstances may be defined and a more suitable goal established—for example, a dietetics practitioner might establish a nutrition prescription for 4,000 mg of sodium per day, and evaluate a patient/client's progress toward this nutrition prescription. A second component of the evaluation is to look at the entire picture of the nutrition care by simultaneously evaluating multiple indicators and determine overall impact on the patient/client outcomes.

The following types of critical thinking skills are essential for the nutrition monitoring and evaluation step:

- Selecting appropriate indicators/measures
- Using appropriate criteria (i.e., previous status, nutrition intervention goals, or reference standards) for comparison
- Defining where patient/client is now in terms of expected outcome
- Explaining variance from expected outcomes
- Identifying factors that help or hinder progress
- Deciding between discharge or continuation of nutrition care

Following is a summary of the three components of the nutrition monitoring and evaluation step.

Nutrition Monitoring and Evaluation Components Summary

Monitor progress

- Check patient/client's understanding and compliance with nutrition intervention
- Determine whether the intervention is being implemented as prescribed
- Provide evidence that the nutrition intervention is or is not changing the patient/client's behavior or status
- Identify other positive or negative outcomes
- Gather information indicating reasons for lack of progress
- Support conclusions with evidence

Measure outcomes

- Select the nutrition care indicator(s) to measure the desired outcome(s)
- Use standardized nutrition care indicator(s) to increase the validity and reliability of the measurements of change

Evaluate outcomes

- Compare monitoring data with the nutrition prescription/goals or reference standard to assess progress and determine future action
- Evaluate impact of the sum of all interventions on overall patient/client health outcomes

---

Edition: 2009

Nutrition Care Indicators

Nutrition care indicators are clearly defined markers that can be observed and measured and are used to quantify the changes that are the result of nutrition care. Selected indicators for nutrition monitoring should be relevant to and reflect a change in the patient/client's nutrition diagnosis and its etiology and signs/symptoms. The indicators selected may also be relevant to the patient/client disease state, quality management goals for nutrition, and health care outcome goals.

Well-chosen indicators enable practitioners to monitor and evaluate progress made toward desired nutrition care outcomes. Nutrition care indicators provide information about the type and magnitude of progress made, when the nutrition problem is resolved, and what aspects of nutrition intervention are working or where adjustments are needed. This is in contrast to data used for nutrition assessment. Many data points may be the same or related; however, dietetics practitioners use additional nutrition assessment data to identify and provide evidence about a nutrition-related problem or diagnosis.

Although not part of the Nutrition Care Process, nutrition care indicators are ideal components of a quality improvement program, which will be discussed further at the end of this chapter. Commonly used indicators vary by practice setting.

Nutrition care outcomes and indicators include:

- Factors that dietetics practitioners can impact directly, such as food and nutrient intake; growth and body composition; food and nutrition-related knowledge, attitudes and behaviors; and food access
- Laboratory values, such as HgbA1c, hematocrit, serum cholesterol
- Functional capabilities, such as physical activity
- Patient perception of nutrition care and results of nutrition care, such as nutrition quality of life

Nutrition monitoring and evaluation reference sheets, now combined with the nutrition assessment reference sheets, define the nutrition care outcome and the indicators that may be appropriate for measuring and evaluating outcomes within a variety of practice settings.

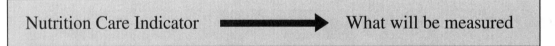

Nutrition Care Indicator ➡️ What will be measured

Measurement and Evaluation of Nutrition Indicators

Dietetics practitioners make judgments about progress toward nutrition-related outcomes by comparing the actual value of the measured indicator to a science-based criteria or an individualized goal/expected outcome.

The dietetics practitioner does this based upon the criteria and scale established for the nutrition care outcome.

Criteria

Two criteria are suggested for nutrition monitoring and evaluation:

- Nutrition prescription or goal/expected outcome (e.g., a behavior change has a goal not a nutrition prescription)
- Reference standard (e.g., national, institutional, and/or regulatory standards)

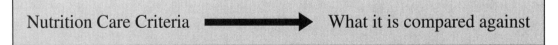

Nutrition Care Criteria ➡️ What it is compared against

The nutrition prescription is the patient/client's individualized recommended dietary intake of energy and/or selected foods or nutrients based on current reference standards or and dietary guidelines and the patient/client's health condition and nutrition diagnosis. For example, a patient of normal body weight has a serum LDL cholesterol of 150 mg/dL. His nutrition prescription is <30% calories from fat with <10% calories from saturated fat. If a behavior change outcome is desired, the patient/client could also have a goal (e.g., take lunch to work at least three times per week and reduce high-fat fast-food intake at lunch to one time per week).

For biochemical outcomes such as LDL cholesterol, the criteria that may be used is the reference standard established by the National Heart Lung and Blood Institute of serum LDL <100 mg/dL. This could also be stated as a goal to reduce baseline LDL by a specific percentage.

> **Special Note:** Laboratory parameters within the nutrition assessment and monitoring and evaluation reference sheets are provided only for guidance.
>
> - Laboratory values may vary depending on the laboratory performing the test.
> - Scientific consensus concerning selection of biochemical tests, laboratory methods, reference standards, or interpretation of data does not always exist.
> - Laboratory findings may be evaluated for their significance or lack of significance depending on the patient/client population, disease severity, and/or treatment goals.
> - Current national, institutional, and regulatory guidelines that affect practice should be applied as appropriate to individual patients/clients.

Reference standards, as noted previously, are national, institutional, and/or regulatory standards. Dietetics practitioners are familiar with reference standards for laboratory measures. Examples of other reference standards include:

- National standards for populations or patient/client groups or disease conditions, e.g., Dietary Reference Intakes (DRIs), Dietary Guidelines or guidelines for specific treatment or disease condition such as those developed by the American Society of Parenteral and Enteral Nutrition and/or the National Kidney Foundation
- Institutional standards, e.g., established guidelines specifying how to evaluate weight change in geriatric patients/clients
- Regulatory standards, e.g., Omnibus Budget Reconciliation Act (OBRA) guidelines for long-term care, the Joint Commission standards

Dietetics practitioners select the most appropriate reference standard or goal based upon the patient/client condition and patient care setting. Further, dietetics practitioners are responsible for understanding any defining parameters or limitations for the reference standard used. The DRIs, for example, have very specific parameters for interpretation of estimated intake.

Monitoring and Evaluation of Nutrient Intake

To begin with, data collection for nutrient intake is imprecise because it relies generally on patient/client estimations and reports of intake. Enteral and/or parenteral nutrition intake can be more precise if it is the sole source of nutrition and accurate records of enteral and/or parenteral nutrition delivery are available.

Once the data are collected, dietetics practitioners compare the estimated nutrient intake to a patient/client goal or a reference standard. Historically, the DRIs have been used for comparison of intake in a variety of populations since other specific reference standards are not always available. Practitioners must keep in mind that the DRIs have the following interpretation parameters:

- For evaluation of nutritional status, nutrient intake data should be combined with biochemical, clinical, anthropometric, medical diagnosis, and clinical data.
- The DRIs are established for healthy individuals. It is not clear how the DRIs should be interpreted in ill patients/clients.
- Estimations consistent with inadequate intake do not necessarily mean there is a nutrient deficiency.
- The following note is part of the definition for the ten reference sheets related to intake. A special note is listed on the next page for bioactive substance intake.

  Note: Whenever possible, nutrient intake data should be considered in combination with clinical, biochemical, anthropometric information, medical diagnosis, clinical status, and/or other factors as well as diet to provide a valid assessment of nutritional status based on a totality of the evidence. (Dietary Reference Intakes. Applications in Dietary Assessment. *Institute of Medicine. Washington, D.C.: National Academy Press; 2000.*)

- Bioactive substances do not have established DRIs. They are not considered to be essential nutrients because inadequate intakes do not result in biochemical or clinical symptoms of a deficiency. However, naturally oc-

Edition: 2009

curring food compounds with potential risk or benefit to health are reviewed by the Food and Nutrition Board of the Institute of Medicine and, if sufficient data exist, reference intakes are established. Further, the nutrition assessment and monitoring and evaluation reference sheet notes that the criteria for evaluation of intake must be the nutrition prescription or goal since there are no established minimum requirements or Tolerable Upper Intake Levels. The nutrition prescription or goal would be based upon an individual goal or research, for example, the ADA Disorders of Lipid Metabolism Evidence-Based Guideline. This guideline considers the evidence supporting intake of plant stanol/sterol esters in the presence of lipid disorders. It is available in the ADA Evidence Analysis Library. Therefore, the note added to the definition of Inadequate Bioactive Substance Intake is:

Note: Bioactive substances are not included as part of the Dietary Reference Intakes, and therefore there are no established minimum requirements or Tolerable Upper Intake Levels. However, RDs can assess whether estimated intakes are adequate or excessive using the patient/client goal or nutrition prescription for comparison.

It is important to reiterate that dietetics professionals are given two criteria for use—the nutrition prescription/goal and reference standards (e.g., national, institutional, and/or regulatory standards). They are not limited to using the DRIs as the criteria for comparison of nutrient intake data. In certain populations where other appropriate scientific information has emerged and reference standards are available, such as in renal disease, it may be appropriate to use an alternate reference standard instead of the DRIs.

Scale

Once the nutrition care indicator is selected and the criteria are established, the next step is evaluating the changes using a scale. Practitioners use the scale to define the degree to which the indicator changed to meet the criteria.

Other professions, such as nursing and speech-language pathology, have developed validated scales for evaluating the changes in a patient/client's status. The dietetics profession has a critical need to have reliable and valid indicators and scales to demonstrate the impact of nutrition care. This need is balanced with the desire to have these measures as soon as is practical to facilitate measuring outcomes and research and to move toward electronic medical records.

This publication locates nutrition care outcomes and indicators, along with the references related to the criteria and sample documentation examples, in nutrition assessment section of the reference manual. A future edition will incorporate recommendations for practitioners to evaluate the degree to which the indicators meet the criteria using scales. While additional time is needed, it is believed that a staged approach will improve the likelihood of developing reliable and valid measures of nutrition care that are critical to the profession.

Selection and Interpretation of the Nutrition Care Indicators

Primary factors affecting indicator selection and interpretation

Although the nutrition monitoring and evaluation reference sheets define the wide variety of indicators that are appropriate for measuring and evaluating outcomes, the reference sheets do not distinguish which nutrition care indicators are best for a particular situation. The dietetics practitioner makes this decision based on the individual situation.

Three primary factors will influence the selection, measurement, and interpretation of the individual nutrition care outcomes indicators:

- Practice setting (e.g., inpatient or outpatient, long-term care, community)
- Age of the patient/client (e.g., pediatrics, geriatrics)
- Disease state and severity (e.g., renal disease, diabetes, critical illness)

National reference standards are available for many indicators; for example, ADA has a Critical Illness Evidence-Based Guideline, which addresses glucose level (indicator) for critically ill patients/clients with hyperglycemia (3). This guideline reads: "Dietitians should promote attainment of strict glycemic control (80-110 mg/dL) to reduce time on mechanical ventilation in critically ill medical ICU patients."

Glucose is the appropriate indicator in a stressed ICU patient and the criteria have been defined. HgbA1c is not used as an indicator in this instance. It is the dietetics practitioner's responsibility to distinguish which indicator is appropriate for the given practice and patient/client situation.

Secondary factors affecting indicator selection and interpretation

The time frame over which a patient/client receives nutrition care influences the selection of the indicator. The previous example illustrates this point. HgbA1c is a measure of glucose status for a 60-90 day period and is not useful in monitoring and evaluation of the ICU patient/client with acute elevation of blood glucose. HgbA1c is appropriate, however, in the outpatient setting when patient/clients are observed over a period of time.

Other considerations

Interpretation of the change seen in particular nutrition care indicators may require evidence or explanation by a dietetics practitioner. For example, if a patient/client attains the goal to reduce overall body fat through nutrition intervention, one may see a negative change or increase in body mass index (BMI) due to the patient/client's increase in muscle mass. Occurrences such as these should be anticipated and appropriate evidence and explanation documented.

The considerations described, along with the examples, illustrate the importance of appropriate indictor selection and interpretation. Each situation will be different depending upon the practice setting, population, and disease state and severity, and the time interval over which the patient/client receives nutrition care. Selection of the incorrect indicator may lead to incorrect conclusions about the impact of nutrition interventions.

Nutrition Monitoring and Evaluation Reference Sheets

The reference sheets for nutrition monitoring and evaluation can be found in the chapter on nutrition assessment. The reference sheets from these two steps have been combined.

Nutrition Monitoring and Evaluation: Documentation

Several components of documentation are recommended throughout the Nutrition Care Process. Documentation is an on-going process that supports all of the steps. Documentation that is relevant and timely is essential, but lacking if it does not include specific statements of where the patient/client is now in terms of expected nutrition outcomes.

Quality documentation for nutrition monitoring and evaluation includes:

- Date and time
- Indicators measured, results, and the method for obtaining the measurement
- Criteria to which the indicator is compared (i.e., nutrition prescription/goal or a reference standard)
- Factors facilitating or hampering progress
- Other positive or negative outcomes
- Future plans for nutrition care, nutrition monitoring, and follow up or discharge

In an initial encounter, it may not be possible to include all of these elements because the nutrition prescription and goals have just been established, and the nutrition intervention may not have occurred. Two complete Case Studies with examples of documentation in various charting formats are available in the Nutrition Care Process and Model Resource section of the ADA website, www.eatright.org, in the Nutrition Care Process section. Brief excerpts of documentation may look like the sample provided on the following page.

Edition: 2009

Initial encounter 7/15

Nutrition assessment: Based upon a three-day food diary, patient/client consumes approximately 120 grams fat per day. Meals are frequently consumed at restaurants where patient often selects high-fat food items. The patient/client's BMI is 29 and serum cholesterol is 190 mg/dL.

Nutrition diagnosis: Excessive fat intake related to frequent restaurant meals with high-fat food choices as evidenced by a current estimated average intake of 120 grams of fat per day.

Nutrition intervention: Nutrition prescription is 60 grams of fat per day. Nutrition counseling provided.

Nutrition monitoring and evaluation: Estimated intake of fat (indicator) is currently 200% of nutrition prescription (criteria). Will monitor change in fat intake at next encounter.

Follow-up encounter 8/10

Nutrition intervention: Patient/client reports difficulty ordering low-fat selections at restaurants. Provided comprehensive education to identify low-fat items on restaurant menus. Patient/client implementing self-monitoring log.

Nutrition monitoring and evaluation: Based upon three-day diet record, some progress toward nutrition prescription as estimated intake of fat is reduced from 120 to 90 grams per day. Will monitor change in restaurant selections (using patient/client's self-monitoring log) and fat intake at next encounter.

Nutrition Monitoring and Evaluation: Data Sources and Tools

To monitor and evaluate a patient/client's progress, the following tools may be used:

- Patient/client questionnaires
- Surveys
- Pretests and posttests
- Patient/client/family member interviews
- Anthropometric measurements
- Biochemical and medical test results
- Food and nutrition intake tools

These tools can be used when patients are seen individually or in groups, or when the encounter is conducted by phone or via computer. Pooled data can be monitored and evaluated using tracking forms and computer software programs.

Nutrition Care Outcome Management System

Nutrition monitoring and evaluation applies to individual patients/clients and to groups of patients/clients. Selecting nutrition monitoring and evaluation data for an individual patient/client depends primarily upon the nutrition diagnosis and the nutrition intervention. An additional consideration when selecting the nutrition monitoring and evaluation indicators for patients/clients is how data may be used when pooled to assess quality of care provided to specific groups of patients. Choosing what to monitor may also be influenced by facility strategic goals and quality improvement plans, regulatory or certifying agency requirements (e.g., American Diabetes Association Self-Management Education certification, Joint Commission regulations).

Aggregate nutrition care indicator data may be reported to administrators, payers, quality improvement organizations, and other decision makers of health care funding.

Potential benefits of the aggregate data include:

- Provide for process improvement and leads to understanding of what works and what does not
- Can be used for outcomes measurement studies and quality improvement initiatives
- Link care processes and resource utilization
- Give an opportunity to identify and analyze causes of less than optimal performance and outcomes

- Define information for inclusion in centralized data systems relevant to nutrition care
- Can be used to quantify the dietetics practitioner's contribution to health care

Various factors that can impact aggregate nutrition care indicator data interpretation and need consideration include:

- Method for collecting the outcome, e.g., three-day diet record versus a 24-hour recall
- Data source, e.g., patient/client, family/caregiver, chart, bedside record
- Intervention components (e.g., type, duration, and intensity)
- Education and skill level of dietetics practitioner
- Nutrition program attributes

A case example integrating nutrition monitoring and evaluation data into a department quality improvement program, Case C, is available in the Nutrition Care Process and Model Resource section of the ADA website, www.eatright.org, in the Nutrition Care Process section.

Summary

Nutrition monitoring and evaluation describes the patient/client's progress through consistent terms that are evaluated based upon carefully selected indicators and criteria. As more and more dietetics practitioners use these tools and share their progress and nutrition care outcomes, the body of literature quantifying the dietetics practitioner's contribution to improving the health of patients/clients and describing effective methods of intervention will grow.

References

1. Lacey K, Pritchett E. Nutrition care process and model: ADA adopts road map to quality care and outcomes management. *J Am Diet Assoc.* 2003;103:1061-1072.

2. Dietary Guidelines for Americans, 2005. Available at: http://www.health.gov/dietaryguidelines/dga2005/document/html/executivesummary. htm. Accessed October 27, 2006.

3. American Dietetic Association. Critical illness evidence-based nutrition guideline, 2006. Available at: http://www.adaevidencelibrary.com/topic.cfm?cat=2809. Accessed November 1, 2006.

Monitoring & Evaluation

Edition: 2009

Map of Nutrition Monitoring and Evaluation Terms in the Combined Nutrition Assessment and Monitoring and Evaluation Reference Sheets

Please refer to the Combined List of Nutrition Assessment and Monitoring and Evaluation Terms for a complete listing of the new terms.

IDNT First Edition Nutrition Monitoring and Evaluation Terms	Term Number	IDNT Second Edition Combined List of Nutrition Assessment and Monitoring and Evaluation Terms	Term Number
DOMAIN: NUTRITION-RELATED BEHAVIORAL-ENVIRONMENTAL OUTCOMES	BE	DOMAIN: FOOD/NUTRITION-RELATED HISTORY	FH
Class: Knowledge/ Beliefs (1)		Class: Knowledge/Beliefs/Attitudes (2)	
Beliefs and attitudes	BE-1.1	Beliefs and attitudes	FH 3.2
Food and nutrition knowledge	BE-1.2	Food and nutrition knowledge	FH 3.1
Class: Behavior (2)		Class: Behavior (3)	
Ability to plan meals/snacks	BE-2.1	Distributed among (depending on the etiology): Food and nutrition knowledge Nutrition-related ADLs and IADLs (physical/cognitive ability) Adherence	FH 3.1 FH 6.2 FH 4.1
Ability to select healthful food/meals	BE-2.2	Distributed among (depending on the etiology): Food and nutrition knowledge Nutrition-related ADLs and IADLs (physical/cognitive ability) Adherence	FH 3.1 FH 6.2 FH 4.1
Ability to prepare food/meals	BE-2.3	Distributed among (depending on the etiology): Food and nutrition knowledge Nutrition-related ADLs and IADLs (physical/cognitive ability) Adherence	FH 3.1 FH 6.2 FH 4.1
Adherence	BE-2.4	Adherence	FH 4.1
Goal setting	BE-2.5	Food and nutrition knowledge Adherence	FH 3.1 FH 4.1

Edition: 2009

Map of Nutrition Monitoring and Evaluation Terms in the Combined Nutrition Assessment and Monitoring and Evaluation Reference Sheets

Please refer to the Combined List of Nutrition Assessment and Monitoring and Evaluation Terms for a complete listing of the new terms.

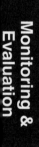

IDNT First Edition Nutrition Monitoring and Evaluation Terms	Term Number	IDNT Second Edition Combined List of Nutrition Assessment and Monitoring and Evaluation Terms	Term Number
DOMAIN: NUTRITION-RELATED BEHAVIORAL-ENVIRONMENTAL OUTCOMES	BE	**DOMAIN: FOOD/NUTRITION-RELATED HISTORY**	FH
Class: Behavior (2)		*Class: Behavior (3)*	
Portion control	BE-2.6	Food and nutrition knowledge	FH32.1
		Adherence	FH 4.1
		Food intake	FH 1.3.2
Self-care management	BE-2.7	Food and nutrition knowledge	FH 3.1
		Adherence	FH 4.1
Self-monitoring	BE-2.8	Food and nutrition knowledge	FH 3.1
		Adherence	FH 4.1
Social support	BE-2.9	Social networking	FH 4.5
Stimulus control	BE-2.10	Divided into:	
		Food and nutrition knowledge (recognition of the stimuli, develop plan, modify environment/behavior)	FH 3.1
		Adherence (adherence to plan for managing stimuli)	FH 4.1
DOMAIN: NUTRITION-RELATED BEHAVIORAL-ENVIRONMENTAL OUTCOMES	BE	**DOMAIN: FOOD/NUTRITION-RELATED HISTORY**	FH
Class: Access (3)		*Class: Factors Affecting Access to Food and Food/Nutrition-Related Supplies (4)*	
Access to food	BE-3.1	Divided into:	
		Food/nutrition program participation	FH 5.1
		Safe food/meal availability	FH 5.2
		Safe water availability	FH 5.3
		Food and nutrition-related supplies availability	FH 5.4

Edition: 2009

424

Map of Nutrition Monitoring and Evaluation Terms in the Combined Nutrition Assessment and Monitoring and Evaluation Reference Sheets

Please refer to the Combined List of Nutrition Assessment and Monitoring and Evaluation Terms for a complete listing of the new terms.

IDNT First Edition Nutrition Monitoring and Evaluation Terms	Term Number	IDNT Second Edition Combined List of Nutrition Assessment and Monitoring and Evaluation Terms	Term Number
DOMAIN: NUTRITION-RELATED BEHAVIORAL-ENVIRONMENTAL OUTCOMES, cont'd	BE	DOMAIN: FOOD/NUTRITION-RELATED HISTORY, cont'd	FH
Class: Physical Activity and Function (4)		*Class: Physical Activity and Function (5)*	
Breastfeeding success	BE-4.1	Breastfeeding	FH 6.1
Nutrition-related instrumental activities of daily living	BE-4.2	Nutrition-related ADLs and IADLs	FH 6.2
Physical activity	BE-4.3	Physical activity	FH 6.3
DOMAIN: FOOD AND NUTRIENT INTAKE OUTCOMES	FI	DOMAIN: FOOD/NUTRITION-RELATED HISTORY	FH
Class: Energy Intake (1)		*Class: Energy Intake (1.2)*	
Energy intake	FI-1.1	Energy intake	FH 1.2.1
Class: Food and Beverage Intake (2)		*Class: Food and Beverage Intake (1.3)*	
Fluid/beverage intake	FI-2.1	Fluid/beverage intake	FH 1.3.1
Food intake	FI-2.2	Food intake	FH 1.3.2
DOMAIN: FOOD AND NUTRIENT INTAKE OUTCOMES	FI	DOMAIN: FOOD/NUTRITION-RELATED HISTORY	FH
Class: Enteral and Parenteral Intake (3)		*Class: Enteral and Parenteral Intake (1.4)*	
Enteral/parenteral nutrition intake	FI-3.1	Enteral/parenteral nutrition intake	FH 1.4.1
Class: Bioactive Substances Intake (4)		*Class: Bioactive Substances Intake (1.5)*	
Alcohol intake	FI-4.1	Alcohol intake	FH 1.5.1
Bioactive substances intake	FI-4.2	Bioactive substances intake	FH 1.5.2
Caffeine intake	FI-4.3	Caffeine intake	FH 1.5.3

Monitoring & Evaluation

Edition: 2009

Map of Nutrition Monitoring and Evaluation Terms in the Combined Nutrition Assessment and Monitoring and Evaluation Reference Sheets

Please refer to the Combined List of Nutrition Assessment and Monitoring and Evaluation Terms for a complete listing of the new terms.

IDNT First Edition Nutrition Monitoring and Evaluation Terms	Term Number	IDNT Second Edition Combined List of Nutrition Assessment and Monitoring and Evaluation Terms	Term Number
DOMAIN: FOOD AND NUTRIENT INTAKE OUTCOMES, cont'd	FI	**DOMAIN: FOOD/NUTRITION-RELATED HISTORY, cont'd**	FH
Class: Macronutrient Intake (5)		*Class: Macronutrient Intake (1.6)*	
Fat and cholesterol intake	FI-5.1	Fat and cholesterol intake	FH 1.6.1
Protein intake	FI-5.2	Protein intake	FH 1.6.2
Carbohydrate intake	FI-5.3	Carbohydrate intake	FH 1.6.3
Fiber intake	FI-5.4	Fiber intake	FH 1.6.4
Class: Micronutrient Intake (6)		*Class: Micronutrient Intake (1.7)*	
Vitamin intake	FI-6.1	Vitamin intake	FH 1.7.1
Mineral/element intake	FI-6.2	Mineral/element intake	FH 1.7.2
DOMAIN: NUTRITION-RELATED PHYSICAL SIGN/SYMPTOM OUTCOMES	S	**DOMAIN: ANTHROPOMETRIC MEASUREMENTS (1)**	AD
Class: Anthropometric (1)			
Body composition/Growth	S-1.1	Body composition/Growth/Weight history	AD 1.1
DOMAIN: NUTRITION-RELATED PHYSICAL SIGN/SYMPTOM OUTCOMES	S	**DOMAIN: BIOCHEMICAL DATA, MEDICAL TESTS AND PROCEDURES (1)**	BD
Class: Biochemical and Medical Tests (2)			
Acid-base balance	S-2.1	Acid-base balance	BD 1.1
Electrolyte and renal profile	S-2.2	Electrolyte and renal profile	BD 1.2
Essential fatty acid profile	S-2.3	Essential fatty acid profile	BD 1.3
Gastrointestinal profile	S-2.4	Gastrointestinal profile	BD 1.4
Glucose profile	S-2.5	Glucose/endocrine profile	BD 1.5

Edition: 2009

Map of Nutrition Monitoring and Evaluation Terms in the Combined Nutrition Assessment and Monitoring and Evaluation Reference Sheets

Please refer to the Combined List of Nutrition Assessment and Monitoring and Evaluation Terms for a complete listing of the new terms.

IDNT First Edition Nutrition Monitoring and Evaluation Terms	Term Number	IDNT Second Edition Combined List of Nutrition Assessment and Monitoring and Evaluation Terms	Term Number
DOMAIN: NUTRITION-RELATED PHYSICAL SIGN/ SYMPTOM OUTCOMES, cont'd	S	**DOMAIN: BIOCHEMICAL DATA, MEDICAL TESTS AND PROCEDURES (1), cont'd**	BD
Class: Biochemical and Medical Tests (2)			
Lipid profile	S-2.6	Lipid profile	BD 1.7
Mineral profile	S-2.7	Mineral profile	BD 1.9
Nutritional anemia profile	S-2.8	Nutritional anemia profile	BD 1.10
Protein profile	S-2.9	Protein profile	BD 1.11
Respiratory quotient	S-2.10	Metabolic rate profile	BD 1.8
Urine profile	S-2.11	Urine profile	BD 1.12
Vitamin profile	S-2.12	Vitamin profile	BD 1.13
DOMAIN: NUTRITION-RELATED PHYSICAL SIGN/ SYMPTOM OUTCOMES	S	**DOMAIN: NUTRITION-FOCUSED PHYSICAL FINDINGS (1)**	PD
Class: Physical Examination (3)			
Nutrition physical exam findings	S-3.1	Nutrition –focused physical findings	PD 1.1
DOMAIN: NUTRITION-RELATED PATIENT/CLIENT-CENTERED OUTCOMES	PC	**DOMAIN: FOOD/NUTRITION-RELATED HISTORY**	FH
Class: Nutrition Quality of Life (1)		*Class: Nutrition-Related Patient/Client-Centered Measures (7)*	
Nutrition quality of life	PC-1.1	Nutrition quality of life	FH 7.1
Class: Satisfaction (2)		Satisfaction: To be added	
To be added			

Edition: 2009

Bibliography and Resources

Publications

International Dietetics and Nutrition Terminology (IDNT) Reference Manual: Standardized Language for the Nutrition Care Process, Second Edition. Chicago, IL: American Dietetic Association; 2009.

Pocket Guide for the International Dietetics and Nutrition Terminology Reference Manual, Second Edition. Chicago, IL: American Dietetic Association; 2009.

International Dietetics and Nutrition Terminology (IDNT) Reference Manual: Standardized Language for the Nutrition Care Process, First Edition. Chicago, IL: American Dietetic Association; 2008.

Pocket Guide for the International Dietetics and Nutrition Terminology Reference Manual, First Edition. Chicago, IL: American Dietetic Association; 2008.

American Dietetic Association. *Nutrition Diagnosis and Intervention: Standardized Language for the Nutrition Care Process*. Chicago, IL: American Dietetic Association; 2007.

American Dietetic Association. *Nutrition Diagnosis: A Critical Step in the Nutrition Care Process*. Chicago, IL: American Dietetic Association; 2006.

Journal articles

Writing Group of the Nutrition Care Process/Standardized Language Committee. Nutrition care process and model part I: The 2008 update. *J Am Diet Assoc*. 2008;108:1113-1117.

Mathieu J, Foust M, Ouellette P. Implementing nutrition diagnosis, step two in the Nutrition Care Process and model: Challenges and lesions learned in two health care facilities. *J Am Diet Assoc*. 2005;105:1636-1640.

Lacey K, Pritchett E. Nutrition care process and model: ADA adopts road map to quality care and outcomes management. *J Am Diet Assoc*. 2003;103:1061-1072.

Web resources

Nutrition Care Process and Model Resources, http://www.eatright.org, select the Nutrition Care Process section

NCP Frequently Asked Questions and Patient/Client Case Studies and Process Improvement Example, http://www.eatright.org, select the Nutrition Care Process section, select Practitioners, then select How Are You Going To Get There, and look under More Resources

Evidence-Based Nutrition Practice Guidelines, available using the Store tab http://www.adaevidencelibrary.com

Scope of Dietetic Practice Framework, Standards of Practice in Nutrition Care and Updated Standards of Professional Performance, and the Standards of Practice in Nutrition Care Appendix, http://www.eatright.org in the Practice Section, Quality Management

Nutrition Care Process and Model Part I: The 2008 Update

The Nutrition Care Process and Model (NCPM) is a systematic problem-solving method that food and nutrition professionals use to think critically and make decisions that address practice-related problems (1). The NCPM provides a consistent structure and framework for food and nutrition professionals to use when delivering nutrition care and is designed for use with patients, clients, groups, and communities of all ages and conditions of health or disease (herein referred to as "patients/clients"). The original model was developed following a review of the literature and was intended to replace other nutrition care processes used in practice and education (1).

This update is the result of a planned, regularly scheduled review of the NCPM to ensure that it reflects current practice. It incorporates the results of a survey of American Dietetic Association groups experienced with the NCPM and incorporates decisions made by the Nutrition Care Process/Standardized Language Committee. Part II of this article, which will appear in an upcoming issue of the *Journal*, describes the official international dietetics and nutrition terminology as outlined in the *International Dietetics and Nutrition Terminology (INDT) Reference Manual* (2), which elaborates on and supports the NCPM. The information in Parts I and II of this article

replaces previous information describing the NCPM.

BACKGROUND

The NCPM contains four distinct but interrelated and connected steps: nutrition assessment, nutrition diagnosis, nutrition intervention, and nutrition monitoring and evaluation (described in Figure 1). In theory, each step informs the subsequent step. However, as new information is obtained, a registered dietitian (RD) may revisit previous steps of the process to reassess, add, or revise nutrition diagnoses, modify interventions, or adjust goals and monitoring parameters. The NCPM is designed to incorporate a scientific base that moves food and nutrition professionals beyond experience-based practice to evidence-based practice. If the NCPM is used consistently by all food and nutrition professionals, improved health outcomes should enhance recognition of RDs and dietetic technicians, registered (DTRs), as the preferred providers of nutrition services.

THE NCPM

Figure 2 is a graphic representation of the NCPM. The outer ring of the Model influences how patients/clients receive nutrition information. The practice setting reflects rules and regulations governing practice, the age and health conditions of particular patients/clients, and how a food and nutrition professional's time is allocated. The health care system mandates the amount of time available to food and nutrition professionals, the type of services provided, and who provides the services. The social system reflects patients'/clients' health-related knowledge, values, and the time devoted to improving nutritional health. The economic aspect incorporates resources allocated to nutrition

care, including the value of a food and nutrition professional's time in the form of salary and reimbursement.

The middle ring of the Model distinguishes the unique professional attributes of food and nutrition professionals from those in other professions. The inner ring illustrates the four steps of the NCPM, which are described in Figure 2. The central core of the model depicts the essential and collaborative partnership with a patient/client. The model is intended to reflect the dynamic nature of relationships throughout the NCPM.

AREAS OUTSIDE THE NCPM
Screening and Referral System

Screening has been defined as "a test or standardized examination procedure used to identify patients requiring special intervention" (3). Nutrition screening is a critical antecedent step of the NCPM that is not typically completed by food and nutrition professionals. Thus, it is not a part of the NCPM. RDs are capable of screening patients and are accountable for developing a screening process that is cost-effective and accurately identifies patients/clients who might have a nutrition problem.

Referral is the act of sending a patient/client to another health professional for care beyond one's own expertise. The term "referral" may also apply to the actual document that authorizes a visit to another health professional and is also a legal requirement for billing purposes. In addition to correctly identifying clients who would benefit from nutrition care, a referral process ensures that patients/clients have identifiable methods of being linked to the RD who is ultimately responsible for the nutrition intervention. Referral mechanisms may be established based on specific medical diagnoses or other agreed upon criteria.

This article was written by the **Writing Group of the Nutrition Care Process/Standardized Language Committee.**

Address correspondence to: Esther Myers, PhD, RD, FADA, Director, Research and Scientific Affairs, American Dietetic Association, 120 South Riverside Plaza, Suite 2000, Chicago, IL 60606-6995. E-mail: emyers@eatright.org doi: 10.1016/j.jada.2008.04.027

Resources

Step 1: Nutrition Assessment

Definition and purpose	Nutrition assessment is a systematic approach to collect, record, and interpret relevant data from patients, clients, family members, caregivers, and other individuals and groups. Nutrition assessment is an ongoing, dynamic process that involves initial data collection as well as continual reassessment and analysis of the patient's/client's status compared to specified criteria.
Data sources/tools for assessment	<ul><li>Screening or referral form.</li><li>Patient/client interview.</li><li>Medical or health records.</li><li>Consultation with other caregivers, including family members.</li><li>Community-based surveys and focus groups.</li><li>Statistical reports, administrative data, and epidemiologic studies.</li></ul>
Types of data collected	<ul><li>Food- and nutrition-related history.</li><li>Anthropometric measurements.</li><li>Biochemical data, medical tests, and procedures.</li><li>Nutrition-focused physical examination findings.</li><li>Client history.</li></ul>
Nutrition assessment components	<ul><li>Review data collected for factors that affect nutrition and health status.</li><li>Cluster individual data elements to identify a nutrition diagnosis as described in diagnosis reference sheets.</li><li>Identify standards by which data will be compared.</li></ul>
Critical thinking	<ul><li>Determining appropriate data to collect.</li><li>Determine the need for additional information.</li><li>Selecting assessment tools and procedures that match the situation.</li><li>Applying assessment tools in valid and reliable ways.</li><li>Distinguishing relevant from irrelevant data.</li><li>Distinguishing important from unimportant data.</li><li>Validating the data.</li></ul>
Determination for continuation of care	If upon completion of an initial or reassessment it is determined that the problem cannot be modified by further nutrition care, discharge or discontinuation from this episode of nutrition care may be appropriate.

Step 2. Nutrition Diagnosis

Definition and purpose	Nutrition diagnosis is a food and nutrition professional's identification and labeling of an existing nutrition problem that the food and nutrition professional is responsible for treating independently.
Data sources/tools for diagnosis	Organized assessment data that is clustered for comparison with defining characteristics of suspected diagnoses as listed in diagnosis reference sheets.
Nutrition diagnosis components	The nutrition diagnosis is expressed using nutrition diagnostic terms and the etiologies, signs, and symptoms that have been identified in the reference sheets describing each diagnosis. There are three distinct parts to a nutrition diagnostic statement: 1. The nutrition diagnosis describes alterations in a patient's/client's status. A diagnostic label may be accompanied by a descriptor such as "altered," "excessive," or "inadequate." 2. Etiology is a factor gathered during the nutrition assessment that contributes to the existence or the maintenance of pathophysiological, psychosocial, situational, developmental, cultural, and/or environmental problems. <ul><li>The etiology is preceded by the words "related to."</li><li>Identifying the etiology will lead to the selection of a nutrition intervention aimed at resolving the underlying cause of the nutrition problem whenever possible.</li><li>Major and minor etiologies may result from medical, genetic, or environmental factors.</li></ul>3. Signs/symptoms (defining characteristics) The defining characteristics are a typical cluster of sings and symptoms that provide evidence that a nutrition diagnosis exists. <ul><li>The signs and symptoms are preceded by the words "as evidenced by."</li><li>Signs are the observations of a trained clinician.</li><li>Symptoms are changes reported by the patient/client.</li></ul>
Nutrition diagnostic statement	A well-written nutrition diagnostic statement should be: <ul><li>Clear and concise;</li><li>Specific to a patient/client;</li><li>Limited to a single client problem;</li><li>Accurately related to one etiology; and</li><li>Based on signs and symptoms from the assessment data.</li></ul>
Critical thinking	<ul><li>Finding patterns and relationships among the data and possible causes.</li><li>Making inferences.</li><li>Stating the problem clearly and singularly.</li><li>Suspending judgment.</li><li>Making interdisciplinary connections.</li><li>Ruling in/ruling out specific diagnoses.</li></ul>
Determination for continuation of care	Because the nutrition diagnosis step involves naming and describing the problem, the determination for continuation of care follows the nutrition diagnosis step. If a food and nutrition professional does not find a nutrition diagnosis, a patient/client may be referred back to the primary provider. If the potential exists for a nutrition diagnosis to develop, a food and nutrition professional may establish an appropriate method and interval for follow-up.

(continued)

Figure 1. The four steps of the Nutrition Care Process and Model.

Step 3. Nutrition Intervention	
Definition and purpose	A nutrition intervention is a purposefully planned action(s) designed with the intent of changing a nutrition-related behavior, risk factor, environmental condition, or aspect of health status. Nutrition intervention consists of two interrelated components: planning and intervention. The nutrition intervention is typically directed toward resolving the nutrition diagnosis or the nutrition etiology. Less often, it is directed at relieving signs and symptoms.
Data sources/tools for interventions	• The American Dietetic Association's Evidence-Based Nutrition Practice Guides or other guidelines from professional organizations. • The American Dietetic Association's Evidence Analysis Library and other secondary evidence such as the Cochrane Library. • Current research literature. • Results of outcome management studies or quality improvement projects.
Nutrition intervention components	Planning • Prioritize diagnoses based on urgency, impact, and available resources. • Write a nutrition prescription based on a patient's/client's individualized recommended dietary intake of energy and/or selected foods or nutrients based on current reference standards and dietary guidelines and a patient's/client's health condition and nutrition diagnosis. • Collaborate with the patient/client to identify goals of the intervention for each diagnosis. • Select specific intervention strategies that are focused on the etiology of the problem and that are known to be effective based on best current knowledge and evidence. • Define time and frequency of care, including intensity, duration, and follow-up. Implementation • Collaborate with a patient/client and other caregivers to carry out the plan of care. • Communicate the plan of nutrition care. • Modify the plan of care as needed. • Follow-up and verify that the plan is being implemented. • Revise strategies based on changes in condition or response to intervention.
Critical thinking	• Setting goals and prioritizing. • Defining the nutrition prescription or basic plan. • Making interdisciplinary connections. • Matching intervention strategies with patient/client needs, nutrition diagnoses, and values. • Choosing from among alternatives to determine a course of action. • Specifying the time and frequency of care.
Determination for continuation of care	If a patient/client has met intervention goals or is not at this time able/ready to make needed changes, the food and nutrition professional may discharge the client from this episode of care as part of the planned intervention.

Step 4. Nutrition Monitoring and Evaluation	
Definition and purpose	Nutrition monitoring and evaluation identifies the amount of progress made and whether goals/expected outcomes are being met. Nutrition monitoring and evaluation identifies outcomes relevant to the nutrition diagnosis and intervention plans and goals.
Data sources/tools for monitoring and evaluation	• Self-monitoring data or data from other records including forms, spreadsheets, and computer programs. • Anthropometric measurements, biochemical data, medical tests, and procedures. • Patient/client surveys, pretests, posttests, and/or questionnaires. • Mail or telephone follow-up.
Types of outcomes measured	• Nutrition-related history. • Anthropometric measurements. • Biochemical data, medical tests, and procedures. • Nutrition-focused physical findings.

Nutrition monitoring and evaluation components	This step includes three distinct and interrelated processes:
	1. Monitor progress:
	  ○ check patient/client understanding and compliance with plan;
	  ○ determine whether the intervention is being implemented as prescribed;
	  ○ provide evidence that the plan/intervention strategy is or is not changing patient/client behavior or status;
	  ○ identify other positive or negative outcomes;
	  ○ gather information indicating reasons for lack of progress; and
	  ○ support conclusions with evidence.
	2. Measure outcomes:
	  ○ Select outcome indicators that are relevant to the nutrition diagnosis or signs or symptoms, nutrition goals, medical diagnosis, and outcomes and quality management goals.
	3. Evaluate outcomes
	  ○ Compare current findings with previous status, intervention goals, and/or reference standards.

Critical thinking	• Selecting appropriate indicators/measures. • Using appropriate reference standard for comparison. • Defining where patient/client is in terms of expected outcomes. • Explaining variance from expected outcomes. • Determining factors that help or hinder progress.
Determination for continuation of care	Based on the findings, the food and nutrition professional may actively continue care or if nutrition care is complete or no further change is expected, discharge the patient/client. If nutrition care is to be continued, reassessment may result in refinements to the diagnosis and intervention. If care does not continue, a patient/client may still be monitored for a change in status and reentry to nutrition care at a later date.

Figure 1. The four steps of the Nutrition Care Process and Model (continued).

Resources

Edition: 2009

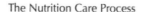

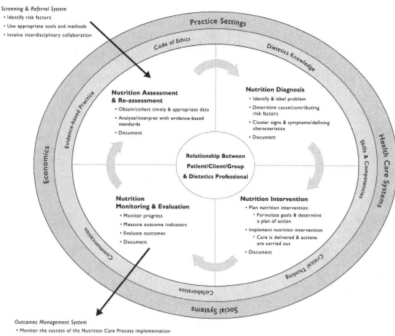

Figure 2. The four distinct but interrelated and connected steps of the Nutrition Care Process and Model.

Outcomes Management System

Outcomes management is based on accumulated data that are collected, analyzed, compared with standards or benchmarks, and the results used to adjust and improve performance. Outcomes management requires an infrastructure to aggregate and manage data documented throughout the NCPM. Results from a large series of patients/clients can be used to determine the effectiveness of intervention strategies and the influence of nutrition care in improving the overall health of individuals and groups. Because an outcomes management system involves data from multiple patients/clients and possibly multiple food and nutrition professionals or sites, it is outside the NCPM.

DISTINCTION BETWEEN MEDICAL NUTRITION THERAPY (MNT) AND THE NCPM

MNT is a term widely used in dietetics. It was defined in the 2001 Medicare benefit legislation as "nutritional diagnostic, therapy, and counseling services for the purpose of disease management, which are furnished by a registered dietitian or nutrition professional" (4). MNT is not synonymous with the NCPM, but is one specific type of nutrition care. The NCPM is used to provide MNT, but also in other forms of nutrition care such as obtaining feeding assistance or referring to another practitioner.

CLARIFICATION FOR PRACTITIONERS

This revised description of the NCPM in Figure 1 makes the following points for practitioners.

- Nutrition assessment has been redefined and the nutrition assessment section has been reformatted to aid in clustering signs and symptoms according to the nutrition diagnoses reference sheets.
- Early examples of nutrition diagnoses included the terminology "potential for" and "risk of" as modifiers of the diagnoses. However, in the absence of data documenting a

cause-and-effect relationship between nutritional risk and nutrition diagnoses, these modifiers are no longer recommended and should not be used.

- The original article on this topic recognized that patients/clients may have more than one nutrition diagnosis. The NCPM continues to accommodate more than one nutrition diagnosis. A nutrition intervention and nutrition monitoring strategy should accompany each nutrition diagnosis.

FUTURE IMPLICATIONS

The NCPM has already begun to influence practice, education, and credentialing of RDs and DTRs, as well as research in the United States and abroad. For example, the American Dietetic Association has developed standards of practice and standards of professional performance that incorporate the NCPM (5). Several groups within the profession have developed practice-specific standards that incorporate the NCPM. The 2008 revised standards of practice in nutrition care for DTRs (6) will more clearly define the role of DTRs relative to the NCPM.

The NCPM is a prominent component of the Commission on Accreditation of Dietetics Education standards released in March 2008 (7,8). It remains to be seen whether educators will reorganize course content to align with the NCPM, but beginning in March 2009, all types of dietetics education programs are required to incorporate NCPM content. Graduates of the Commission on Accreditation for Dietetics Education–accredited programs should be prepared to assume an appropriate role in nutritional assessment but also in nutrition diagnosis and nutrition intervention, monitoring, and evaluation.

RDs entering the profession since 2006 have taken a revised and updated Registration Examination for Dietitians. The nutrition assessment, nutrition diagnosis, nutrition intervention, and nutrition monitoring and evaluation steps of the NCPM comprise 40% of the examination (9). NCPM education for practicing food and nutrition professionals has been made available at affiliate meetings in almost all states. A number of educational materials are available to American Dietetic

Association members at no charge from the American Dietetic Association Web site (www.eatright.org). In addition, the Commission on Dietetic Registration has developed a continuing education module available to all food and nutrition professionals.

EVIDENCE-BASED PRACTICE AND THE NCPM

Evidence-based practice involves using the highest quality of available information to make practice decisions. It combines the experience of clinicians with a critical evaluation of primary and secondary knowledge sources to support the decision-making process. The American Dietetic Association's electronic Evidence Analysis Library (www.adaevidencelibrary.com) contains thousands of documents that support the steps of the NCPM. These documents have been rigorously evaluated by trained evidence analysts, ranked for quality, and compiled into Evidence-Based Guidelines and Toolkits. The Guidelines and Toolkits elaborate the NCPM as it applies in adult and pediatric weight management, critical illness, disorders of lipid metabolism, and other topics are in preparation. The Dietetics Practice-Based Research Network has been involved in validating nutrition diagnosis terms and will no doubt participate in further studies incorporating and elaborating the NCPM.

CONCLUSIONS

Since it was accepted by the House of Delegates, the NCPM has been elaborated, refined, and updated to reflect current practice. The NCPM is being incorporated into education, credentialing, and materials supporting evidence-based practice. As these initiatives continue, the NCPM will be more widely understood and adopted within the profession.

References

1. Lacey K, Pritchett E. Nutrition Care Process and Model: ADA adopts road map to quality care and outcomes management. *J Am Diet Assoc.* 2003;103:1061-1071.
2. *International Dietetics and Nutrition Terminology (INDT) Reference Manual.* Chicago, IL: American Dietetic Association; 2007.
3. US Preventive Services Task Force. *Guide to Clinical Preventive Services.* 2nd ed. Washington, DC: US Department of Health and Human Services, Office of Disease Prevention and Health Promotion; 1996.
4. Medicare Program; Revisions to Payment Policies and Five Year Review of and Adjustments to the Relative Values Units Under the Physician Fee Schedule for Calendar Year 2002; Final Rule. Subpart G—Medical nutrition therapy. 66 *Federal Register* 55331 (2001) (codified at 42 CFR §405, 410, 411, 414, and 415).
5. Kieselhorst KJ, Skates J, Pritchett E. American Dietetic Association: Standards of practice in nutrition care and updated standards of professional performance. *J Am Diet Assoc.* 2005;105:641-645.
6. The American Dietetic Association 2007-2008 and 2006-2007 Quality Management Committees. American Dietetic Association Revised Standards for Dietetic Practice and Professional Performance: 2008 Standards of Practice for Registered Dietitians in Nutrition Care; 2008 Standards of Professional Performance for Registered Dietitians; 2008 Standards of Practice for Dietetic Technicians, Registered in Nutrition Care; 2008 Standards of Professional Performance for Dietetic Technicians, Registered. American Dietetic Association Web site. http://www.eatright.org/ada/files/3_-_2008_Document_SOP_SOPP_APPROVED_FINAL_4.18.08.pdf. Accessed May 12, 2008.
7. Commission on Accreditation for Dietetics Education. 2008 eligibility requirements and accreditation standards for didactic programs in dietetics. American Dietetic Association Web site. http://www.eatright.org/cps/rde/xchg/ada/hs.xsl/CADE_16149_ENU_HTML.htm. Accessed March 19, 2008.
8. Commission on Accreditation of Dietetics Education. 2008 eligibility requirements and accreditation standards for dietetic internships. American Dietetic Association Web site. http://www.eatright.org/cps/rde/xchg/ada/hs.xsl/CADE_16149_ENU_HTML.htm. Accessed March 19, 2008
9. Registration examination for dietitians. Commission on Dietetic Registration Web site. http://www.cdrnet.org/certifications/rddtr/rdcontent.htm. Accessed January 4, 2007.

The writing group was composed of: Jennifer Bueche, PhD, RD; Pam Charney, PhD, RD; Jessie Pavlinac, MS, RD, CSR; Annalynn Skipper, PhD, RD, FADA; Elizabeth Thompson, MPH, RD; and Esther Myers, PhD, RD, FADA.

Additional members of the Nutrition Care Process/Standardized Language Committee were: Nancy Lewis, PhD, RD—Chair; Elise Smith, MA, RD—Vice-Chair; Donna Israel, PhD, RD, FADA; Judy Beto, PhD, RD, FADA; Claudia A. Conkin, MS, RD; Melinda Zook-Weaver, MS, RD; and Constance J. Geiger, PhD, RD.

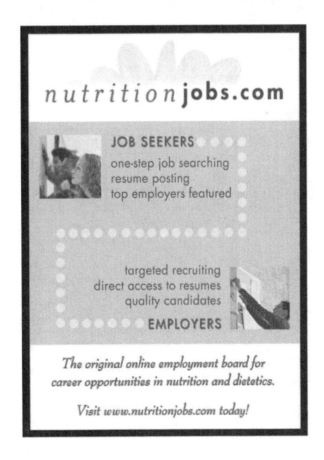

Feedback Form

Name: _____

Book: _____

Publication year: _____

Please provide feedback on the revisions you would suggest to the next edition of the *International Dietetics and Nutrition Terminology (IDNT) Reference Manual: Standardized Language for the Nutrition Care Process*, Second Edition. Please indicate whether each section should be included and identify what questions you would like answered in the next edition as well as additional materials that you would find helpful.

The following items should be included in the next edition:

	YES	NO
	Please Check	

Nutrition Care Process Summary

Step 1: Nutrition Assessment *SNAPshot*

Introduction

Combined Nutrition Assessment and Monitoring and Evaluation Terminology

Combined Nutrition Assessment and Monitoring and Evaluation Terms/Definitions

Combined Nutrition Assessment and Monitoring and Evaluation Reference sheets

Step 2: Nutrition Diagnosis *SNAPshot*

Introduction

Terminology

Terms and Definitions

Reference Sheets

Step 3: Nutrition Intervention *SNAPshot*

Introduction

Terminology

Terms and Definitions

Reference Sheets

Step 4: Nutrition Monitoring and Evaluation *SNAPshot*

Introduction

Bibliography

Other

What questions would you like answered in the next edition?

What additional materials would be helpful in the next edition?

Please mail form or e-mail information to: Scientific Affairs and Research, American Dietetic Association, Nutrition Care Process/Standardized Language Committee, 120 South Riverside Plaza, Suite 2000, Chicago, IL 60606-6995. emyers@eatright.org; lornstein@eatright.org

Edition: 2009